COMBINING WORK AND CARE

Sustainable Care

Series Editors: **Sue Yeandle**, CIRCLE, University of Sheffield, **Jon Glasby,** University of Birmingham, **Jill Manthorpe**, King's College London and **Kate Hamblin**, CIRCLE, University of Sheffield

---

This series provides novel contributions to understanding care systems, care work and care relationships. Focusing on the concept of 'sustainable care', it makes an innovative and distinctive contribution to understandings of future care challenges and how care arrangements could be made more sustainable.

Scan the code below to discover new and forthcoming titles in the series, or visit:

policy.bristoluniversitypress.co.uk/
sustainable-care

COMBINING WORK AND CARE

Carer Leave and Related Employment Policies in International Context

Edited by
Kate Hamblin, Jason Heyes and Janet Fast

First published in Great Britain in 2024 by

Policy Press, an imprint of
Bristol University Press
University of Bristol
1-9 Old Park Hill
Bristol
BS2 8BB
UK
t: +44 (0)117 374 6645
e: bup-info@bristol.ac.uk

Details of international sales and distribution partners are available at policy.bristoluniversitypress.co.uk

British Library Cataloguing in Publication Data
A catalogue record for this book is available from the British Library

ISBN 978-1-4473-6570-9 paperback
ISBN 978-1-4473-6571-6 ePub
ISBN 978-1-4473-6572-3 OA PDF

Cover design: Robin Hawes
Front cover image: iStock/ Andrey Danilovich
Bristol University Press and Policy Press use environmentally responsible print partners.
Printed and bound in Great Britain by CPI Group (UK) Ltd, Croydon, CR0 4YY

FSC
www.fsc.org
MIX
Paper | Supporting
responsible forestry
FSC® C013604

Contents

List of figures and tables

Figures

Tables

Notes on contributors

Linnéa Aldman holds a Master's degree in Political Science and has extensive experience of carrying out evaluations, assessments and pilot studies within different contexts, such as human rights, gender equality and the empowerment of seldom-heard groups (for example, people with migration, refugee and asylum-seeking experiences). She currently works at the Swedish Family Care Competence Centre (SFCCC/Nka), where she takes part in carrying out literature reviews and report writing on a range of carers' topics, including carer support and carer leave policies.

Camille Allard is research fellow in Sociology at the University of Milan. Her research interests include unpaid care, care ethics, inequalities at work and their impact on workers' health and well-being. Her current research examines how organisations make decisions to invest in health and well-being promotion for their employees.

Jacquie Eales, as Research Manager of Research on Aging, Policies and Practice (RAPP) in the Department of Human Ecology at the University of Alberta for nearly three decades, bridges research, policy and practice to make a meaningful difference in the lives of older adults and their family caregivers. Jacquie successfully implements transdisciplinary research projects, working collaboratively with an array of valued partners to ensure research projects are relevant to their needs and mentoring graduate students in the process. She has co-authored numerous academic articles, book chapters and conference papers, including two Top 5 published articles and one Editors' Choice journal article. She is passionate about translating research knowledge into useful formats to facilitate its uptake by policy, practice and community partners. She makes a meaningful difference in her community by serving on the Age-Friendly Edmonton Leadership Table (2018–23) and the Board of Directors of GEF Seniors Housing (2016–22), by championing the Cycling Without Age grassroots programme, and by co-hosting four-generation family suppers every week. In 2022, Jacquie was nominated for a Minister of Seniors Service Award for her outstanding commitment and contribution to Alberta Seniors.

Janet Fast is Professor in the Department of Human Ecology at the University of Alberta, and Co-director of the Research on Aging, Policies and Practice research programme. She holds a PhD in Family and Consumer Economics from Cornell University. Major themes of her research are the economics of ageing and the paid and unpaid care work of family members. She is a member of the leadership team of the AGE-WELL National Centres of Excellence, Canada's ageing and technology network.

Kate Hamblin is Professor at the Centre for International Research on Care, Labour and Equalities, University of Sheffield. She leads the Economic and Social Research Council (ESRC) Centre for Care's Digital Care research theme and is a member of the leadership team for the ESRC and Health Foundation-funded IMProving Adult Care Together (IMPACT) Implementation Centre. She joined the University of Sheffield in 2018 to work on the ESRC-funded Sustainable Care programme. Her research has focused on technology and its role in the care of older people with complex needs as well as issues related to employment, including the balance between unpaid care and paid work; self-employment and ageing; and 'active ageing' employment and pension policies.

Elizabeth Hanson is Professor of Health Care Sciences at the Linnaeus University (LNU) in Sweden and Research Director at the Swedish Family Care Competence Centre (Nka), a national centre of excellence on informal care. She heads up the Informal Carers, Care and Caring research group at LNU, which acts as the research arm of Nka. Elizabeth is a board member and past president of Eurocarers, the European association working for informal carers. She established the Eurocarers Research Working Group, whose aim is to feed into the definition of evidence-based policy making on the role and added value of informal carers. She acts as expert advisor to the National Board of Health and Welfare Sweden on carer issues. Elizabeth recently led an EU Horizon 2020 young carers project ('ME–WE') comprising Eurocarers members in six European countries. She has a long-standing interest in carer issues and over the last 25 years has led a variety of national and international projects in partnership with informal carers, service users, health and social care practitioners, decision makers, policy makers and non-governmental organisations, the goal being to strengthen the knowledge base and stimulate evidence-based policies and practices for and with carers across the lifecourse.

Jason Heyes is Professor of Employment Relations in the Management School at the University of Sheffield and director of the Management School's Centre for Decent Work. He has published on topics including underemployment, vocational training, work intensity and European labour market policy. He is currently leading a project on young workers' transitions in the labour market, which is being funded by the Economic and Social Research Council. He has also undertaken research projects on behalf of, among others, the International Labour Organization, the European Commission, the Low Pay Commission and the European Trade Union Institute.

Valentina Hlebec, PhD, is a full professor at the Faculty of Social Sciences, University of Ljubljana. She holds extensive knowledge of social methodology, especially regarding cognitive laboratory techniques, and the development and evaluation of the measurement quality of survey measurement instruments. She has lately been focused on social welfare and informal/formal social care.

Andreas Hoff is Professor of Social Gerontology at Zittau/Görlitz University of Applied Sciences and Director of the research institute Gesundheit, Altern, Arbeit, Technik (GAT; English translation: Health, Ageing, Labour, Technology), Germany. His research over the past 25 years has focused on family care/informal care in the context of different European welfare states, more specifically on the use and co-creation of assistive technologies in older people's homes and in home care, the reconciliation of employment and family care, as well as intergenerational relations in family, community and society.

Maša Filipovič Hrast, PhD, is Associate Professor at the Faculty of Social Sciences, University of Ljubljana. Her research topics include changes in the welfare state, social policy, housing policy, quality of life of vulnerable groups in society, social exclusion and ageing and care policies.

Shingou Ikeda, PhD, is Vice Research Director (Professor) on human resource management at the Japan Institute for Labor Policy and Training (JILPT). He was a member of working group for amendment of care leave policy in 2016 and 2024 at Ministry of Health, Labor and Welfare in Japan. He has published extensively on issues related to work and care in Japan. His latest book on Japanese care leave policy was awarded the highest prize on labor studies in Japan in 2023.

Katja Knauthe has a Master's degree in social policy. She is researching her dissertation on the reconciliation of care and work from the perspective of companies. From 2018 to 2021, she was a visiting researcher at the University of Sheffield in the Economic and Social Research Council-funded *Sustainable Care* programme. She is the author of several reports on the economic and social impact of the lack of reconciliation of family, care and work. Since 2020 she has volunteered on the presidium of the German Red Cross for the expansion of social services for people with family care responsibilities. In addition, she holds a staff position for gender equality in the city of Görlitz. Her research focuses on the sociology of ageing, social policy and the welfare state, gender dimensions of care work and work–life balance as a topic of the future.

Emilia Leinonen has a PhD in social and public policy, works as a postdoctoral researcher and coordinator in the Centre of Excellence in Research on Ageing and Care at the University of Jyväskylä and is an affiliated researcher at the University of Helsinki, Finland. She defended her doctoral dissertation, 'Locating adult foster care: adult foster care for older people in between formal and informal', in 2020. Her main research interests include care, housing, temporalities and the interplay between policies and the everyday life of older persons.

Kate O'Loughlin, Associate Professor (Honorary), is a health sociologist in the School of Health Sciences, The University of Sydney, Australia and Investigator at the Centre of Excellence in Population Ageing Research. Kate's research focuses on mature-age workforce participation and ageing-related health and care policies. Her current research is in three key areas: the socioeconomic and political context of combining paid work and carer responsibilities; attitudes to ageing and age discrimination; and use of technology for ageing in place. Published books/chapters include *Ageing in Australia: Challenges and Opportunities* (2017; co-editors Colette Browning and Hal Kendig), 'Older Adults and Digital Technologies' (2019; with Meryl Lovarini and Lindy Clemson) and 'Ageing and Health' (2022; editors Alphia Possamai-Inesedy and Peta Cook). Kate is an associate editor of the *International Journal of Care and Caring* and *Frontiers in Public Health (Aging)*.

Jolanta Perek-Białas, PhD, is Associate Professor at the Jagiellonian University, Cracow in Poland. She is the Director of the Center for Evaluation and Public Policies Analysis, and works also at the Institute of Statistics and Demography of the Warsaw School of Economics. Her research interest focuses on the socioeconomic situation of older persons in Central and Eastern Europe, including active ageing, ageism in the labour market policy, old-age social exclusion, age-friendly approach and the organisation of care for older persons, including looking for effective measures to support working caregivers. She has been coordinator of various research projects as well as an expert consultant to policy makers at the local (Cracow), regional (Małopolska), national (Ministry of Family, Labour and Social Policy) and international levels (such as Organisation for Economic Co-operation and Development, European Commission, United Nations Economic Commission for Europe, World Health Organization).

Tatjana Rakar, PhD, is Associate Professor of Sociology at the Faculty of Social Sciences, University of Ljubljana. Her fields of research encompass studies in social policy, welfare systems, family and care policies as well as third sector and social economy developments.

Anna Ruzik-Sierdzińska, PhD, is Professor at the Warsaw School of Economics. Her research interests include social security systems, labour economics and health economics. She has participated in various research projects, among others with Organisation for Economic Co-operation and Development, the World Bank and the United Nations Development Programme.

Eva Sennemark is a facilitator and project leader at the Swedish Family Care Competence Centre (Nka). She is a registered nurse, trained in public healthcare and holds a Master's degree in Applied Social Anthropology. Eva has more than 20 years of experience in working with evaluations, audits and applied research within health and social care and education. She has an active interest in carers' issues and has written articles, reports and literature reviews in this area. Eva is currently project leader of Nka's 'database' project, which involves the development and piloting of a national database of municipal support to informal carers and to test indicators to follow up perceived quality of carer support as perceived by carers themselves.

Alison Williams is a research associate with the Mature Workers in Organisations Stream of the Australian Research Council Centre of Excellence in Population and Ageing Research, University of Sydney, undertaking research into mature-aged workers and organisations. She also teaches in employment relations and human resource management.

Acknowledgements

The editors gratefully acknowledge the support of the (UK) Economic and Social Research Council for the *Sustainable Care: connecting people and systems* programme (grant reference: ES/P009255/1, 2017–21, principal investigator: Professor Sue Yeandle, University of Sheffield).

We also thank the anonymous reviewer for their helpful comments, and Professors Sue Yeandle, Jill Manthorpe and Jon Glasby for their feedback on the book. Our thanks also go to Dr Kelly Davidge for her assistance in the preparation of the final manuscript, and Laura Vickers-Rendall and Jay Allan from Policy Press for their support throughout the publication process.

Series editors' preface

Jon Glasby, Kate Hamblin,
Jill Manthorpe and Sue Yeandle

The *Sustainable Care* book series arises from a large grant programme, *Sustainable Care: connecting people and systems*, delivered by a multidisciplinary partnership of 35 scholars in eight universities, funded by the UK's Economic and Social Research Council. It provides novel, interdisciplinary and internationally informed contributions based on work by linked research teams studying care systems, care work and care relationships.

Our focus is timely and important. The series is presenting the findings from a distinctive programme of new research on social care. Our main aims for the series are that it will make an innovative and distinctive contribution to understandings of future care challenges and how they could be addressed. The series offers new empirical, conceptual and methodological writing, in scholarly but accessible form, aimed to inform and inspire scholars, policy makers, employers, practitioners and citizens interested in care.

The Sustainable Care programme's book series with Policy Press brings together data, practices, systems, structures, narratives and actions relevant to social care, particularly our ageing populations. While much of our subject matter is distinct and specific to the UK's unique policy, demographic, cultural and socioeconomic circumstances, it also has clear global relevance. Similar concerns are salient around the world and especially relevant in other advanced welfare states: population ageing is profoundly changing age structures; developments in technology and in healthcare mean more people who are ill or have long-term conditions need support at home; and 'traditional' gendered sources of daily caring labour are dwindling, as levels of female labour force participation rise and family networks become more dispersed. The COVID-19 pandemic has amplified such challenges.

Subject areas, disciplines and themes

The series critically engages with fierce contemporary debates about care infrastructure; divisions of caring labour and the political economy of care; care ethics, rights, recognition and values; care technologies and human–technology interactions; and care relations in intergenerational, emotional, community and familial context. Within its overarching concept, sustainable care, its subject areas span social and welfare policy and systems; family and social gerontology; ageing and disability studies; employment and workforce organisation; diversity (including gender and ethnicity); social work and human resources; migration and mobility; and technology studies.

We all have the potential to benefit from new multidisciplinary work on care that embraces progress in global scholarship on diversity, culture and the uses of technology, and engages with issues of inequality, political economy and the division of labour. These were the distinctive features of our programme and they are highlighted and developed in this book series. We are grateful to all who have contributed as researchers, programme administrators and research participants, to our funders, our advisory group and to members of the public who have engaged with our studies so far. We hope this series of books reflects the quality of their contributions. We thank each book's editors, authors and our publisher for their commitment to spreading ideas, knowledge and experiences.

Introduction: comparing carer leave policies cross-nationally

Kate Hamblin, Jason Heyes and Janet Fast

This book examines and compares, for the first time, the origins, content and implications of national policies and policy instruments intended to enable people to provide care to family members and friends while remaining in paid employment. It focuses particularly on the emergence of legislated opportunities to take temporary leaves of absence from work to permit employees to fulfil care responsibilities – referred to throughout as 'carer leave'.

In all countries included in this comparative book – Australia, Canada, Finland, Germany, Japan, Poland, Slovenia, Sweden and the United Kingdom – the proportion of employees with caring responsibilities is growing. Population ageing and global trends in economic conditions, among other factors, have produced rising labour force participation rates, especially among women, and dual-earner households have increasingly become the norm (Ortiz-Ospina et al, 2018). In many countries across the globe, although life expectancy is increasing, disability-free and healthy life expectancies have remained stable, increasing demand for care (Beard et al, 2016; GDB Ageing Collaborators, 2022). Health and long-term care systems are presented as being 'in crisis' due to concerns about financial and social sustainability (UN, 2018). In this context, many governments around the world are seeking to reduce or minimise expected growth in expenditure on health and care services. Increasingly, some argue, national policies rely ever more heavily on carers, with states 'bringing the family in [to caring arrangements] through the back door' (Kodate and Timonen, 2017: 291). As a result, there is now substantial evidence that family members and friends are providing high levels – and indeed the vast majority – of care around the world (Cès et al, 2019; Dykstra and Djundeva, 2020; Fast et al, 2023). Carers, it is argued, are conceived of as 'background resources' within welfare systems (Lloyd, 2023: 134), with their own needs and well-being marginalised.

Reflecting these trends, the number of 'working carers' has grown rapidly and is predicted to continue to rise as societies age (Addati et al, 2018; Wimo et al, 2018). As Bouget et al (2016) highlight, demographic, social and cultural trends are increasing the likelihood of having to combine paid work and care. There is ample evidence too that many working carers experience negative financial, health and social consequences linked to their 'double duties'; numerous studies show these threaten the sustainability of both the 'caringscape' (Kodate and Timonen, 2017: 291) and the care sector (Jacobs et al, 2013; Bauer and Sousa-Poza, 2015; Feinberg and Spillman, 2019). The effects spill-over beyond the care sector, affecting other stakeholders, including employers, other labour market actors and the broader economy.

In all the countries included here, this situation is increasingly acknowledged as a challenge to the well-being of people receiving and providing care as well as to the sustainability of national health and care systems, individual enterprises and national economies. The International Labour Organization (ILO) reports that, globally, 647 million people of working age are outside the labour force due to caring responsibilities (Addati et al, 2018) and that policies that support working carers are seen as increasingly important by national governments and enterprises. Policy makers and some employers have sought to address the consequences of this confluence of trends in recent years, drawing attention to a pressing need for guidance on how the evolving demands on carers can be reconciled with their participation in paid work (Eurofound, 2015; Brimblecombe et al, 2018).

Initiatives aimed at helping working carers reconcile their paid work and caring responsibilities have been implemented in most European Union (EU) countries (Eurofound, 2015), as well as in North America (Feinberg, 2019), Oceania (Temple et al, 2019) and Asia (Lorenz et al, 2021). Kodate and Timonen (2017) assert that measures to facilitate 'ageing in place' (outside of residential or hospital settings) are coupled with national policies that are 'enabling extremely flexible forms of care labour that necessitate the constant active involvement of family members in the broader "caringscape"' (Kodate and Timonen, 2017: 291), including legislating for temporary leave from paid work for employed carers, that is, for an arrangement whereby carers can combine paid employment and care with fewer negative consequences (Feinberg, 2019). Statutory leaves of short duration, intended to help employees deal with family emergencies, are now available in 127 countries, 101 of which provide for such leave to be paid (Addati et al, 2022). In contrast, far fewer countries have more sophisticated leave provisions, such as longer-term leaves, the right to return to the same job or (partial) income replacement while taking leave. Only 55 countries globally offer a statutory right to long-term care leave, and in only 34 of these is this leave paid (Addati et al, 2022). Most countries that have legislated for long-term care leave entitlements are in Europe, Central Asia and other high-income countries. In some, leave is available only to enable care for a child with a serious illness or disability. Elsewhere, as in Japan, Norway and Canada, employees can take paid leave to care for a broad range of family members.

Little is known about the efficacy of these initiatives; evidence is often drawn from small-scale studies, based on the experience of a small number of companies or individuals. One recent review of the literature on support for carers concluded that 'there are significant gaps in the evidence base with regards to interventions, outcomes and types of caring situation studied', calling for more evaluation of the efficacy and cost-effectiveness of recent policy initiatives (Brimblecombe et al, 2018: 35). Studies addressing this could help to establish whether the desirable and multiple outcomes identified by Feinberg (2019) are in fact being realised. In theory, carer leave should reduce carer strain, improve working carers' financial security, reduce older and disabled people's moves into residential care and contribute to workforce productivity. A recent review of work–care reconciliation policies for carers in eight countries nevertheless found that 'many of the measures governments have introduced have been modified or adapted within a few years of initial implementation. [...] suggest[ing] they are experimenting with ... policies, seeking to find what is acceptable to employers or workers, [or] responding "ad hoc" to the pressure of opinion, campaigns or perceived problems' (Yeandle, 2017: 39).

The purpose of this book is to help fill knowledge gaps about the development, implementation and outcomes of carer leave policies. It is the first to examine in detail the development, implementation and implications of carer leave policies (and related policy instruments) and to situate these within the social, economic, labour market and political contexts of nine countries in different parts of the world. The countries included offer contrasting examples of efforts to support working carers, in differing contexts in terms of employment, care, welfare and labour policies and social values, yet share certain structural characteristics. To facilitate cross-national comparative analysis, chapter authors describe their own country's particular policy contexts – the set of political, social, economic and cultural factors that shape policy processes. These 'non-shared' attributes (Sartori, 1994) vary from one country to another and have been shaped by history and by social, political and economic change over time. The policy orientation of national governments and the advocacy roles of carers' organisations, trade unions and employer bodies are discussed where applicable. Chapter authors describe the carer leave policies and policy instruments in place in their own country, aiming to assess their equity/inclusivity, flexibility, job protection and income security properties, and to reflect on 'what works' with regard to policies to support carers in employment, highlighting examples of innovative policies. Differences in the arrangements they describe offer new information for cross-national comparative policy analysis and transfer, helping to unravel the issues that lie behind both policy success and failure, and any persistent differences or emerging similarities between countries.

The book comprises 11 chapters: this first, introductory chapter sets out the book's objectives, approach and organisation. Nine country-specific chapters follow, each discussing carer leave and related developments in its country-specific context. The final chapter concludes the book with an international comparative analysis of the evidence presented in the country chapters; a discussion of how far national social, political and economic contexts may explain national variations in carer leave policies and policy instruments; and some final comments on what contributors' findings contribute to understanding and analysis of international policy transfer.

Aims of the book: cross-national policy comparison and learning

This book has two principal aims. First, it aims to provide comprehensive overviews of nine nations' carer leave policies, examining their origins and evolution, the wider context within which they are situated and their implications and impacts. The country chapters share a similar structure, beginning with an overview of the national economic, political and social background; then presenting a detailed description of the content and development of carer leave policies (and other support) for working carers; and concluding with an appraisal of the adequacy of the policies described, including issues such as their implications for equity, inclusivity and flexibility, and the level of income and job protection offered.

Exploring the impact of carer leave and other related policies is particularly important, given widespread attention in the literature to negative outcomes arising from combining work and care. Studies highlight that working carers spend less time with family members, on themselves or engaging in social and networking events with colleagues (Mooney et al, 2002; Phillips et al, 2002) and report fatigue, stress and poorer mental health linked to the dual demands of employment and caring (Mooney et al, 2002; Lero et al, 2012; Gaugler et al, 2018). Evidence also indicates that working carers who give up work to care often regret doing so and find it very difficult to return to work (Yeandle et al, 2007). Working carers have also been found to have limited opportunities for career progression and training, compared with co-workers without caring responsibilities (Phillips et al, 2002); and to face pressure to reduce their working hours, which can endure beyond the end of the caring role (Evandrou and Glaser, 2005) and with immediate effects on carers' incomes as well as longer-term consequences for pension accrual (Daly and Rake, 2003; Evandrou and Glaser, 2003). Working carers who lack workplace support are more likely to report poor mental well-being and to be planning to quit their jobs than other working carers (Austin and Heyes, 2020). Benefits working carers have reported, related to their dual roles, nevertheless include maintaining a good relationship with the person they care for and personal satisfaction (Mooney et al, 2002; Eldh and Carlsson, 2011); and deriving a source of identity, self-worth and a 'buffer' (or escape) from demanding care situations by being in paid work (Keck and Saraceno, 2009; Masuy, 2009; Sakka et al, 2016; Heitink et al, 2017).

An important issue to underscore is the continuing and highly gendered nature of care – with consequential inequities and inequalities – which could be addressed by appropriate policies. As has been claimed, 'the "invisible hand" of modern economic activity is utterly reliant upon the "invisible heart" of unpaid care work' (Foley and Cooper, 2021: 467), and the care largely undertaken by women means they are also disproportionately exposed to negative outcomes of combining work and care. As Lloyd (2023) emphasises the shift away from care in institutional settings in the UK as part of the 'care in the community' policy agenda reinforced the idea that the family and home were the 'natural sites' of care, and women the 'natural' providers. Similar arguments have been made about policies to facilitate 'ageing in place' (Kodate and Timonen, 2017). However, policy agendas such as these and gender norms that make women the 'natural' providers of care remain at odds with established notions of the 'ideal worker' (Williams, 2000; Foley and Cooper, 2021), and female carers have been found to be more likely than their male counterparts to opt for part-time employment, give up paid work entirely, be absent, take leave and retire early (Boise and Neal, 1996; Dentinger and Clarkberg, 2002; Matthews and Fisher, 2013; Carr et al, 2018; Stanfors et al, 2019; Urwin et al, 2023). Yet gender is not the sole site of inequality for those combining work and care. Studies have shown how other intersecting characteristics, including race, ethnicity, age and socioeconomic status influence the intensity and impact of caring (Anderson et al, 2013; Do et al, 2014; Cohen et al, 2017, 2019).[1]

Each country chapter in this book thus offers both a standalone source of information about its national context and can be read as part of our comparative analysis, highlighting cross-national similarities and differences in the construction and characteristics of carer leave policies and their consequences. This provides valuable new knowledge for academics and policy makers, as knowledge of our social world is produced through comparison (Dogan and Pelassy, 1990; Rose, 1991). This links to the second aim of the book: to highlight areas of promising policy '[b]y making the researcher [or policy maker] aware of unexpected differences, or even surprising similarities, between cases, [and] … [bringing] a sense of perspective to a familiar environment and discourag[ing] parochial responses to political issues' (Hopkin, 2002: 249).

To achieve this aim, we draw on the 'third tradition' of cross-national comparative analysis (Hantrais, 1999). Alongside the first (mainly descriptive) and second (culturalist) traditions of comparative analysis Hantrais identifies, the third approach highlights that 'social reality is … context dependent, but the context itself serves as an important explanatory variable and an enabling tool' (Hantrais, 1999: 94). This 'societal approach' specifically addresses the consequences of differences and similarities, as a means, among other aims, to define good practice with regard to policy.

Carer leave and associated policies

In any cross-national analysis it is important that the area of policy subjected to comparison is explicit (Hopkin, 2002), and that authors focus on an area or concept that 'travels', resonating across different contexts without falling into 'concept stretching' and 'definitional sloppiness' (Sartori, 1970, 1991). All the country chapters in this book consider carer leave, defined as the paid and unpaid leave available to those in employment or work who also support an adult family member or child, or a friend or neighbour, with illness, disability or other daily needs (our choice of language is explained in Box 1.1).[2] To provide vital context, authors also present an overview of other national policies in their country designed to support working carers, including state benefits/financial transfers, tax breaks, loan schemes, rights relating to flexible working arrangements and job-protection measures.

Box 1.1: A note on language

This English-language volume covers evidence about different countries where many other languages are spoken. We recognise that, ultimately, 'Words matter. The language we use to describe the human experience is essential to understanding individuals' lived experiences and how we can best care for their well-being' (Applebaum, 2022: 621). It is thus vital, from the outset, to be clear about the language used in this book. There is considerable debate, and sometimes confusion, over how care and those who provide it are described. It can sometimes be unclear, in the English language, whether terminology refers to people caring in a paid or unpaid capacity (or both). In speech, the term 'carer' is often used interchangeably with 'care worker'. Distinguishing between 'paid' and 'unpaid' carers to address this is, we feel, unsatisfactory; it puts carers who receive state financial benefits or who are funded in some way to support them to care in an ambiguous position. In striving for clarity, authors sometimes differentiate between 'formal' and 'informal' carers, with the latter to include those providing care outside any professional role they may have. Some academics (Stall et al, 2019; Applebaum, 2022; Castro et al, 2022) and carer advocacy organisations (Care Alliance Ireland, 2017) challenge or object to this distinction. Applebaum, for example, states, 'The word *formal* suggests official, proper, qualified, while *informal* suggests casual, unofficial, easy' (original emphasis, Applebaum, 2022: 621). For this reason, in this book we decided to use the term 'carer' to include 'unpaid individual[s], such as a family member, neighbour, friend or other significant individual, who takes on a caring role to support someone with a diminishing physical ability, a debilitating cognitive condition or a chronic life-limiting illness' (IACO, nd). We acknowledge that this term is not fully satisfactory, and brings its own challenges of resonance and self-identification (Caregivers Nova Scotia, nd).

We have, however, chosen to retain the language used in the titles of legislation in country chapters, where the term 'informal carers' is sometimes used.

Selecting and clustering countries: care and employment regimes

Carer leave and other forms of support for working carers intersect the 'care' and 'employment' policy spheres. Just as it is part of human nature to make sense of our world through comparison (Dogan and Pelassy, 1990; Rose, 1991), so categorisation according to similarities and differences between institutions and/or policies has also been a preoccupation within the social sciences, especially among scholars of welfare provision, gender equality, care and employment. Some researchers have explored how countries may be clustered into 'welfare regimes' (Esping-Andersen, 1990, 1999), care regimes (Langan and Ostner, 1991; Lewis, 1992, 1997; Anttonen and Sipilä, 1996; Millar, 1999; Pfau-Effinger, 1999, 2005a, 2005b; Yeandle, 1999; Leitner, 2003; Kröger, 2011) and 'employment regimes' (Gallie, 2007), mainly in European countries, and how these regimes may influence the extent or specificities of work–family conflict (Scherer and Steiber, 2007; McGinnity and Calvert, 2009). Regime approaches offer a useful heuristic mechanism, informing the selection of countries and the ordering of chapters in this book. There are limitations in these approaches, which we discuss in more detail later in this chapter (Falkingham and Hills, 1995; Arts and Gelissen, 2002; Meyer and Pfau-Effinger, 2006; Mahon et al, 2012), but we agree with Clark's assertion that (2009: 273) 'countries do not necessarily fall nicely into one or the other category, and if they do, they might not stay there over time. It is easy to be somewhat caustic about this kind of categorisation. However, it arguably provides more structure than noting that Spain is not the same as Sweden'.

Care regimes

Care regime approaches strive to take a less 'gender-blind' attitude to the categorisation of countries than more traditional analyses of welfare regimes (Esping-Andersen, 1990, 1999). Various approaches sit within the broad framework of care regimes, with demarcations made between 'breadwinner models' (Lewis, 1992); 'maximum private/public responsibility models' (Sainsbury, 1996: 96) and the level of autonomy over labour market participation facilitated by care policy (Millar, 1999). The care regimes literature, broadly speaking, groups countries according to the division of responsibility for care between the 'welfare triangle' of state, market and households (Leitner, 2003), or 'care diamonds' which add the voluntary sector as a fourth point (Razavi, 2007). Kröger (2011) points out that care regime theory emerged as a critique of typologies of national welfare approaches focused on the provision of benefits to allow individuals to withdraw from the labour market and become 'decommodified', as in the work of Esping-Andersen (1990). Some authors claim that welfare regime approaches have tended to ignore gender and unpaid work in the private sphere of the home, thereby 'decommodifying' women engaged in unpaid care work (Langan and Ostner, 1991; Lewis, 1997; Pfau-Effinger, 2005a, 2005b). Responding to this, the most widely used approach within the care regimes literature has explored the opportunities for 'defamilialisation' offered by national welfare provision (Kröger, 2011), that is, 'the degree to which individual adults can uphold a socially acceptable standard of living, independently of family relationships, either through paid work or through the social security system' (Lister, 1994: 37).

Care regime literature emphasises the varying roles states play in providing care, and their implications for the family or the market as the provider of care, with the interplay between state, market and family in part shaped by cultural attitudes about the family. Some authors have contrasted this 'welfare-resourcing' perspective on care with an 'ethico-political' strand (Conradi, 2020), while others (Tronto, 1993; Daly, 2021) present this as less of a dichotomy, 'as socio-economic conditions and ideologies often shape the ethics of care and are used to explain its absence' (Moore and Price, 2023: 204). Thus, the care regime literature offers several examples of typologies that classify nations according to how care is provided for children or adults with support needs (or both) and/or the degree to which nations have departed from a male-breadwinner model. Though some authors factor maternity, paternity and parental leaves into their clustering of countries (for example, Bettio and Plantenga, 2004; Saraceno, 2016), leaves for carers are not always included (an example that does is Frericks et al, 2014). In this book, however, we use a broad care regimes approach in selecting countries for comparison and in ordering the chapters, grouping nations that could reasonably be expected to have adopted similar approaches to care, carer leave and other policies that support working carers.

Although there is no universally accepted typology (Peng and Yeandle, 2017), the care regime literature broadly aligns with the notion that Scandinavian countries (for example, Finland and Sweden) have adopted a 'defamilialistic' approach, with a dual-breadwinner labour market model. For this reason, we include chapters on these nations first, and together.

More specifically, Finland and Sweden have been characterised by scholars exploring care regimes as offering:

- a dual breadwinner model, where the state assumes the role of carer and where both male and female partners work (Lewis, 1992; Pfau-Effinger, 1999);
- universal support for care, funded from taxation with a limited role for the market (Anttonen and Sipilä, 1996);
- emphasising 'individual autonomy', with care as the state's responsibility (Millar, 1999);
- 'optional familialism', with provision of care services but also support for caring (Leitner, 2003).

The next grouping we present includes countries characterised as adopting policies aligned with familialism, with limited statutory care provision and either a male-breadwinner or dual-earner model if families are able to purchase care on the market. Here, the UK is often included as an exemplar (Lewis, 1992; Anttonen and Sipilä, 1996; Millar, 1999; Pfau-Effinger, 1999; Yeandle, 1999; Leitner, 2003). Contributors to the care regime literature have often categorised Australia and Canada with the UK, based on the view that, in each of these nations, the state mainly provides care support for those who are least able to afford private care services. Brennan et al (2012) nevertheless see key differences among them, based on their specific policy histories and political structures. In Canada's federal system of government, provision of care services is mainly the responsibility of provinces and territories, meaning there is no single care 'system', although some services – including residential care facilities, palliative care, respite, rehabilitation and personal care services – are provided throughout Canada on a needs-based and income-tested basis. There is strong reliance on carers in Canada, with at least 75 per cent of all care provided by family members or friends (Stall, 2019). It has been argued that Australia has shifted towards a care model that is increasingly reliant on the private market (Brennan et al, 2012). Fine and Davidson (2018: 508) identify 'a consumer-driven, market-based system', with carers 'filling gaps' in provision (O'Loughlin and Williams, Chapter 4, this volume). For these reasons, the UK, Australia and Canada are the next three chapters presented. The key features of the care regimes in each of these three countries are summarised in Table 1.1.

Next, we consider Germany and Japan. Germany's approach is strongly influenced by the 'subsidiarity principle' (Anttonen and Sipilä, 1996), in that families are first and foremost responsible for providing care to their members, with support available, where needed, from the state, funded by a Long-Term Care Insurance (LTCI) system. Prior to introducing its LTCI scheme, Germany was widely seen as a 'strong male breadwinner' regime,

Table 1.1: Australia, the UK and Canada vis-à-vis the care regime literature

Country	Care regime typology and characteristics
Australia	'a consumer-driven, market-based system' (Fine and Davidson, 2018: 508)
UK	• Means and needs-tested model: targeted public support for those most in need; state contracts services out to market (Anttonen and Sipilä, 1996) • Dual-breadwinner/marketised carer (Pfau-Effinger, 1999)/dual-earner/marketised-female-domestic-economy (Yeandle, 1999) • Explicit familialism: no/limited formal care provision and pro-familialistic policies (Leitner, 2003)
Canada	• Fragmented federal/provincial/territorial 'system' with heavy reliance on familial provision (Stall, 2019)

with a clear division between the public and private spheres, its lack of care provision contributing to the strong concentration of women in part-time jobs (Lewis, 1997) and exemplifying 'explicit familialism' in its limited formal care provision and pro-familialistic policies (Leitner, 2003). Japan, which has similarly adopted an LTCI scheme, has undergone significant changes in how care is provided and funded by the state, shifting away from a model based predominantly on family within the 'filial piety' tradition. Influenced by Germany's LTCI arrangements, Japan's compulsory system provides universal support on a needs-tested basis to people over age 65 (and to younger people with age-related disabilities). Peng and Yeandle (2017) argue that this changed public attitudes towards wider acceptance of use of formal care services. In introducing its LTCI system, Japan became the first nation in East Asia where the state shoulders partial responsibility for care (Soma and Yamashita, 2011).

Despite the similarities between the insurance-based systems introduced in Germany and Japan, there is one crucial difference. The German system permits use of LTCI funds as payments to unpaid (family) carers, an arrangement that some argue stimulates family members (primarily women) to take up caring roles. In Japan, this is not permitted – payments can be used only for the purchase of care services on the market (Rhee et al, 2015).

Next, we couple our chapters on Slovenia and Poland, countries that exhibit tendencies to 'implicit familialism' in Slovenia (Hlebec et al, 2016; 2017; Filipovič Hrast et al, 2020), 'family-by-default' arrangements in Poland (Radziwinowiczówna and Rosińska, 2022), and offer limited opportunities for 'defamilialisation'. In Slovenia, statutory provision was traditionally focused on care in residential institutions, with families legally obliged to contribute to the cost of this care. Home care services are developing, but residential care still predominates, and families remain the main providers of care (Hlebec et al, 2016, 2017; Filipovič Hrast et al, 2019). Poland, too, has limited statutory care provision. Citing reductions in funding and the requirement that people contribute to their own care, Radziwinowiczówna and Rosińska (2022) describe the Polish approach as 'neoliberalisation of familialism by default', rather than 'refamilialisation'. Slovenia and Poland can thus be seen as examples of the 'family care model' (Anttonen and Sipilä, 1996) that has also been a feature in many southern European nations, with their historically limited state provision of care (Bettio and Platenga, 2004).

Employment regimes

As highlighted already, carer leave provision spans the policy domains of both care and employment. Policy on care shapes the division of caring labour between the state, the market and (working) carers, and affects the extent to which carers are financially compensated for providing care; employment policy is, however, often where leave policies are situated. Just as scholars have grouped countries according to their welfare (and specifically care) provision, so attention has turned to states' differential role in policies related to employment. Most relevant to carer leave are those that, under the broad umbrella of 'employment' or 'production' regimes (in turn part of a wider school of institutional approaches [Holman, 2013b]), consider aspects relevant to working carers. In scope here are flexibility and measures to support work–life balance (Anttila et al, 2015), seen by some as indicators of broader issues, such as job quality (Gallie, 2007; Scherer and Steiber, 2007; Holman, 2013a, 2013b).

While Holman (2013b) does not include carer leave as a measure of flexibility or work–life balance in his empirical exploration of employment regimes (or 'institutional regimes' in Holman's work) and job quality, the clustering of countries in the typology he presents and empirically examines aligns with the care regimes previously discussed. Holman (2013b) drew on the work of Whitely (1999), Amable (2003), Gallie (2007) and Goergen et al (2009) to explore job quality in five institutional regimes. He proposed that social democratic regimes such as Sweden and Finland, labelled 'inclusivist' by Gallie (2007), are more likely to promote job quality by including organised labour in decision making and in policies to enhance employment and employment rights. Dualist (Gallie, 2007) or continental (Holman, 2013b) regimes (such as Germany) offer strong employment rights to a core workforce, with weaker rights for those on the margins. Overall job quality is consequently (on average) high, but lower than in social democratic regimes. In another analysis, Japan (not included in Holman's 2013b work) has been identified as adopting a 'dualist' regime (Lee, 2011). In 'market' (Gallie, 2007) or 'liberal' (Holman, 2013b) regimes, as the terminology suggests, the market leads, with relatively low employment regulation and worker voice. In this analysis, countries in this regime such as the UK (Holman, 2013b and Canada (Holman, 2013a) are seen as exhibiting low job quality.

Other analyses see 'southern' and 'transitional' regimes (including Poland and Slovenia) as characterised by rather weak labour movements and low levels of state invention in working conditions, also resulting in poor job quality (Whitely, 1999; Amable, 2003; Goergen et al, 2009; Holman, 2013a, 2013b).

A potential area of divergence from the care regime grouping of nations is Australia (not included in Holman's 2013b analysis). Other scholars see Australia as closer to a dualist than to a market regime, with a relatively strong labour movement, albeit one historically focused mainly on male-dominated sectors which has 'often ignored or over-ridden the interests of working women in pursuit of the interests of men' (Pocock, 2005: 40), a gender balance that some claim is shifting (Foley and Cooper, 2021). Nonetheless, in exploring both care and employment regime literatures, it is apparent that the clustering identified in both contains a great deal of overlap, and therefore provides a structure for the country-focused chapters.

Some caveats on regime theory

It is, however, worth noting that approaches that focus on identifying welfare/care/employment regimes have been criticised for a number of reasons. First, they are argued to extrapolate to the point where nuance and differences among countries within regimes are missed (Mahon et al, 2012). As Arts and Gelissen (2002: 137) note, states rarely are 'pure' types, and indeed, authors in this book identify areas of divergence from where their country of focus has been placed within care regime theory (for example, Leinonen, Chapter 2; Aldman et al, Chapter 3). Also, regime approaches are attuned to identifying differences and similarities between nations, but they are less adept at addressing policy change and therefore provide a 'snapshot' of policy at a particular point in time (Falkingham and Hills, 1995; Meyer and Pfau-Effinger, 2006).

Other approaches have sought to situate care provision within a broader analysis of workers' lifecourses, and in doing so add a dynamic element to the analysis of national policies. The transitional labour market (TLM) framework developed by Schmid (2011, 2017), for example, focuses on transitions workers might make between different employment statuses during their lifetimes, including between work and unpaid care, or an employment status that involves a combination of work and unpaid care. With regard to policies to support transitions, the TLM approach calls for employment, social protection and vocational education and training policies. Schmid et al find such policies:

> *empower individuals* to switch from one work-situation to another according to changes in the economy as well as according to individuals' changing preferences, other obligations, or work capacities over the

life course. *Citizens should therefore have the right to transitions.* '*Work*', in this context, includes all activities of social obligatory character, whether paid or not. Typical and commonly used examples are the right to family-related furloughs such as parental or other care leave. (emphasis in original, Schmid et al, 2023: 16)

While studies have shown that welfare, employment and care regimes interact to shape outcomes for families, especially for women, the evidence on how work–family conflict is affected by regime type is mixed. Clustering according to policies, rather than real-world outcomes, raises questions, perhaps, about the explanatory value of regimes analyses. Crompton and Lyonette (2006) found work–life conflict to be lower in Finland and Norway (both social democratic welfare regimes with relatively well-developed 'family-friendly' policies) than in Great Britain, France and Portugal. Scherer and Steiber (2007), however, found that while more developed family-friendly policies, such as parental leave and affordable childcare, increase women's ability to engage in paid work, they may not prevent work–family conflict. Such conflict was found to be lower when provision of family-friendly policies coincided with workers having a significant control over their working time. Similarly, in comparing outcomes for women in Australia, France and Sweden, Anxo et al (2017) concluded that relatively low maternal employment rates and relatively high rates of female part-time employment in Australia reflect the legacy of an 'industrial male breadwinner' tradition with weak support for parental leave and childcare. By contrast, high employment rates and longer working hours for women in Sweden reflect the greater support for parental leave and childcare in that country. Despite this, in all three countries women remain the primary caregivers, and gender pay gaps persist. Indeed, issues of equity and equality are explored in the country-specific chapters, allowing for a comparison not only of the carer leave and associated policies cross-nationally, but also their outcomes.

Analysis of carer leave in nine countries

The empirical evidence is this book is presented in nine 'country chapters'. Each starts with a description and assessment of carer leaves. We begin with two Nordic states. For Leinonen (Chapter 2), Finland emphasises widespread labour force participation alongside a contradictory social expectation that families will provide significant care. Finns can access three short-term temporary unpaid leaves to care for a family member or friend who needs help with Activities of Daily Living (ADLs) or because of serious illness or injury. A longer break (100–180 days) is also available, subject to strict eligibility criteria, in which case an allowance calculated at 70 per cent of Finland's statutory unemployment allowance is payable.

Leinonen finds these unpaid/low-paid leaves problematic, arguing that they put employees' income, career development and pensions at risk. She points out that support for employees caring for adult family members or for friends with care needs falls far short of what is provided for working parents, an observation repeated in many of the subsequent country-specific chapters in the book.

In Chapter 3, Aldman, Sennemark and Hanson describe Sweden as a Nordic welfare state with collectivist values and a fundamental philosophy that social services should maximise an individual's independence from family. Unfortunately, an upshot of this is that, at least until recently, carers and their challenges were not prioritised in Swedish health and social care policy. Provisions in Sweden include leave for urgent family reasons (illness or an accident) implemented through collective agreements between national unions and employers. This mode of implementation means the length of leave varies (from part of a working day to several days), as does compensation (from 0 to 100 per cent of pay). Parents of a child aged under 23 years with a serious illness may take between 10 and 120 days off to attend to their child's care, while parents of children under 16 may take between 60 and 120 days. They are also entitled to a temporary parental allowance. Sweden provides longer-term leaves to care for a family member, relative, friend or neighbour with a life-threatening illness too (up to a maximum of 100 days, or 240 days if caring for someone with HIV). Aldman et al conclude that the support offered is not sufficiently flexible to meet the needs of individual carers but nevertheless note indications that political willingness to address the needs of Swedish carers is growing, exemplified by the launch of a national carers strategy in Sweden in 2022.

We then move to Australia (Chapter 4) as an example of a liberal welfare state with selected universal benefits and targeted support for those with specific needs. O'Loughlin and Williams observe shifts to more individual responsibility and to recently implemented market-based aged and disability care systems, characterised by a consumer-directed funding model intended to reduce pressure on public expenditure and offer service users better choice and control. They note increased casualisation of the labour market, with growing numbers of workers ineligible for paid leave. Unsurprisingly, this has increased pressure on family carers. Legislation on workplace rights nevertheless gives Australian employed carers access to paid personal and/ or carer leave, as well as to paid compassionate leave and unpaid carer leave. Australia's 'long-term' leave is short compared to other countries, however, at ten days, but with the option to accrue leave and often more days available to those in different employment sectors. The authors describe Australia's system of leaves as rather flexible, in that employees can use such leave for their own needs (including sickness) as well as for caring responsibilities. The system is quite complex, however, as entitlements are determined by a mix of labour legislation, workers' compensation arrangements, industry- and occupation-specific awards and enterprise-level agreements.

Hamblin, Heyes and Allard report in Chapter 5 that addressing the support needs of working carers has become critically important in the United Kingdom (UK) in recent years. The UK's approach to the provision of care services nevertheless focuses on extensive privatisation and marketisation, with limited direct state provision. Rights for working carers are governed by legislation, including the Employment Relations Act 1999, which protects employees from dismissal if they respond to an emergency involving a dependant. In 2023 a Carer's Leave Act was passed, to give employees the right to up to five days of unpaid carer leave. Non-governmental organisations and carer advocacy groups have, since the 1960s, played a notable and unique role in the evolution of carer support policies, raising the profile of carers and awareness of care work as a legitimate public policy issue. Their attention continues to focus on support for working carers as part of wider lobbying for the 'right to a life outside caring', including in paid employment.

In Chapter 6, Fast and Eales describe Canada as a liberal welfare state with a political ideology that emphasises labour force sustainability. Multiple short- and longer-term carer leaves have been legislated as a result of this. The leaves are job protected, relatively generous in duration (3–12 days and 17–28 weeks, respectively) and based on inclusive definitions of family. In addition, multiple carers can share the longer-term leaves. Carers who qualify for longer-term leaves are also eligible for partial income replacement (55 per cent of pre-leave earnings, up to a fixed maximum amount). The authors nevertheless note important geographical differences for Canadians, arising from how jurisdiction over labour and care policy in Canada is split, and in some instances overlaps with legislation introduced by the nation's various federal, provincial and territorial governments. Age inequalities are also present in the Canadian system, with greater entitlements for those caring for children than for people who care for adults in need of care. Despite their apparent generosity, Canada's longer-term leaves are available only to those caring for family members or friends with medically documented critical, life-threatening and terminal conditions, resulting in carers of someone with a chronic condition being eligible for only a few days per year of Family Responsibility Leave. Canada also lacks some carer supports available in other countries (such as carer benefits, pension protections and carers' ability to apply for and receive social care services in their own right).

In Chapter 7, Knauthe and Hoff describe Germany's sociopolitical context as a conservative or familialist welfare regime in which it is assumed families hold primary responsibility for caring for their members. LTCI is, however, a central feature of Germany's current approach to meeting care needs. Compulsory employee and employer insurance contributions fund the statutory LTCI scheme. When long-term care is needed, carers, including family members, may be paid to provide this care, although the payment they receive is substantially lower than the wage paid to professional care workers. Employed carers in Germany have access to three unpaid carer leave schemes: short-term leave of up to ten working days; longer-term full- or part-time leave of up to six months; and partial leave of absence (reduction in working hours) for up to two years. Carers taking the short-term carer leave are entitled to an allowance amounting to 90 per cent of net foregone pay, and there are loans available for longer-term leave. All employees are entitled to the short-term leave, but carers working for small and medium-sized companies have no legal entitlement to the longer-term leaves, a significant omission, as 56 per cent of private sector employees in Germany work in small and medium-sized enterprises (Statista, 2022).

In Chapter 8, the focus turns to Asia, and to Japan. Ikeda describes Japan as one of the most aged societies globally, with many older people (albeit in declining numbers) co-residing with their adult children. He observes a waning familialist approach to welfare, exemplified by the introduction in 2000 of LTCI. This expanded formal care services, aiming to reduce pressure on family members to provide high levels of care for older people. Financial constraints within the LTCI scheme have resulted in rather few Japanese working carers actually taking long-term carer leave. Rather, they tend to take time off or to change their working hours, providing care themselves. Ikeda describes Japan's statutory carer leave system as well established, with unpaid short-term leave of five days per year, and a longer-term leave of 93 days (which, under recent iterations of the scheme, can be split into three periods), plus exemption from compulsory overtime. Employees taking long-term leave, aimed particularly at the care of their elderly parents, are compensated through employment insurance, up to 67 per cent of their normal salary and (in both cases) are protected from dismissal.

In Chapter 9, Rakar, Filipovič Hrast and Hlebec describe Slovenia as a former socialist society in which the state played a dominant role. After gaining its independence in 1991, Slovenia's welfare system evolved as a hybrid conservative-corporatist and social democratic model. Compulsory social insurance is the main social protection mechanism and a strong state sector the main service provider, with equal access for all. Slovenia has a mixed approach to family policy, which is highly de-familialised as it pertains to care for children, but highly familialised with respect to supporting older people. The authors report that while Slovenia's history of high female labour force participation rates gave rise to robust childcare services and generous maternity and parental leave, they have left it without a similar response to carers' growing responsibilities for their older relatives. Slovenia has one legislated carer leave, in place since Slovenia's socialist period, available when an employed carer needs to care for a co-resident sick spouse or child. Each episode of carer leave may be of up to 10 days (20 days for children aged under seven years or with special needs, or in exceptional circumstances, up to 40 days). Those taking such leave are paid at 80 per cent of their average gross earnings during this time. A new Long Term Care Act was passed in 2021 and is intended to improve this situation, but labour market segmentation, austerity, cost-containment measures and political instability have delayed its implementation.

In Poland, the working carers received little policy attention until recently. Indeed, Perek-Białas and Ruzik-Sierdzińska report in Chapter 10 that in 2015 Eurofound ranked Poland last among EU countries with respect to support for combining paid work and care work. Like Slovenia, Poland has transitioned from a socialist regime in which state institutions and state-owned employers met many social needs, to a more liberal welfare state with multiple free-market economy and personal responsibility characteristics. This transition, together with traditional views on family and a gendered division of roles and inadequate publicly funded care services (and unaffordable private care), has made family members the 'first line of defence' in meeting care needs. The authors describe substantial regional variation in social services and social security, responsibility for which is divided among Poland's national, regional and local governments. As in several other countries discussed in this book, family policy in Poland provides more support for people with childcare responsibilities than for those helping adults with support needs, although proposals to align Polish labour law with EU minimum standards on work–care reconciliation (to include five days of unpaid carer leave per year) were implemented in April 2023, creating two new, short-term leaves for carers.

Having set out in detail the background, specific features and specificities of carer leave in each of the nine countries, the book concludes by offering a critical comparative analysis of the foregoing material. Our concluding chapter highlights commonalities and differences in the nine countries' policies and policy instruments; considers to what extent these represent policy successes and failures; and aims to account for these by reference to the countries' different political, social and economic contexts.

We close with high-level observations about future directions for research, policy and practice, with the aspiration that these, and the detailed material presented elsewhere in the book, may inspire positive change, both in our nine selected countries and more widely, creating policy settings that evolve and grow and enable more carers to successfully combine caring with paid work in coming decades.

Notes
[1]   Albeit beyond the specific scope of this book, we also acknowledge that the relationship between paid work and providing unpaid care has crucial dimensions linked to global

inequalities. As female labour force participation rates in the global North have grown, women workers from the global South have increasingly been drawn upon to address 'care deficits' in affluent societies (Pocock, 2014), often further exacerbating inequalities in the global division of labour.

[2] Thus policies and provision associated with parenthood more generally – such as maternity, paternity and adoption leaves and benefits, and the provision of childcare services – are beyond the scope of this book.

References

Addati, L., Cattaneo, U. and Pozzan, E. (2022) *Care at work: Investing in care leave and services for a more gender equal world of work*, Geneva: International Labour Organization.

Addati, L., Cattaneo, U., Esquivel, V. and Valarino, I. (2018) *Care work and care jobs for the future of decent work*, Geneva: International Labour Organization.

Amable, B. (2003) *The diversity of modern capitalism*, Oxford: Oxford University Press.

Anderson, L.A., Edwards, V.J., Pearson, W.S., Talley, R.C., McGuire, L.C. and Andresen E.M. (2013) 'Adult caregivers in the United States: characteristics and differences in well-being, by caregiver age and caregiving status', *Preventing Chronic Disease: Public Health Research*, 15:10:E135. https:// doi.org/10.5888/pcd10.130090

Anttila, T., Oinas, T., Tammelin, M. and Nätti, J. (2015) 'Working-time regimes and work–life balance in Europe', *European Sociological Review*, 31(6): 713–24.

Anttonen, A. and Sipilä, J. (1996) 'European social care services: is it possible to identify models?' *Journal of European Social Policy*, 6(2): 87–100.

Anxo, D., Baird, M. and Erhel, C. (2017) 'Work and care regimes and women's employment outcomes: Australia, France and Sweden compared', in D. Grimshaw, C. Fagan, G. Hebson and I. Tavora (eds), *Making work more equal: A new labour market segmentation approach*, Manchester: Manchester University Press, pp 309–29.

Applebaum, A.J. (2022) 'There is nothing informal about caregiving', *Palliative and Supportive Care*, 20: 621–2, https:// doi.org/10.1017/S1478951522001092.

Arts, W. and Gelissen, J. (2002) 'Welfare states, solidarity and justice principles: does the type really matter?' *Acta Sociologica*, 44: 283–99.

Austin, A. and Heyes, J. (2020) *Supporting working carers: How employers and employees can benefit*, research report, CIPD/University of Sheffield.

Bauer, J.M. and Sousa-Poza, A. (2015) 'Impacts of informal caregiving on caregiver employment, health, and family', *Population Ageing*, 8: 113–45.

Beard, J.R., Officer, A., De Carvalho, I.A., Sadana, R., Pot, A.M., Michel, J.P., and Chatterji, S. (2016) 'The world report on ageing and health: a policy framework for healthy ageing', *The Lancet*, 387(10033): 2145–54.

Bettio, F. and Plantenga, J. (2004) 'Comparing care regimes in Europe', *Feminist Economics*, 10(1): 85–113.

Boise, L. and Neal, M. (1996) 'Family responsibilities and absenteeism: Employees caring for parents versus employees caring for children', *Journal of Managerial Issues*, 8(2): 218–38.

Bouget, D., Spasova, S. and Vanhercke, B. (2016) *Work–life balance measures for persons of working age with dependent relatives in Europe. A study of national policies*, European Social Policy Network (ESPN), Brussels: European Commission.

Brimblecombe, N., Fernandez, J.-L., Knapp, M., Rehill, A. and Wittenberg, R. (2018) 'Review of the international evidence on support for unpaid carers', *Journal of Long-Term Care*, September, 25–40. https://doi.org/10.21953/lse.ffq4txr2nftf

Care Alliance Ireland (2017) *The right not to be called an informal carer; Care Alliance Ireland: Position statement on language use*. Available from: https://www.carealliance.ie/userfiles/files/CAI_Position_Paper_On_Language_Use_(2017).pdf [Accessed 16 November 2023].

Caregivers Nova Scotia (nd) *Caregiving language*. Available from: https://caregiversns.org/who-we-are/caregiving-language/ [Accessed 16 November 2023].

Carr, E., Murray, E.T., Zaninotto, P., Cadar, D., Head, J., Stansfeld, S. and Stafford, M. (2018) 'The association between informal caregiving and exit from employment among older workers: prospective findings from the UK household longitudinal study', *The Journals of Gerontology: Series B*, 73(7): 1253-1262. https://doi.org/10.1093/geronb/gbw156

Castro, A.R., Arnaert, A., Moffatt, K., Kildea, J., Bitzas, V. and Tsimicalis, A. (2022) '"Informal caregiver" in nursing: an evolutionary concept analysis', *Advances in Nursing Science*, 10: 1097.

Cès, S., Hlebec, V. and Yghemonos, S. (2019) *Valuing informal care in Europe: Analytical review of existing valuation methods*, Brussels: Eurocarers. Available from: https://eurocarers.org/publications/valuing-informal-care-in-europe/ [Accessed 16 November 2023].

Clark, A. (2009) Review: 'Employment Regimes and the Quality of Work – Edited by Duncan Gallie', *British Journal of Industrial Relations*, 47: 793–795. https://doi.org/10.1111/j.1467-8543.2009.00753_4.x

Cohen, S.A., Cook, S.K., Sando, T.A., Brown, M.J. and Longo, D.R. (2017) 'Socioeconomic and demographic disparities in caregiving intensity and quality of life in informal caregivers: a first look at the National Study of caregiving', *Journal of Gerontological Nursing*, 43(6): 17–24.

Cohen, S.A., Sabik, N.J., Cook, S.K., Azzoli, A.B. and Mendez-Luck, C.A. (2019) 'Differences within differences: gender inequalities in caregiving intensity vary by race and ethnicity in informal caregivers', *Journal of Cross-Cultural Gerontology*, 34, 245–63.

Conradi, E. (2020) 'Theorising care: attentive interaction or distributive justice?', *International Journal of Care and Caring*, 4(1): 25–42, https://doi.org/10.1332/239788219X15633663863542.

Crompton, R. and Lyonette, C. (2006) 'Work–life "balance" in Europe', *Acta Sociologica*, 49(4): 379–93.

Daly, M. (2021) 'The concept of care: insights, challenges and research avenues in COVID-19 times', *Journal of European Social Policy*, 31(1): 108–18.

Daly, M. and Rake, K. (2003) *Gender and the welfare state: Care, work and welfare in Europe and the USA*, Hoboken, NJ: John Wiley & Sons.

Dentinger, E. and Clarkberg, M. (2002) 'Informal caregiving and retirement timing among men and women: gender and caregiving relationships in late midlife', *Journal of Family Issues*, 23: 857–79. https://doi.org/10.1177/019251302236598

Do, E.K., Cohen, S.A. and Brown, M.J. (2014) 'Socioeconomic and demographic factors modify the association between informal caregiving and health in the Sandwich Generation', *BMC Public Health*, 14: 1–8.

Dogan, M. and Pelassy, D. (1990) *How to compare nations: Strategies in comparative politics*, London: Chatham House Publishers Inc.

Dykstra, P.A. and Djundeva, M. (2020) 'Policies for later-life families in a comparative European perspective', in R. Nieuwenhuis and W. Van Lancker (eds), *The Palgrave handbook of family policy*, Cham, Switzerland: Palgrave Macmillan, pp 331–66.

Eldh, A.C. and Carlsson, E. (2011) 'Seeking a balance between employment and the care of an ageing parent', *Scandinavian Journal of Caring Sciences*, 25(2): 285–93.

Esping-Andersen, G. (1990) *The three worlds of welfare capitalism*, Cambridge: Polity Press.

Esping-Andersen, G. (1999) *Social foundations of postindustrial economies*, Oxford: Oxford University Press.

Eurofound (2015) *Working and caring: Reconciliation measures in times of demographic change*, Luxembourg: Publications Office of the European Union.

Evandrou, M. and Glaser, K. (2003) 'Combining work and family life: the pension penalty of caring', *Ageing and Society*, 23(5): 583–601.

Evandrou, M. and Glaser, K. (2005) *Family, work and quality of life: Changing economic and social roles*, Full Research Report ESRC Award No. L480254036: Available from: http://www.esrcsocietytoday.ac.uk/ESRCInfoCentre/ViewAwardPage.aspx?AwardId=839 [Accessed 12 March 2019].

Falkingham, J. and Hills, J. (1995) 'Introduction', in J. Falkingham and J. Hills (eds), *The dynamic of welfare: The welfare state and the life cycle*, London: Harvester Wheatsheaf, pp 1–10.

Fast, J., Duncan, K.A., Keating, N.C. and Kim, C. (2023) 'Valuing the contributions of family caregivers to the care economy', *Journal of Family and Economic Issues*, 1–14, online first.

Feinberg, L.F. (2019) 'Paid family leave: an emerging benefit for employed family caregivers of older adults', *Journal of the American Geriatrics Society*, 27(7): 1336–41.

Feinberg, L.F. and Spillman, B.C. (2019) 'Shifts in family caregiving – and a growing care gap', *Generations: Journal of the American Society on Aging*, 43(1): 73–7.

Filipovič Hrast, M., Schoyen, M.A. and Rakar, T. (2019) 'A comparative analysis of people's views on future policies for the elderly', *Revija za socijalnu politiku*, 26(2): 153–69.

Filipovič Hrast, M., Hlebec, V. and Rakar, T. (2020) 'Sustainable care in a familialist regime: coping with elderly care in Slovenia', *Sustainability*, 12(20): 84–98.

Fine, M. and Davidson, B. (2018) 'The marketization of care: global challenges and national responses in Australia', *Current Sociology*, 66(4): 503–16.

Foley, M. and Cooper, R. (2021) 'Workplace gender equality in the post-pandemic era: where to next?' *Journal of Industrial Relations*, 63(4): 463–76.

Frericks, P., Jensen, P.H. and Pfau-Effinger, B. (2014) 'Social rights and employment rights related to family care: family care regimes in Europe', *Journal of Aging Studies*, 29: 66–77.

Gallie, D. (2007) 'Production regimes, employment regimes, and the quality of work', in D. Gallie (ed), *Employment regimes and the quality of work*, Oxford: Oxford University Press, pp 1–33.

Gaugler, J.E., Pestka, D.L., Davila, H., Sales, R., Owen, G., Baumgartner, S.A. and Kenney, M. (2018) 'The complexities of family caregiving at work: a mixed-methods study', *The International Journal of Aging and Human Development*, 87(4): 347–76.

GBD Ageing Collaborators (2022) 'Global, regional, and national burden of diseases and injuries for adults 70 years and older: systematic analysis for the Global Burden of Disease 2019 Study', *British Medical Journal*, 376: e068208.

Goergen, M., Brewster, C. and Wood, G. (2009) 'Corporate governance and training', *Journal of Industrial Relations*, 51(4): 459–87.

Hantrais, L. (1999) 'Contextualization in cross-national comparative research', *International Journal of Social Research Methodology*, 2(2): 93–108.

Heitink, E., Heerkens, Y. and Engels, J. (2017) 'Informal care, employment and quality of life: barriers and facilitators to combining informal care and work participation for healthcare professionals', *Work*, 58(2): 215–31.

Hlebec, V. and Rakar, T. (2017) 'Ageing policies in Slovenia: before and after austerity', in L. Tomczyk (ed), *Selected contemporary challenges of ageing policy*, Krakow, Poland: Uniwersytet Pedagogiczny w Krakowie, pp 27–51.

Hlebec, V., Srakar, A. and Majcen, B. (2016) 'Care for the elderly in Slovenia: a combination of informal and formal care', *Revija za socijalnu politiku*, 23(2): 159–79.

Holman, D. (2013a) 'An explanation of cross-national variation in call centre job quality using institutional theory', *Work, Employment and Society*, 27(1): 21–38.

Holman, D. (2013b) 'Job types and job quality in Europe', *Human Relations*, 66(4): 475–502.

Hopkin, J. (2002) 'Comparative methods', in D. Marsh and G. Stoker (eds), *Theory and methods in political science* (2nd edn), Basingstoke: Palgrave Macmillan, pp 249–70.

IACO (International Association of Carers Organizations) (nd) 'Recognising carers'. Available from: https://internationalcarers.org/carer-facts/ [Accessed 16 November 2023].

Jacobs, J.C., Lilly, M.B., Ng, C. and Coyte, P.C. (2013) 'The fiscal impact of informal caregiving to home care recipients in Canada: how the intensity of care influences costs and benefits to government', *Social Science and Medicine*, 81: 102–9.

Keck, W. and Saraceno, C. (2009) *Balancing elderly care and employment in Germany* (No. SP I 2009–401). WZB Discussion Paper.

Kodate, N. and Timonen, V. (2017) 'Bringing the family in through the back door: the stealthy expansion of family care in Asian and European long-term care policy', *Journal of Cross-Cultural Gerontology*, 32: 291–301.

Kröger, T. (2011) 'Defamilisation, dedomestication and care policy: Comparing childcare service provisions of welfare states', *International Journal of Sociology and Social Policy*, 31(7/8): 424–40.

Langan, M. and Ostner, I. (1991) 'Gender and welfare: towards a comparative framework', in G. Room (ed), *Towards a European welfare state?* Bristol: SAUS, pp 127–50.

Lee, S.Y.S. (2011) 'The evolution of welfare production regimes in East Asia: a comparative study of Korea, Japan, and Taiwan', *Journal of Policy Studies*, 26(1): 49–75.

Leitner, S. (2003) 'Varieties of familialism: the caring function of the family in comparative perspective', *European Societies*, 5(4): 353–75.

Lero, D., Spinks, N., Fast, J. and Tremblay, D.-G. (2012) *The availability, accessibility and effectiveness of workplace supports for Canadian caregivers*, Final report to Human Resources and Skills Development Canada, Gatineau, PQ.

Lewis, J. (1992) 'Gender and the development of welfare regimes', *Journal of European Social Policy*, 2(3): 159–73.

Lewis, J. (1997) 'Gender and welfare regimes: further thoughts', *Social Politics: International Studies in Gender, State and Society*, 4(2): 160–77.

Lister, R. (1994) ' "She has other duties": women, citizenship and social security', in S. Baldwin and J. Falkingham (eds), *Social security and social change: New challenges*, Hemel Hempstead: Harvester Wheatsheaf, pp 31–44.

Lloyd, L. (2023) *Unpaid Care Policies in the UK: Rights, Resources and Relationships*, Bristol: Policy Press.

Lorenz, F., Whittaker, L., Tazzeo, J. and Williams, A. (2021) 'Availability of caregiver-friendly workplace policies: an international scoping review follow-up study', *International Journal of Workplace Health Management*, 14(4): 459–76.

Mahon, R., Anttonen, A., Bergqvist, C., Brennan, D. and Hobson, B. (2012) 'Convergent care regimes? Childcare arrangements in Australia, Canada, Finland and Sweden', *Journal of European Social Policy*, 22(4): 419–31.

Masuy, A.J. (2009) 'Effect of caring for an older person on women's lifetime participation in work', *Ageing and Society*, 29(5): 745–63.

Matthews, R.A. and Fisher, G.G. (2013) 'The role of work and family in the retirement process: A review and new directions', in M. Wang (ed), *The Oxford handbook of retirement*, New York: Oxford University Press, pp 354–70.

McGinnity, F. and Calvert, E. (2009) 'Work–life conflict and social inequality in Western Europe', *Social Indicators Research*, 93: 489–508.

Meyer, T. and Pfau-Effinger, B. (2006) 'Gender arrangements and pension systems in Britain and Germany: tracing change over five decades', *International Journal of Ageing and Later Life*, 1(2): 67–110.

Millar, J. (1999) 'Obligations and autonomy', in R. Crompton (ed), *Restructuring gender relations and employment: The decline of the male breadwinner*, Oxford: Oxford University Press, pp 26–40.

Milligan, C. (2012) *There's no place like home: Place and care in an ageing society*, Farnham: Ashgate.

Mooney, A., Statham, J. with Simon, A. (2002) *The Pivot Generation: Informal Care and Work after Fifty*, Bristol: Policy Press for the Joseph Rowntree Foundation. Available from: https://www.jrf.org.uk/report/informal-care-and-work-after-fifty [Accessed 25 June 2022].

Moore, E. and Price, D. (2023) 'Editorial', *International Journal of Care and Caring,* 7(2): 201–11.

Ortiz-Ospina, E. Tzvetkova, S. and Roser, M. (2018) *'Women's employment'*. Available from: https://ourworldindata.org/female-labor-supply [Accessed 16 November 2023].

Peng, I. and Yeandle, S.M. (2017) *Eldercare policies in East Asia and Europe: Mapping policy changes and variations and their implications,* UN Women's Discussion Paper Series, United Nations Entity for Gender Equality and the Empowerment of Women (UN Women): New York.

Perek-Białas, J. and Slany, K. (2015) 'The elderly care regime and migration regime after the EU accession: The case of Poland', in U. Karl, and S. Torres (eds), *Ageing in contexts of migration*, London: Routledge, pp 27–38.

Pfau-Effinger, B. (1999) 'The modernization of family and motherhood', in R. Crompton (ed), *Restructuring gender relations and employment: The decline of the male breadwinner*, Oxford: Oxford University Press, pp 60–80.

Pfau-Effinger, B. (2005a) 'Culture and welfare state policies: reflections on a complex interrelation', *Journal of Social Policy*, 34(1): 3–20.

Pfau-Effinger, B. (2005b) 'Welfare state policies and the development of care arrangements', *European Societies*, 7(2): 321–47.

Phillips, J., Bernard, M. and Chittenden, M. (2002) *Juggling work and care: The Experiences of working carers of older adults*, Bristol: The Policy Press for the Joseph Rowntree Foundation.

Pocock, B. (2005) 'Work/care regimes: institutions, culture and behaviour and the Australian case. Gender', *Work and Organization*, 12(1): 32–49.

Pocock, B. (2014) 'Work, bodies, care: gender and employment in a global world', in A. Wilkinson, G. Wood and R. Deeg (eds), *The Oxford handbook of employment relations*, Oxford: Oxford University Press, pp 495–521.

Radziwinowiczówna, A. and Rosińska, A. (2022) 'Neoliberalization of familialism by default: the case of local organization of elder care in Poland', in L. Näre and L. Widding Isaksen (eds), *Care loops and mobilities in Nordic, Central, and Eastern European welfare states*, Cham: Springer International Publishing, pp 41–62.

Razavi, S. (2007) *The political and social economy of care in a development context: conceptual issues, research questions and policy options*, #Gender and Development Programme Paper No. 3, United Nations Research Institute for Social Development, Geneva: UNRISD.

Rhee, J.C., Done, N. and Anderson, G.F. (2015) 'Considering long-term care insurance for middle-income countries: comparing South Korea with Japan and Germany', *Health policy*, 119(10): 1319–29.

Rose, R. (1991) 'Comparing forms of comparative analysis', *Political Studies*, 39(3): 446–62.

Sainsbury, D. (1996) *Gender, Equality and Welfare States*, Cambridge, UK: Cambridge University Press.

Sakka, M., Sato, I., Ikeda, M., Hashizume, H., Uemori, M. and Kamibeppu, K. (2016) 'Family-to-work spillover and appraisals of caregiving by employed women caring for their elderly parents in Japan', *Industrial Health*, 54(3): 272–81.

Saraceno, C. (2016) 'Varieties of familialism: comparing four southern European and East Asian welfare regimes', *Journal of European Social Policy*, 26(4): 314–26.

Sartori, G. (1970) 'Concept misformation in comparative politics' *American Political Science Review*, 64(4): 1033–53.

Sartori, G. (1991) 'Comparing and miscomparing', *Journal of Theoretical Politics*, 3(3): 243–57.

Sartori, G. (1994) 'Compare why and how: comparing, miscomparing and the comparative method', in M. Dogan and A. Kazancigil (eds), *Comparing nations: Concepts, strategies, substance*, London: Basil Blackwell, pp 14–34.

Scherer, S. and Steiber, N. (2007) 'Work and family in conflict? The impact of work demands on family life', in D. Gallie (ed), *Employment regimes and the quality of work*, Oxford: Oxford University Press, pp 1–33.

Schmid, G. (2011) 'Flexibility and security on the labour market: managing and sharing parental risks', *Journal of Economic and Social Policy*, 14(1): 62–95.

Schmid, G. (2017) 'Transitional labour markets: theoretical foundations and policy strategies', *The new Palgrave dictionary of economics*, Basingstoke: Palgrave Macmillan, pp 1–15.

Schmid, G., Bellmann, L., Gazier, B. and Leschke, J. (2023) *Governing sustainable school to work transitions: lessons for the EU,* IZA Policy Paper No. 197.

Soma, N. and Yamashita, J. (2011) 'Child care and elder care regimes in Japan', *Journal of Comparative Social Welfare*, 27(2): 133–42.

Stall, N. (2019) 'We should care more about caregivers', *Canadian Medical Association Journal*, 191(9): E245–E246.

Stall, N.M., Campbell, A., Reddy, M. and Rochon, P.A. (2019) 'Words matter: the language of family caregiving', *Journal of the American Geriatrics Society*, 67(10): 2008–10.

Stanfors, M., Jacobs, J.C. and Neilson, J. (2019) 'Caregiving time costs and trade-offs: Gender differences in Sweden, the UK, and Canada', *SSM-Population Health*, 9: 100501.

Statista (2022) *Kleine und mittlere Unternehmen (KMU) in Deutschland.* https://de.statista.com/statistik/studie/id/46952/dokument/kleine-und-mittlere-unternehmen-kmu-in-deutschland/ [Accessed 23 January 2024].

Temple, J., Dow, B. and Baird, M. (2019) 'Special working arrangements to allow for care responsibilities in Australia: availability, usage and barriers', *Australian Population Studies*, 3(1): 13–29.

Tronto, J. (1993) *Moral boundaries: A political argument for an ethic of care*, New York and London: Routledge.

United Nations (UN) (2018) *'Global care crisis' set to affect 2.3 billion people warns UN labour agency.* Available from: https://news.un.org/en/story/2018/06/1013372 [Accessed 21 December 2021].

Urwin, S., Lau, Y.S., Grande, G. and Sutton, M. (2023) 'Informal caregiving and the allocation of time: implications for opportunity costs and measurement', *Social Science and Medicine*, 334: 116164.

Whitley, R. (1999) *Divergent Capitalisms: The Social Structuring and Change of Business Systems,* Oxford: Oxford University Press.

Williams, J.C. (2000) *Unbending Gender: Why Family and Work Conflict and What to Do about It,* New York: Oxford University Press.

Wimo, A., Gauthier, S. and Prince, M. (2018) *Global estimates of informal care.* Available from: https://www.alz.co.uk/adi/pdf/global-estimates-of-informal-care.pdf [Accessed 16 November 2023].

Yeandle, S. (1999) 'Women, men and non-standard employment: Breadwinning and caregiving in Germany, Italy and the UK', in R. Crompton (ed), *Restructuring gender relations and employment: The decline of the male breadwinner*, Oxford: Oxford University Press, pp 80–105.

Yeandle, S. (2017) *Work-care reconciliation policy: legislation in policy context in eight countries, background paper for German Federal Ministry for Families*, Senior Citizens, Women and Youth (Bundesministerium für Familie, Senioren, Frauen und Jugend) Available from: http://circle.group.shef.ac.uk/wp-content/uploads/2018/11/yeandle-WCR-v2.pdf [Accessed 23 January 2024].

Yeandle, S. and Buckner, L. (2007) *Carers, Employment and Services: time for a new social contract?* Report No. 6 Carers, Employment and Services Report Series. Available from: http://circle.group.shef.ac.uk/wp-content/uploads/2018/04/CES-6-EWS4031Time-for-a-new-social-contract.pdf [Accessed 13 April 2019].

Yeandle, S., Bennett, C., Buckner, L., Fry, G. and Price, C. (2007) *Managing Caring and Employment*, Carers Employment and Services Report No. 2, London: Carers UK.

2

Finland

Emilia Leinonen

Introduction

In this chapter, Finnish care leave and related employment policies are described and assessed. In Finland, there are currently two types of short-term leave available for employees, namely 'Absence for compelling family reasons' (*Poissaolo pakottavista perhesyistä*) and 'Absence for taking care of a family member or someone close to the employee' (*Poissaolo perheenjäsenen tai muun läheisen hoitamiseksi*). In addition, a new amendment to the Employment Contracts Act, called 'Carer's Leave' (*Omaishoitovapaa*), came into force on 1 August 2022. There is also a form of long-term leave called Job Alternation Leave (*Vuorotteluvapaa*), although initially this was not developed for caring purposes. Other support measures for working carers include flexible working arrangements such as flexible working hours, flexible working time, working time bank and reduced working hours. Employees with caring responsibilities can also apply for informal Carer's Leave, even if the employee does not have a formal agreement with a municipality or does not receive an Informal Care Allowance.

In 2022, Finnish social and health policies underwent several changes and reforms, all of which also have implications for working carers' capacity to combine work and care. The first major change is a health and social services reform, which will transfer the responsibility for organising social and health services from municipalities to 'well-being services counties' (Act on Organising Healthcare and Social Welfare Services, 2021: 612). This will also change how these services are organised and funded. A second major reform is the family leave reform, which aims to allocate family care responsibilities more equally between parents and to strengthen equality in working life (Ministry of Social Affairs and Health, 2022a, 2022b). Finally, the implementation of the Directive of the European Parliament and of the Council on work–life balance for parents and carers took place in 2022 (European Parliament, 2019), resulting in a new form of carer's leave (Finnish Ministry of Justice, 2022).

Analysis of the adequacy of carer leave policies shows that despite existing legislation, working arrangements, available care leaves and future reforms, Finnish working life has elements that make combining paid work and care responsibilities difficult, especially for women. Finland's labour market is characterised by a persistent gender pay gap, a gender-segregated labour market and uneven distribution of care responsibilities between parents. Furthermore, despite women's greater caring responsibilities, their opportunities to utilise flexible working arrangements are more limited than men's, partly because of the gender-segregated labour market. Although job protection is at a high level, most leave schemes available for people caring for an adult family member are unpaid. In addition, many available flexible working arrangements reduce the employee's monthly income. Thus, while Finnish legislation on employment and care prohibits unequal treatment of employees based on gender, in Finnish working life and in care policies there is still a need for more standardised practices that ensure equal treatment of employees, regardless of their age, gender or caring responsibilities.

National context

Political context

Finland is a parliamentary republic with 19 regions and over 300 municipalities and is a member of the European Union. The Parliament consists of 200 representatives who are elected for a four-year term. The government formed in 2019 (by the Social Democratic Party, the Centre Party, the Greens, the Left Alliance and the Swedish People's Party of Finland) was led by Prime Minister Sanna Marin from the Social Democratic Party until June 2023. From June 2023, the new government (formed by the National Coalition Party, Finns Party, the Christian Democrats and the Swedish People's Party of Finland) has been led by Prime Minister Petteri Orpo from the National Coalition Party. Until recently, governance has been quite decentralised; all municipalities are self-governing, with the right to levy taxes, and have been responsible for local administration of many community services, such as schools, infrastructure and care services. In 2021, however, the first stage of the new health and social services reform came into effect and changed how services are organised, produced and funded. The objectives of the reform are to ensure that everyone has equal access to health and social services, regardless of their place of residence, but also to decrease the costs of social and health care sector. Since the 2000s and 2010s, several Finnish governments have been trying to make a major reform of the structures of social and health care because of the growing costs (Kröger, 2019). In 2023, the reform transferred responsibility for organising health, social and emergency services from municipalities to the new regional level, that is, to 21 new health and social services counties ('well-being services counties', or 'county councils'). At first, these counties will not have a right to levy taxes, although there is already political discussion on this. The counties' activities will mainly be funded by central government. The first county elections were held in January 2022 and county councils started their work in March 2022 (Ministry of Finance, 2022; Ministry of Social Affairs and Welfare, 2022b).

Economic and labour market context

Finland is a highly developed country. The largest sector of the Finnish economy is the service sector (69 per cent of GDP in 2020), followed by industry and construction (28 per cent) and agriculture, forestry and fishery (3 per cent) (Statistics Finland, 2021a). Finland can be seen as a dual-earner regime that encourages both men and women, including mothers of young children, to engage in both unpaid care and paid work (Sihto, 2019; Mesiäislehto et al, 2022). In December 2021, 73.3 per cent of people of employment age (from 15 to 64) residing in Finland were in the labour force, up from 70 per cent in December 2020. At that time, the unemployment rate stood at 6.7 per cent, having been 7.6 per cent a year earlier (December 2020) (Statistics Finland, 2022). In 2021, the employment rate was 71.7 per cent for women and for men 72.8 per cent. Of all employees, men more often had a permanent full-time work contract than women (in 2020, 40.2 per cent and 34.4 per cent, respectively), while women had a permanent part-time work contract or a fixed-term work contract more often than men (7.1 per cent and 3.4 per cent; 8.8 per cent and 6.1 per cent, respectively, Statistics Finland, 2021c).

There are several laws in Finland that prohibit unequal treatment or discrimination of employees based on gender, parenthood or caring responsibilities (Act on Equality between Women and Men, 1986; Employment Contracts Act, 2001; Non-discrimination Act, 2014). The Act on Equality between Women and Men 1986, for instance, states that the employer's duty is to 'facilitate the reconciliation of working life and family life for women and men by paying attention especially to working arrangements'. Furthermore, in 2022, the Directive of the European Parliament and of the Council on work–life balance for parents and carers (European Parliament, 2019) was implemented in Finnish legislation. Nevertheless, although Finland has established gender-equality policies and is a relatively gender-equal society, there are some gender-equality problems, such as a persistent gender pay gap, a gender-segregated labour market and uneven distribution of care responsibilities between parents (Mesiäislehto et al, 2022).

Social context

Finland's total population is 5.5 million, and its population density is 16/km^2 (41.4/sq mi), which makes it a geographically large, rather sparsely populated country. There are two official languages in Finland – Finnish and Swedish – and Sami is also a recognised national language. Finland is considered a Nordic welfare state with universally available comprehensive publicly funded welfare services and a relatively strong social security system. However, on certain issues it lags somewhat behind its Nordic neighbours; it also displays some features of marketisation and (re)familialism. In Finland, women predominantly do full-time work but, as highlighted earlier, there are elements in Finnish social policy and the labour market that generate gender inequalities and make reconciliation of work and care difficult for women. Notably, the care of small children is more often women's responsibility: for instance, 92 per cent of women use the (subsidised) child home-care leave, which allows a parent to care for children under the age of three at home (Finnish Social Insurance Institution, 2021). The Finnish labour market is also rather gender segregated: 70 per cent of jobs in the public sector are occupied by women, affecting the pay gap between the genders as salaries are lower in the public sector than in the private sector (Statistics Finland, 2018). In August 2022, however, Finland's family leave system was reformed. The main goals of the reforms were to allocate family leave entitlements more equally between parents, strengthen equality in working life and reduce the gender pay gap. In the new reform, in addition to pregnancy leave (total of 40 working days), both parents get parental leave with parental benefits for 160 working days (320 days in total, Finnish Social Insurance Institution, 2022b).

Familialistic features are also visible in arrangements for care of older persons. Finland is one of the most rapidly ageing countries in the world. In 2000, the proportion of individuals in Finland aged 65 years and older was 15 per cent; it had increased to 22.7 per cent in 2020, and is projected to reach 28 per cent by 2050 (Statistics Finland, 2021a). Family members in Finland are not legally responsible for caring for their ageing parents or other adult family members. Instead, according to the Constitution of Finland (section 19), welfare services should be available for all in need for care. Despite this, there have been major changes in provision of care for older persons in recent years: today, only older persons with the most extensive care needs receive services, and most older people with care needs receive less formal help than before (Kröger and Leinonen, 2012; Kröger, Puthenparambil and Van Aerschot, 2019). An ageing-in-place policy also emphasises home care instead of institutional care, which has led to a further increase in the responsibilities of families, in particular in arranging care for their ageing relatives.

In fact, in Finnish care policy legislation there seems to be an underlying assumption that older people have family members or friends helping them arrange the care services they need (Kalliomaa-Puha, 2017). Moreover, family members are also seen as a potential care resource in Finnish eldercare policies and municipal strategies (Ahosola, 2018). Thus, 'informal' care has been, and still is, a significant element of care in Finland. Approximately

50,000 carers have a contract with their municipality and receive the Informal Care Allowance and support services, but it is estimated that Finland also has an additional 350,000 carers providing care to relatives who are ill, disabled or ageing. There are no exact statistics available on how many employees give support, care and help to their close ones, but it has been estimated that 1.4 million regularly provide help for family members and relatives (Vilkko et al, 2014) and that over 700,000 employees are combining paid work with family care (Carers Finland, 2022). Other estimates suggest that without the care provided by family members, the cost of long-term care would be €2.8 billion higher (Kehusmaa, 2014).

In the next section, the available care leave policies are introduced and briefly described. One of the reasons for developing these leaves has been the growing need for options for care leaves for employees caring for an older family member (Jolanki, Szebehely and Kauppinen, 2013). In Finland, there are currently two types of short-term leave available for employees, Absence for compelling family reasons (*Poissaolo pakottavista perhesyistä*) and Absence for taking care of a family member or someone close to the employee (*Poissaolo perheenjäsenen tai muun läheisen hoitamiseksi*). In addition, a new amendment to the Employment Contracts Act called Carer's leave (*Omaishoitovapaa*) came into force on 1 August 2022. There is also a form of long-term leave called Job alternation leave (*Vuorotteluvapaa*).

Carer leave policies

Short-term leaves

Absence for compelling family reasons

The Employment Contracts Act (section 7) permits an employee's absence for compelling family reasons. An employee is entitled to temporary absence from work because of unforeseeable and compelling reasons due to an illness or accident suffered by a family member. The law does not specify who is considered a family member, but the Ministry of Economic Affairs and Employment of Finland has defined a family member as an employee's relative in ascending or descending line or his/her spouse's/live-in spouse's relative in ascending or descending line.

The leave is available to all workers with an employment contract in Finland. Employees must notify their employer of their absence and its reason as soon as possible. On request, the employee must present proof of the reasons for the absence (for instance, a medical certificate) and for its discontinuation. Duration of leave and other arrangements are based on necessity and agreement between the employer and the employee. The duration is not specified in the Act, but should be only temporary: some collective agreements specify a duration of one or two days. The Employment Contracts Act does not require the employer to pay the employee remuneration for the duration of the absence, but in some collective agreements this is required.

Absence for taking care of a family member or someone close to the employee

A new amendment to the Employment Contracts Act's Section 7 was made in 2011. If it is necessary for an employee to be absent in order to provide special care for a family member or someone else close to them, the employee is entitled to a temporary absence from work. The amendment differs from the absence for compelling family reasons in that it allows a longer absence from work and does not specify the family members as strictly as the Act's original Section 7. The employee must be caring for a family member or 'someone else close' to the employee, including more distant relatives and friends. According to the Employment and Equality Committee report on changing the Employment Contracts Act 2010, a 'family member' or 'someone close' usually refer to an employee's relatives or friends, or their spouse or live-in partner's relatives.

The underlying reason for care is 'special care needs', which means that the care receiver needs the employee's help with their activities of daily living. The leave is available to all workers with an employment contract in Finland and is based on agreement between the employer and employee. The employer must try to arrange the work so that the employee may be absent from work for a fixed period, which is specified in some collective agreements to be one week. The employer is not required to pay the employee remuneration during the absence, and no other compensation for loss of earnings during the leave is available. The employee has a right to return to their former position/duties, but if this is not possible, the employee is offered equivalent work in accordance with their work contract.

The duration of leave is based on 'necessity', that is, how long the family member needs the employee's help, and agreement between the employer and the employee. As such, there are no limits as to how often the leave may be taken, as it is based on necessity. Returning to work in the middle of a period of leave must be agreed by both employer and employee. If an agreement cannot be reached, the employee may discontinue their leave for a justifiable reason by informing their employer of their return no later than one month before the date of return to work. On request, the employee must present proof of the grounds for the absence (for example, a medical certificate about a family member's illness).

Carer's Leave

Carer's Leave is a new amendment to the Employment Contracts Act which came into effect on 1 August 2022. According to this amendment, an employee has a right to have up to five days off during a calendar year if the employee's immediate presence is needed because their relative or someone else close to them needs a considerable amount of support or assistance because of serious illness or injury. In addition, an employee has a right to Carer's Leave in the case of palliative care of their relative. Here the amendment specifies that 'relative' refers to an employee's child, parent, spouse, live-in partner or a person who is in a registered partnership with the employee. 'Someone else close' to the employee refers to 'a person who lives with the employee'.

The employee must notify their employer about the Carer's Leave and its estimated duration as soon as possible. On request, the employee must present proof of the reason for the leave. The leave is unpaid but entails more rights than the 'absence' policy outlined earlier. For Carer's Leave, the employee's job and position are protected and, in contrast to the absence, the leave is a subjective right and does not require negotiation with their employer. The amendment is a part of the implementation of the Directive of the European Parliament and of the Council on work–life balance for parents and carers (European Parliament, 2019). The aim of the Directive is to promote gender equality in work life and reconciliation between work and family. In Finland, the Carer's Leave includes only the minimum requirements of the Directive. For example, the Directive recommends that the leave should be paid, but doesn't require it. In Finnish legislation, family leaves are generally unpaid but there are many exceptions to this in different collective agreements – for instance, in some collective agreements the first three months of parental leave are paid.

Long-term leave

Job alternation leave

Job alternation leave is an arrangement designed to allow employees to have career breaks while also improving the employment potential of unemployed jobseekers through a fixed-term work experience. An employee, in accordance with a job alternation agreement made with the employer, is released for a fixed period from their work duties covered by their service relationship, and the employer agrees to hire, for a corresponding period, a person registered as an unemployed jobseeker for a fixed-term work experience in the job alternator's place.

While the job alternation leave was not initially designed for care leave purposes, nowadays the programme is described as an opportunity to have a longer leave that can be used for studying, leisure or taking care of children or other relatives (Finnish Employment Office, 2022). All employees with an employment or a service contract have the right to take the leave, but there are certain conditions that an employee must meet. The employee needs to have worked for at least 20 years prior to the leave (family leaves are included in the work–history calculations), have a continuous work contract with the same employer for at least 13 months prior to the leave (with no more than 30 days of unpaid leave), and their working hours must be at least 75 per cent of full-time working hours. An employee cannot retire right after the leave; the upper age limit is three years below the old-age pension age. After the leave, an employee must have at least a five-year employment period before applying for a new job alternation leave.

The employee is entitled to a job alternation allowance (70 per cent of the unemployment allowance). The allowance is earnings related if the employee is a member of an unemployment fund. However, if the employee is not a member of an unemployment fund the job alternation allowance is 70 per cent of the basic unemployment allowance and is paid by the Finnish Social Insurance Institution. In Finland, most employees receiving job alternation allowances are members of an unemployment fund: in 2013, only 171 employees received the allowance from the Finnish Social Insurance Institution (2022c). While the home care allowance reduces the amount of job alternation allowance, a housing allowance, child allowance or Informal Care Allowance does not affect the amount of job alternation allowance. The job alternation allowance also accrues pension.

The minimum duration of a job alternation leave is 100 successive calendar days, up to a maximum of 180 calendar days. The leave ends immediately if the employee becomes eligible for a parental allowance or parental leave. The employee has the right to return to their former position and duties, but if this is not possible, the employee is offered equivalent work in accordance with their work contract. In this sense the employee's job is protected – however, if grounds for dismissal are fulfilled, an employee can also be dismissed.

Table 2.1 summarises the carer leave options available in Finland as of November 2023.

Other support measures

Flexible working arrangements

Other important and quite widely used support measures applicable to many working carers are connected to flexible arrangements for work and working time. Compared to other European countries, Finland stands out as regards the number of different kinds of flexible arrangements available for employees (Toppinen-Tanner and Kirves, 2016). The Finnish Working Hours Act recognises four types of working time flexibility: flexible working hours, flexible working time, working time bank and reduced working hours, all of which can be used to reconcile work and care. In 2020, 71 per cent of employees reported having a flexible working hours system in

Table 2.1: Carer leave schemes, Finland (November 2023)

| Leave details | | | | Eligibility | | | | |
Leave name and introduced	Time period	Compensation	Worker/employee status	Qualifying period	Person needing care	Evidence	Notice period and process
Absence for compelling family reasons, 2001	Unspecified but short term	Unpaid	All with an employment contract	–	Family member	Employer can ask for medical certification	Notify employer ASAP
Absence for taking care of a family member or someone close to the employee, 2011	Unspecified but short term	Unpaid	All with an employment contract	–	Family member or someone close	Employer can ask for medical certification	Notify employer ASAP
Carer's Leave, 2022	5 days per annum	Unpaid	All with an employment contract	–	Family member or someone close	Employer can ask for medical certification	Notify employer ASAP
Job Alternation Leave, 2003	100–180 days	70% of one's unemployment benefit for a maximum of 180 days	Contracted employees working at least 75%	20-year work history; 13 months with employer	Family member or someone close	Employer can ask for medical certification	Notify employer ASAP

use at their workplace, and 64 per cent had a working time bank system (Keyriläinen, 2021).

Flexible working hours can be agreed between an employer and an employee, allowing the employee to determine the beginning and end of daily working hours, to a certain extent. A flex-period, which either shortens or lengthens the daily working time, can be up to four hours per day. During a four-month follow-up period, the total number of flexible working hours used to shorten the regular working hours cannot exceed 20 hours, and overtime hours cannot exceed 60 hours (Act on Working Hours 872/2019, 12 §). Flexible working time means that an employer and an employee can agree that an employee may determine where and when they work. At least half of regular working hours can be used in a flexible working time arrangement. On average, regular working hours cannot exceed 40 hours per week (Act on Working Hours 872/2019, 13 §). If a working time bank system is used in a workplace, employees can save their extra working hours, overtime hours and other working hours based on flexible working hours (up to 60 hours during a four-month period) to be used later as flexi-leaves. Employees can also change their overtime pay to flexi-leaves, but the maximum number of saved hours cannot exceed 180 hours per calendar year (Act on Working Hours 872/2019, 14 §). Reduced working hours means that for social or health reasons, an employee can also ask for reduced working hours, that is, to work less than the regular working hours, in which case the employer must seek to arrange work so that the employee can work part time. The agreement on reduced working hours is valid for 26 weeks (Act on Working Hours 872/2019, 15 §).

Carer leave and tax deductions

The Act on Support for Informal Carers 2006 recognises family care. The support includes: an 'Informal Care Allowance'; respite and substitute care during the respite; necessary social and health care services; and other supportive services such as training and health and well-being check-ups. Employees with caring responsibilities can apply for 'Informal Carer's Leave', even if the employee does not have a formal agreement with a municipality or does not receive an Informal Care Allowance. The Informal Care Allowance varies from the minimum amount of €423 to a maximum of €847 (in 2022). The maximum allowance is paid if the carer is unable to participate in employment. According to the Social Welfare Act (1301/2014), municipalities can arrange leave for working carers without a formal agreement under the same principles that are available to informal carers with a formal agreement, that is, at least two or three days off per month depending on the intensity of care. Furthermore, an employee who has a child with a long-term illness or disabilities can receive partial childcare leave until the child turns 18. The employee must have been employed by the same employer for at least six months during the previous 12 months in order to be eligible for the partial leave.

The tax credit for household expenses means that a person is entitled to a tax credit if they are using for-profit or non-profit services and paying for care work done in the person's own home or in their relative's home. The care work includes caring for children, persons with disabilities or older persons, and can include washing, feeding and other care tasks such as assisting a person, for instance, with visiting the bank. The maximum credit for household expenses is €2,250 per person per year. A person who receives an Informal Care Allowance cannot receive a tax credit for household expenses that are based on paid care work (Finnish Tax Administration, 2022).

COVID-19 pandemic response and implications for employed carers

Compared to other European countries, Finland has been relatively successful in restricting the spread of the coronavirus. During the first wave of the pandemic in 2020, schools and all public cultural venues were shut. Although these restrictions were lifted in June 2020, during the second and third waves, public services such as libraries were closed, secondary and tertiary education were mostly delivered via distance learning and remote work increased significantly. In 2021, the proportion of employees doing remote work was 41 per cent (Mesiäislehto et al, 2022). Mesiäislehto et al (2022) assessed the impact of COVID-19 on gender equality in Finland in terms of employment, income, family life and working conditions. The restriction measures particularly affected specific employment sectors, such as the service industry (restaurants, bars) and tourism, which are female dominated. Employment decreased by over 75,000 persons, among whom 46,000 were women and 29,000 men, but employment figures recovered for both men and women in the spring of 2021 and in fact were then higher than at any point since the financial crisis of 2008 (Mesiäislehto et al, 2022).

Some adjustments to unemployment benefits were made at the beginning of the pandemic (Räsänen, Jauhiainen and Pyy-Martikainen, 2020), but no additional financial support was targeted specifically at families apart from a temporary flat-rate benefit to parents unable to work due to school closures. Families were hit by the crisis, but women's work and care reconciliation were particularly affected during the first wave of the pandemic, albeit temporarily (Mesiäislehto et al, 2022). However, it was not only families with children who were impacted by the crisis – the situation of older persons was also difficult, especially during the first wave of the pandemic. As in many other countries, the Finnish Government recommended that all persons aged 70 years or over should stay in quarantine-like conditions from March 2020 onward. According to Aaltonen et al (2021), the situation of older persons living at home and receiving family care and support was more difficult compared to those older persons living in intensive service housing (institutional care): to receive the care or support they needed, they could not follow the social distancing recommendations and were, in that sense, more vulnerable to the virus and possible infection. Aaltonen et al (2021) further argue that older persons who received help, care and support from their families were forgotten in the crisis preparation and management plans. During the pandemic, governmental budget allocations were made to eldercare services, but most of these were for healthcare services: support was given to healthcare districts to fund equipment costs, and municipalities received additional subsidies for arranging basic services (Mesiäislehto et al, 2022).

Sihto, Leinonen and Kröger (2022; also Eurocarers/IRCCS-INCRA, 2021) found that the impacts of the pandemic on the situation of carers were also quite severe. Finnish carers suffered from a lack of services for themselves and those they cared for, a lack of contact with other people and an overall lack of support measures, such as the protective masks available to professional care workers. The report highlighted that the situation was especially difficult for carers whose caring responsibilities were most intense: their services were cancelled more often, and they more often reported a decline in their mental well-being compared to other carers. Younger carers worried more about their financial situation than others. Overall, carers did not receive enough support or services, nor was their situation adequately acknowledged in the government's policy responses to the crisis.

Adequacy of carer leave policies

Short-term and long-term leaves

There are no recent statistics on the number of employees using the two forms of short absences: for compelling family reasons and for taking care of a family member. In 2013, a report was made for the Ministry of Economic Affairs and Employment of Finland by the Finnish Institute of Occupational Health (Kauppinen, 2013). One of the report's aims was to evaluate the right of absence for taking care of a family member or someone close to the employee, which was at that time a new amendment to the Employment Contracts Act (Section 7a). The report was based on a follow-up survey of employees (450 respondents) and health and safety representatives and heads of occupational health and safety (3,185 respondents). Approximately 20 per cent of the employee respondents cared for a family member or someone close to them. Of those with caring responsibilities, 24 per cent felt that it would be difficult to raise the need for leave or an absence with their supervisor. These respondents felt that the new amendment would facilitate work and care reconciliation at least 'quite a lot' (45 per cent). However, there was little knowledge of the amendment (only 15 per cent of the employees were aware of it). Moreover, employee respondents felt that the amendment could potentially increase inequality between men and women because women have more caring responsibilities. In addition, 70 per cent of employee respondents felt that, because it was unpaid, the absence based on the amendment was not used. In total, 40 per cent of safety representatives were aware of the amendment. However, in most cases the amendment was not applied because there were other ways to organise absence from work and reconcile work and care. These included the possibility of agreeing a temporary absence with the supervisor, use of flexible or reduced working hours, use of a working hours bank, use of job alteration leave, changing the holiday bonus for days off and the possibility to work from home.

According to another survey (n=435) (Kauppinen and Silfver-Kuhalampi, 2015), unpaid absence from work and flexible working hours were the two most common arrangements when an employee's family member needed help or assistance. Those respondents who received the Informal Care Allowance more often used unpaid absence and other arrangements, which reduced the number of their working hours (such as part-time work and work time bank). Absence for taking care of a family member or someone else close to the employee has been criticised because the law does not guarantee an absolute right to such absence (Kalliomaa-Puha, 2019). Since the absence is based on an agreement between the employee and the employer, the employer can refuse to agree to the absence and is under no obligation to state the reason for doing so. One way of reinforcing the right to an absence is to oblige the employer to give a statement of reasons for declining it. Another major problem is that the absences are unpaid (Kalliomaa-Puha, 2019), including those enabled by the recently adopted European Union (EU) Directive on carer's leave (European Parliament, 2019). In Finland, most informal carers, both with and without an official agreement, are women, which means that taking advantage of the leave provisions associated with the new Directive will negatively affect women's income. Furthermore, employees may not be able to afford to take unpaid absences.

In Finland, the opportunities to take long-term care leaves are quite limited. Only 8 per cent of the respondents of the earlier mentioned survey study (Kauppinen and Silfver-Kuhalampi, 2015) reported that they used job alternation leave. It is worth noting changes in the eligibility criteria for job alternation leave in the past decade. Two significant changes have been to the duration of the leave and to the duration of the employee's work history: before 2016, the eligibility criteria included only a ten-year work history with the possibility to have a 360-day leave (Finnish Social Insurance Institution, 2016). Between 2005 and 2012, the number of employees receiving a job alternation allowance rose from 16,800 to 22,500 (HE,

2014: 36). Most users were women from the municipal social and health care sector. In 2021, the number of employees receiving the allowance from unemployment funds dropped to 5,000, mainly because of tighter eligibility criteria (The Federation of Unemployment Funds in Finland, 2022). Thus, a longer absence from work is not a realistic option for many employees. Furthermore, the new government has suggested abolishing the job alternation leave in 2024 to reduce public spending.

In 2010, the amendment to the absence for taking care of a family member was opposed: it was feared that it would increase employment costs and have negative consequences for women's participation in working life (Jolanki et al, 2015). The same concerns that were addressed in discussions on the right to absence for taking care of a family member are also addressed in the government's proposals for the new carer's leave. It is estimated that, on one hand, the leave may facilitate the reconciliation of work and family life in difficult and stressful situations, since the carer's leave is a subjective right; on the other hand, since the leave is unpaid, low-income employees may not be able to use it at all. Although the new carer's leave is part of the implementation of the EU Directive that aims to promote better work–life balance for parents and carers (European Parliament, 2019), the assumption in the legislative work seems to be that the majority of users will be women. The governmental proposal for carer's leave includes an impact assessment of the new leave, and it is stated there that carer's leave will not promote women's participation in working life (HE, 2021: 129). However, in the same governmental proposal it is suggested that since male employees have more possibilities for flexible working hours, the opportunity for carer's leave could enhance female employees' possibilities to care for their family members. In other words, the government proposal suggests that carer's leave would bring flexibility to female employees' working lives, but only in terms of flexibility to *care*, which echoes the old story of women's double duty, not better work–life balance for all genders.

All in all, it is reasonable to argue that the length of the carer's leave is not adequate in the most intensive caring situations, such as in palliative care, even if it could be combined with the absences for compelling family reasons and for taking care of a family member. It is probable that, in the case of an accident or a sudden illness, the absence for compelling family reasons will be used first, and if the need for an employee's presence with their family member continues, the carer's leave could be used. It is nevertheless important to recognise that all legislative measures related to the absences in question require joint agreement between employee and employer, which can also increase openness in workplaces about employees' caring responsibilities (Kauppinen and Silfver-Kuhalampi, 2015), regardless of their age or gender. Furthermore, the Directive on work–life balance requires all EU member states to ensure that their legislation prohibits discrimination and unequal treatment on the basis of taking the carer's leave or parental leaves, using the flexible working arrangements or using the right for absence for compelling family reasons or taking care of a family member (European Parliament, 2019). In Finland, the Act on Equality between Women and Men 1986 prohibits that kind of discrimination as indirect gender-based discrimination.

Other support measures

The development of the quality of working life in Finland is assessed in the Working Life Barometer, conducted annually by the Ministry of Economic Affairs and Employment of Finland. It seems that, in terms of overall availability of flexible working time arrangements, there are some differences between male and female employees. According to the latest Working Life Barometer (Keyriläinen, 2021), 71 per cent of all employees reported having a flexible working time system in their workplace in 2020, male employees (73 per cent) reporting this slightly more often than female employees (69 per cent). In total, 64 per cent of employees reported having a working time bank system in their workplace. Male employees (68 per cent) reported more often than female employees (59 per cent) that it was possible for them to use their overtime hours as days off. In addition, 63 per cent of all employees reported that they could 'always' run their own or family errands during working hours, again men more often (68 per cent) than women (58 per cent). Employees in the municipal sector had fewer possibilities to run their errands (42 per cent) than others.

Overall, in terms of gender equality, work–care reconciliation seems to be more difficult for female employees, since they usually have more caring responsibilities but their possibilities for flexible working time are not as good as those of male employees. However, flexible working arrangements are not solely positive, as their use might be a result of a forced necessity, not of a voluntary choice. Furthermore, flexible working arrangements, and reduced working hours in particular, also have negative consequences on working carers' economic situation, especially if the employee is forced to refuse the possibility to do full-time work. In addition, the need for flexibility in work might have more nuanced effects on the employee's situation: they might need to turn down new work assignments, work trips and other social events at the workplace (Kauppinen and Silfver-Kuhalampi, 2015).

In 2017, three out of four family carers with a formal family care agreement were women (Leppäaho et al, 2019). Out of those aged under 68 years with formal family care agreement, approximately 28 per cent had a full-time job and 10 per cent had a part-time job, whereas out of those aged from 30 to 60, approximately 50 per cent had a full-time or a part-time job (personal communication from Tillman, 2019 cited in Kalliomaa-Puha, 2019). There are some indications that male family carers (aged 18–62) are more often unemployed than female family carers (Mikkola et al, 2016). If the carer has a full-time job, usually they receive only two days off from family care work per month (Kalliomaa-Puha, 2019). It is interesting that only half of family carers with a formal agreement used their statutory days off (Leppäaho et al, 2019). This is partly explained by the quality of the substitute carers and the difficulties in receiving substitute care in the care receiver's own home: in 2017, only 5 per cent of leaves were organised as home care (Kalliomaa-Puha and Tillman, 2016; Leppäaho et al, 2019; Kalliomaa-Puha, 2019). Since the Informal Care Allowance is discretionary, however – that is, the municipality decides how much funding is allocated to informal care per year, how many formal agreements can be concluded and for how long (Association of Finnish municipalities, 2022) – it is unlikely that municipalities will offer days off from family care to family carers without an agreement. According to Noro (2019), only 500 carers without an agreement have received discretionary days off (there are no statistics on how many of these carers were working carers).

It has been argued that the Informal Care Allowance is turning into an income support option for retired carers who care for their partner, since the number of retired informal carers is rising (Jolanki et al, 2015). In 2019, in total 48,700 persons had a formal agreement on informal care, among whom 57 per cent were aged over 65 (Association of Finnish Municipalities, 2022). However, the Informal Care Allowance could compensate some of the working carer's earnings loss, although the level of the allowance is quite modest (the minimum allowance is €423.61 per month, Ministry of Social Affairs and Health [2022b]) If a working carer receives the Informal Care Allowance, the municipality also has to grant certain services to the allowance receivers: these services include annual health checks, and the previously mentioned carer leaves with substitute care (in an institution or done by a substitute carer) (Act on Support for Informal Carers, 2006). In addition to these services, the municipalities can offer services for working carers that support them in combining work and care; for instance, municipalities can offer home care and day care or grant a personal assistant (Noro, 2019). This depends, however, on the municipality.

Conclusion

The Nordic welfare states rely heavily on high labour force participation, but at the same time the expectation that families will provide informal care is embedded in Finnish social and care policies (Rostgaard et al, 2022). The growing emphasis on home care of older adults is accompanied by the growing responsibilities of informal networks and carers, which means that family care has been brought into long-term care policy 'through the back door' (Kodate and Timonen, 2017). The emphases on high labour force participation and informal care provision are contradictory, especially from the gender perspective. Still, in Finland, working female carers often combine care with full-time work (Sihto, 2018). There are many aspects of Finnish working life that have an impact on gender equality, in particular the persistent gender pay gap, the gender-segregated labour market and uneven distribution of care responsibilities between parents. What is most alarming in terms of gender equality is that female employees, despite having more caring responsibilities, have fewer possibilities for flexible working arrangements. This is further amplified by the 'refamilialisation' process of care, which has increased the care responsibilities of families, especially women.

Attitudes in workplaces in general also have an effect on gender equality: according to the Equality Barometer (Attila et al, 2018), only one quarter of respondents felt that men are encouraged to use their parental leaves. If it is difficult for men to use the right for parental leave, staying on a longer care leave is probably even more difficult (Kalliomaa-Puha, 2019). Furthermore, although Finland stands out its large number of flexible working arrangements, it seems that the right to flexibility is not as widely known, or at least not as widely implemented, as one might assume (Kalliomaa-Puha, 2019). There is particularly low awareness of the right to an absence, even among safety representatives in workplaces. Overall, flexibility in working time is important, as it acknowledges different family and care situations; but it should not be the only way of supporting employees with care responsibilities, as it has several downsides, especially if the employee's caring responsibilities are intense. Using flexible working arrangements may reduce an employee's monthly salary or increase feelings of inferiority as an employee compared to other employees. Also, the use of absences, especially if the need for absence happens often, may lead to a fear of being labelled as a difficult employee (Kauppinen and Silfver-Kuhalampi, 2015; Kalliomaa-Puha, 2019), even though the job is quite well protected.

Since the population of Finland is ageing, the family responsibilities of caring or arranging care for ageing family members are likely to rise. Finnish employment legislation has thus far barely recognised the position of employees caring for their ageing relatives, especially when compared to the opportunities provided to working parents (Jolanki et al, 2013). Of course, flexible working arrangements also help those employees who are caring for their older relatives, but compared to the number and variety of leaves and other support measures available for working parents caring for their children, the situation of carers of older people is rather poor. In that sense, the new Carer's Leave, despite being unpaid and modest in length, is an important reform. However, if a longer care leave is needed for more intensive care, there is only one option available – the Job Alternation Leave – and only if the employee meets the strict eligibility criteria.

Gender equity and renewal of the social and health care system and the parental leave system have been two major goals of the current government, but their effects on regional and gender equality remain to be seen. The COVID-19 pandemic has without doubt increased the use of flexibility in working life, but not equally: remote working is more common among managers and upper-level office workers than among lower-lever office workers or in the female-dominated care sector. All in all, the most problematic issue in terms of Finnish care leaves is that they are predominantly unpaid; this endangers the employee's income level, career development and pension level if the care responsibilities force the employee to reduce their working hours in the long term. To enhance employees' ability to combine work and care without sacrificing their income level too much, especially in the situation of palliative care, policy makers should consider broadening the use of the Informal Care Allowance. The Act on Support for Informal Carers 2006 already allows such use, but it seems that too often the decision-making process in the municipalities takes too much time or it does not fit the criteria of the municipalities (Kalliomaa-Puha, 2019). Although Finnish legislation on employment and care prohibits unequal treatment of employees based on gender, in Finnish working life and care policies there still is a need for more standardised practices that ensure equal treatment of employees, regardless of their age, gender or caring responsibilities.

Overall, the available forms of flexibility in work and possibilities to take leaves in Finland are important and could be transferable to other countries. However, all available policies lean towards a familialistic approach. People are living longer and healthier lives than ever, but that does not change the fact that many need support and services at some point. There are indications of policy changes in the content of care provided and in the division of responsibilities: what part of care is a public responsibility and what is intended to be provided by the families (Rostgaard et al, 2022). As the coverage of formal services for older people especially is declining, families are expected to take more responsibility in arranging and providing care – 'leaving the informal carers to pick up where the public sector left' (Rostgaard et al, 2022: 208). In Finland, the carer is usually a woman, making familialism a gender issue.

References

Aaltonen, M., Pulkki, J., Teräväinen, P. and Forma, L. (2021) 'Ikääntyneiden kokemukset hoivan ja avun saamisesta koronapandemian aikana' ['Older persons' experiences on receiving care and help during the Covid-19 pandemic'], *Gerontologia*, 35(4): 326–41.

Act on Organising Healthcare and Social Welfare Services (2021: 612). Available from: https://www.finlex.fi/fi/laki/alkup/2021/20210612 [Accessed 10 May 2023].

Act on Equality between Women and Men (1986: 609) Available from: https://www.finlex.fi/en/laki/kaannokset/1986/en19860609_20160915. pdf [Accessed 3 April 2024]

Act on Working Hours (2019: 872) Available from: https://www.finlex. fi/en/laki/kaannokset/2019/en20190872.pdf [Accessed 3 April 2024].

Act on Support for Informal Carers 2006 (2005: 937) Available from: https://www.finlex.fi/en/laki/kaannokset/2005/en20050937 [Accessed 3 April 2024].

Non-discrimination Act (2014: 1325) Available from: https://www.finlex. fi/en/laki/kaannokset/2014/en20141325.pdf [Accessed 3 April 2024].

Ahosola, P. (2018) *Vanhushoivapolitiikan uusfamilismi. Omaisettomat hoivan tarvitsijat institutionaalisen hallinnan kohteena [The Refamilisation of Eldercare Policies]*, Tampere: Tampere University.

Association of Finnish Municipalities (2022) 'Iäkkäiden palvelut, omaishoito' ['Services for older people, family care']. Available from: https://www.kunt aliitto.fi/sosiaali-ja-terveysasiat/sosiaalihuolto/iakkaiden-palvelut/omaisho ito [Accessed 14 February 2022].

Attila, H., Pietiläinen, M., Keski-Petäjä, M., Hokka, P. and Nieminen, M. (2018) 'Tasa-arvo barometri 2017' ['Equality barometer 2017'], Helsinki: The Ministry of Social Affairs and Health.

Carers Finland (2022) *'Omaishoidon tietopaketti. Ansiotyö ja omaishoito' ['Information package of family care. Employment and family care']*. Available from: https://omaishoitajat.fi/mita-on-omaishoito/tietoa-omaishoidosta/ [Accessed 31 January 2022].

Employment Contracts Act (2001: 55) Available from: https://www.finlex.fi/ en/laki/kaannokset/2001/en20010055.pdf [Accessed 3 April 2024].

Eurocarers/IRCCS-INRCA (2021) 'Impact of the COVID-19 outbreak on informal carers across Europe – Final report', Brussels/Ancona. Available from: https://eurocarers.org/wp-content/uploads/2021/05/EUC-Covid-study-report-2021.pdf [Accessed 12 October 2023].

European Parliament (2019) 'Directive (EU) 2019/1158 of the European Parliament and of the Council of 20 June 2019 on work–life balance for parents and carers and repealing Council Directive 2010/18/EU', Brussels: European Parliament. Available from: https://eur-lex.europa.eu/legal-cont ent/EN/TXT/?uri=celex%3A32019L1158 [Accessed 30 June 2023].

Finnish Employment Office (2022) 'Job alternation leave guidelines'. Available from: https://www.te-palvelut.fi/documents/43002293/43009 923/vuorotteluvapaa_pdf_337_kt.pdf/d3c57392-2ab3-d60f-2198-a7efa f3231cb?t=1616545734491 [Accessed 16 March 2022].

Finnish Social Insurance Institution (2016) 'Vuorotteluvapaan ehdot muuttuvat' ['Eligibility criteria for job alternation leave will be changed']. Available from: https://www.kela.fi/-/vuorotteluvapaan-ehdot-muuttuv-1?inheritRedirect=true [Accessed 29 March 2022].

Finnish Social Insurance Institution (2021) 'Tilasto lastenhoidon tuista' ['Statistics on childcare subsidies']. Available from: https://www.kela.fi/tilastot-aiheittain-lastenhoidon-tuet [Accessed 20 March 2022].

Finnish Social Insurance Institution (2022a) 'Family leave reform'. Available from: https://www.kela.fi/web/en/family-leave-reform-2022 [Accessed 9 February 2022].

Finnish Social Insurance Institution (2022b) 'Parental allowances after 4 September 2022'. Available from: https://www.kela.fi/web/en/parental-allowances-after-4-9-2022 [Accessed 9 February 2022].

Finnish Social Insurance Institution (2022c) 'Vuorottelukorvauksen saajien määrä' ['The number of employees receiving job alternation allowance']. Available from: https://bit.ly/38uO5qY [Accessed 14 February 2022].

Finnish Tax Administration (2022) 'Tax credit for household expenses'. Available from: https://www.vero.fi/en/individuals/tax-cards-and-tax-returns/income-and-deductions/Tax-credit-for-household-expenses/ [Accessed 22 February 2022].

HE (2014: 36) 'Hallituksen esitys eduskunnalle laiksi vuorotteluvapaalain muuttamisesta' ['Government proposition to the Parliament on changing the job alternation leave act']. Available from: https://www.eduskunta.fi/FI/vaski/HallituksenEsitys/Documents/he_36+2014.pdf [Accessed 20 March 2022].

HE (2021: 129) 'Hallituksen esitys eduskunnalle laeiksi sairausvakuutuslain, työsopimuslain ja varhaiskasvatuslain muuttamisesta sekä niihin liittyviksi laeiksi' ['Government proposition to the Parliament on hanging the Sickness insurance act, Employment contracts act and Early childhood education and care act']. Available from: https://www.eduskunta.fi/FI/vaski/HallituksenEsitys/Sivut/HE_129+2021.aspx [Accessed 20 March 2022].

Jolanki, O. (2015) 'To work or to care? Working women's decision-making', *Community, Work and Family*, 18(3): 268–83.

Jolanki, O., Szebehely, M. and Kauppinen, K. (2013) 'Family rediscovered? Working carers of older people in Finland and Sweden', in T. Kröger and S. Yeandle (eds), *Combining paid work and care: Policies and experiences in international perspective*, Bristol: Policy Press, pp 53–69.

Kalliomaa-Puha, L. (2017) 'Vanhuksen oikeus hoivaan ja omaisolettama' ['Older person's right for care and assumption of a family member'], *Gerontologia*, 31(3): 227–42.

Kalliomaa-Puha, L. (2019) 'Omaishoidon ja ansiotyön yhteensovittaminen' ['Reconciliation of family care and paid work'], Helsinki: Ministry of Social Affairs and Health. Available from: https://julkaisut.valtioneuvosto.fi/bitstream/handle/10024/161286/R_60_2018_Omaishoidon_ja_ansiotyo_WEB.pdf?sequence=1&isAllowed=y [Accessed 24 January 2024].

Kalliomaa-Puha, L. and Tillman, P. (2016) 'Äiti on aina äiti. Lasten omaishoitajien arjen haasteet' [Mom is always a mom. The everyday life challenges of children's informal carers', in A. Haataja, I. Airio, M. Saarikallio-Torp and M. Valaste (eds), *Laulu 573 566 perheestä. Lapsiperheet ja perhepolitiikka 2000luvulla [Families with children and family policies in the 2000s]*, Helsinki: Kelan tutkimus, pp 322–54.

Kauppinen, K. (2013) 'Omais- ja läheishoitovapaan käytön tilanneselvitys' ['The situation of the use of family care leaves and absence for compelling family reasons'] Helsinki: Finnish Institute of Occupational Health.

Kauppinen, K. and Silfver-Kuhalampi, M. (2015) 'Työssäkäynti ja läheis- ja omaishoiva – työssä jaksamisen ja jatkamisen tukeminen' ['Employment and family care. How to support well-being and continuation in working life']. Helsinki: University of Helsinki.

Kehusmaa, S. (2014) 'Hoidon menoja hillitsemässä. Heikkokuntoisten kotona asuvien ikäihmisten palvelujen käyttö, omaishoito ja kuntoutus' ['Controlling the costs of care. The use of services, family care and rehabilitation of frail older persons living at home']. Tampere: Juvenes Print.

Keyriläinen, M. (2021) 'Working life barometer 2020'. Helsinki: Ministry of Economic Affairs and Employment of Finland. Available from: https://julkaisut.valtioneuvosto.fi/bitstream/handle/10024/163200/TEM_2021_36.pdf?sequence=1&isAllowed=y [Accessed 18 February 2022]

Kodate, N. and Timonen, V. (2017) 'Bringing the family in through the back door: the stealthy expansion of family care in Asian and European long-term care policy', *Journal of Cross Cultural Gerontology*, 32: 291–301.

Kröger, T. (2019) 'Looking for the easy way out: Demographic panic and the twists and turns of long-term care policy in Finland', in T.-K. Jing, S. Kuhnle, Y. Pan and S. Chen (eds), *Aging welfare and social policy: China and the Nordic countries in comparative perspective*, International Perspectives on Aging 20, Cham: Springer International Publishing, pp 91–104, https://doi.org/10.1007/978-3-030-10895-3_6.

Kröger, T. and Leinonen, A. (2012) 'Transformation by stealth: the retargeting of home care services in Finland', *Health Social Care Community*, 20(3): 319–27.

Kröger, T., Puthenparambil, J.M. and Van Aerschot, L. (2019) 'Care poverty: unmet care needs in a Nordic welfare state', *International Journal of Care and Caring*, 3(4): 485–500.

Leppäaho, S., Jokinen, S., Kehusmaa, S., Luomala, O. and Luoma, M.-L. (2019) 'Iäkkäiden perhehoidon tilanne – Omais- ja perhehoidon kysely 2018' ['The situation of adult foster care'], in A. Noro (ed), *Omais- ja perhehoidon kehitys vuosina 2015–2018. Päätelmät ja suositukset jatkotoimenpiteiksi [The development of family care and adult foster care in 2015–2018. Conclusions and recommendations for further actions]* Helsinki: Ministry of Social Affairs and Health, pp 37–44.

Mahon, R., Anttonen, A., Bergqvist, C., Brennan, D. and Hobson, B. (2012) 'Convergent care regimes? Childcare arrangements in Australia, Canada, Finland and Sweden', *Journal of European Social Policy*, 22(4): 419–31.

Mesiäislehto, M., Elomäki, A., Närvi, J., Simanainen, M., Sutela, H. and Räsänen, T. (2022) 'The gendered impacts of the Covid-19 crisis in Finland and the effectiveness of the policy responses. Findings of the project "The impact of the Covid-19 crisis in Finland"', Helsinki: Finnish Institute of Health and Welfare.

Mikkola, H., Komu, M., Räsänen, T., Ahola, E. and Tillman, P. (2016) 'Omaishoitajien tulorakenne ja –kehitys – onko tuella merkitystä? Esitys Omaishoito tänään ja huomenna –seminaarissa' ['The income level and income development of family carers']. Presentation at Family Care Today and Tomorrow seminar]. Available from: https://www.slideshare.net/kelantutkimus/mikkola-et-al-omaishoitajien-tuloraken-ne-ja-tulokehitys [Accessed 23 February 2022].

Ministry of Finance (2022) 'Health and social services reform will transform the structure of government and the tasks of municipalities'. Available from: https://vm.fi/en/-/health-and-social-services-reform-will-red uce-the-functions-of-local-government-and-halve-municipal-personnel [Accessed 31 January 2022].

Ministry of Social Affairs and Health (2022a) 'Family leave reform enters into force in August 2022'. Available from: https://stm.fi/en/-/family-leave-reform-enters-into-force-in-august-2022 [Accessed 10 May 2023]

Ministry of Social Affairs and Health (2022b) 'Omaishoidon palkkiot 2022' ['Informal Care Allowances in 2022']. Available from: https://stm.fi/-/kuntainfo-omaishoidon-tuen-hoitopalkkiot-vuonna-2022 [Accessed 16 March 2022].

Noro, A. (2019) 'Omais- ja perhehoidon kehitys vuosina 2015–2018. Päätelmät ja suositukset jatkotoimenpiteiksi' ['The development of family care and adult foster care in 2015–2018. Conclusions and recommendations for further actions'] Helsinki: Ministry of Social Affairs and Health.

Räsänen, T., Jauhiainen, S. and Pyy-Martikainen, M. (2020) 'Sosiaaliturvan stressitesti' ['Stress test of the social insurance system'], Helsinki: Social Insurance Institution of Finland.

Rostgaard, T., Jacobsen, F., Kröger, T. and Peterson, E. (2022) 'Revisiting the Nordic long-term care model for older people – still equal?' *European Journal of Ageing*, 19: 201–10.

Sihto, T. (2018) 'Distances and proximities of care: analysing motion-spatial distances in informal caring', *Emotion, Space and Society*, 29: 62–8.

Sihto, T. (2019) *Placing women? How locality shapes women's opportunities for reconciling work and care*, Jyväskylä: University of Jyväskylä.

Sihto, T., Leinonen, E. and Kröger, T. (2022) *Omaishoito ja COVID-19-pandemia: omaishoitajien arki, elämänlaatu ja palveluiden saatavuus koronapandemian aikana [Family care and the COVID-19 pandemic. Family carers everyday life, quality of life and access to services during the pandemic].* Jyväskylä: University of Jyväskylä. Available from: https://jyx.jyu.fi/han dle/123456789/80448 [Accessed 12 October 2023].

Statistics Finland (2018) 'Gender equality in Finland'. Available from: https://www.stat.fi/tup/julkaisut/tiedostot/julkaisuluettelo/yyti_gef_201800_201 8_19723_net.pdf [Accessed 29 March 2022].

Statistics Finland (2021a) 'Finland in Figures. National accounts'. Available from: https://www.stat.fi/tup/suoluk/suoluk_kansantalous_en.html# Structuralper cent20changeper cent20ofper cent20theper cent20economy [Accessed 18 February 2022]

Statistics Finland (2021b) 'Äidit tilastoissa' ['Mothers in statistics']. Available from: https://www.stat.fi/tup/tilastokirjasto/aidit-tilastoissa.html [Accessed 18 February 2022].

Statistics Finland (2021c) 'Työelämä. Naisten ja miesten työmarkkina-asema' ['Working life. Labour force status of men and women']. Available from: https://www.stat.fi/tup/tasaarvo/tyoelama/index.html [Accessed 20 March 2022].

Statistics Finland (2022) 'Clearly more employed persons in December than one year before'. Available from: https://www.stat.fi/til/tyti/2021/12/ tyti_2021_12_2022-01-25_tie_001_en.html [Accessed 18 February 2022].

The Federation of Unemployment Funds in Finland (2022) 'Muut kassojen maksamat etuudet, vuorottelukorvaus' ['Other benefits paid by the unemployment funds, job alternation allowance']. Available from: https://www.tyj.fi/tilastot/ muut-kassojen-etuudet/#vuorottelukorvaus [Accessed 16 March 2022].

Tillman, P. (2019) Sähköpostiviesti 3.1.2019 Kelan omaishoitotutkimuksen työikäisiä koskevista tuloksista. [*Email message on January 3, 2019 about the results of Kela's family care survey for working-age people.*]

Toppinen-Tanner, S. and Kirves, K. (2016) 'Työn ja muun elämän yhteensovittamista tukevat käytännöt ja kulttuuri suomalaisilla työpaikoilla' ['The practices and work culture in the Finnish workplaces that support the reconciliation of work and other aspects of life'], *Työelämän tutkimus*, 14(3): 276–94.

Vilkko, A., Muuri, A., Saarikalle, K., Noro, A., Finne-Soveri, H. and Jokinen, S. (2014) 'Läheisavun moninaisuus' [The diversity of informal care and informal help], in M. Vaarama, S. Karvonen, L. Kestilä and P. Moisio (eds), *Suomalaisten hyvinvointi 2014 [The wellbeing of Finnish people in 2014]*, Tampere: Suomen yliopistopaino, pp 222–237.

3

Sweden

Linnéa Aldman, Eva Sennemark and Elizabeth Hanson

Introduction

Approximately one in five people in Sweden provide regular help, care and/or support to a family member or friend. Indeed, 'informal' carers provide most of the care for people with health and/or care needs living at home (Magnusson et al, 2022). Carers have been relatively invisible in Sweden due to the political system and the assumption that the welfare state provides for its citizens from the cradle to the grave. The underlying philosophy is that social services should maximise the individual's independence from both next of kin and family, regardless of their situation (Esping-Andersen, 1990). This view, however, means that carers and issues surrounding them have neither been prioritised nor paid significant attention within national health and social care policy until more recently. A growing awareness of carers' situations among policy makers is largely a result of ageing demographic trends, continued municipal cutbacks of long-term care, a strong focus on community care and care at home and, more lately, the impact of the COVID-19 pandemic.

The aim of this chapter is to outline and discuss the range of care leave and employment policies that relate to working carers. Examples are provided of both short-term leave and long-term leave available. However, the circumstances where the main forms of leave are accessible by all groups of working carers currently remain rather limited. For example, in accordance with the Act on the Right to Leave for Urgent Family Reasons (The Swedish Parliament, 1998: 209), an employee is entitled to unpaid leave from paid employment for urgent family reasons that are solely related to illness or an accident that make the employee's immediate presence absolutely necessary. The maximum length of the leave, as well as possible compensations, are mostly decided in central agreements between national unions and employers. Parents of children who require special support and services (The Swedish Parliament, 1993: 387) are eligible for certain economic benefits and paid contact days. Additionally, parents with an eligible disabled child/ren are entitled to reduce their working hours if they so wish. The Compassionate Care Leave (SSIA, 2018) gives employees the right to take paid time off work to care for a family member or significant other due to a serious, life-threatening illness. Overall, mainly due to the local autonomy that allows regions and municipalities to decide on the type and range of health and care services and how best to deliver them, the supports available for working carers vary considerably across the country.

We conclude that the existing supports and leave available in their current form do not sufficiently address the needs and preferences of working carers. Nevertheless, there is a growing political will to recognise the situation of carers in Sweden, marked by the launch of the first national carers strategy by the previous government in April 2022 (MHSA, 2022). Along with the strategy, the government commissioned the National Board of Health and Welfare Sweden (NBHWS) to develop support aimed at decision makers and practitioners within health and social care and other stakeholders (including employers) to strengthen a carer perspective, make carer support less variable across the country and implement reviews to follow up the support more effectively (MHSA, 2022). Parliament also approved the implementation of the EU Work–life Balance Directive for parents and working carers (European Parliament, 2019) in June 2022 (SOU, 2020: 81).

National context

In this section we describe the political, economic and social contexts that influence policy making in Sweden to help readers understand the context in which the policies and laws are applied. Throughout the chapter, what some term 'informal carers' are referred to as 'carers'.

Political context

Sweden is a parliamentary democracy with four levels of government, consisting of the supranational (EU-level), national, regional (21 counties) and local (290 municipalities) levels. At the national level, general laws and guidelines are enacted. Municipalities are responsible for a large part of the community and social services (school, social services, care for older people), while regions are responsible for healthcare, regional development, transport, communication and infrastructure. Hence, responsibilities and issues overlap at times between the different governmental levels (SALAR, 2014). As national laws and guidelines are enacted at the national level and interpreted at the regional and local levels, this leads to varying outcomes from the same policies around the country (SALAR, 2014; Liljeqvist, 2021). Likewise, varying outcomes are also created as strong local autonomy allows regions and municipalities to decide about the range of health and care services and how best to produce and deliver them.

Historically, Sweden is considered to be built on the Nordic model with the welfare state at its core, guided by collectivist values. In the post-war era, responsibilities that were previously the responsibility of the family were taken over by the state (Johansson, Sundström and Malberg, 2018). As the participation of women in the labour force increased during this time, public childcare, care for older people and other social services expanded accordingly. Additionally, individual independence is highly valued in Swedish culture and spouses do not have a legally binding duty of care (The Swedish Parliament, 1987: 230), except for parents' duties to care for their child/children (The Swedish Parliament, 1949: 381). Children, however, do not have a duty of care towards their parents (Ulmanen, 2015). Spouses do, however, have a legal obligation to contribute to the best of their ability to meet the common needs of the shared household and have a joint responsibility for economy and household chores. Thus, each spouse is, in theory, able to decide to what extent (if any) they want to help their partner with instrumental and personal care tasks (The Swedish Parliament, 1987: 230), as it is the public sector's duty to meet the health and care needs of older, sick and/or disabled people.

The underlying philosophy is that social services are to maximise the individual's independence from both next of kin and family, regardless of their situation (Esping-Andersen, 1990). As a result, carers' situations have not been given much attention by policy makers until at least the late 1990s. It has been assumed that the state cares for its citizens in need, but in reality, families continue to play an important role in the care of older, sick and/or disabled people. A key factor was the deregulation and privatisation of public services that started in the early 1990s (Svallfors and Tyllström, 2017) and accelerated after the Alliance government took over in 2006, which led to threats to the 'safety net' of equal care on equal terms, regardless of geographic location, that Sweden is often said to have (IVO, 2021). Although financing of the care system is predominantly based on taxation, the actual delivery of services within healthcare and care for older people has, to an increasing extent, been by private for-profit providers (OECD, 2013).

Between 1999 and 2001, the government earmarked SEK300 million for the municipalities to increase their support for carers, leading to multiple development projects and the strengthening of the carer advocate role.[1] However, the municipalities simultaneously cut down on state-funded care for older people (for example, closing of some nursing homes), in part due to an in-country financial crisis. In 1993, the Act Concerning Support and Service for Certain Functional with Impairments (1993: 387) (Law on Special Support and Service to Certain Persons with Disabilities – LSS) was implemented. This legislation is a rights-based law which entitles people with multiple and/or profound disabilities to access special support and services and aims to make disabled people as independent as possible, possibly relieving some of the pressure that carers might experience (Magnusson et al, 2017).

Since 2009, municipalities have a statutory obligation to support carers according to the Social Services Act 2001: 453 (2009: 549). However, the type of support is not specified, which leads to significant variation in the type and extent of support offered by municipalities across the country. In the last few years, a major systemic change in Sweden's healthcare system has been taking place towards integrated, people-centred healthcare (MHSA, 2022). In effect, this will lead to more healthcare being provided at home, which will most likely translate to more care by family members/ significant others (Vicente et al, 2022). A growing awareness of the role of carers among policy makers and politicians is evidenced by the launch of the first national Carers Strategy by the previous government in April 2022. This focused on the importance of a carer perspective within health and social care and included the role of employers in supporting carers (MHSA, 2022).

Economic and labour market context

Sweden generally has a stable and healthy economy, although it is not immune to global economic crises (Finansinspektionen, 2022). Currently Sweden's economy is negatively affected by high inflation and interest rates and an extremely weak Swedish krona (Ministry of Finance, 2023). The state's main income source is taxes paid by citizens and corporations (Ekonomifakta, 2020). As a member of the European Union (EU), over 50 per cent of the agenda in Swedish municipalities and regions is directly or indirectly affected by EU legislation (SALAR, 2021).

The employment rate of women in full-time work in Sweden is among the highest in the EU (Eurostat, 2021). In 2021, almost 80 per cent of women were participating in the Swedish labour force. Nevertheless, this figure falls to 55.3 per cent for non-EU born women. Most (74 per cent of women and 89 per cent of men) were working full time, with 26 per cent of women and 11 per cent of men in paid employment working part time (Akademikernas A-kassa, 2021). The second-most common reason for women to work part time (after not being able to secure a full-time job) is care of children (Skandia, 2021). For men, the second-most common reason is that they are studying (Akademikernas A-kassa, 2021). Women's labour force participation is thus more affected by care responsibilities, as compared to men's. Further, the segregation within and between different professions in Sweden is among the highest globally (Hedström, 2020). For example, in 2020, around 90 per cent of nurses and home care staff in Sweden were women and about 99 per cent of skilled craftspeople were men (SCB, 2020). In 2018, the total unemployment rate was 6.3 per cent, rising to 6.6 per cent in 2022 due to the pandemic (SCB, 2022a).[2]

Social context

Sweden is a relatively small country with 10,554,692 inhabitants in August 2023 (SCB, 2023). The population is projected to exceed 11 million by 2034. In 2021, almost 20 per cent of the Swedish population was born in another country, with Syria and Iraq being the most common countries of origin, followed by Finland, Poland and Iran (SCB, 2021).

The Swedish population has a high life expectancy (81.2 years for men and 84.8 for women) (SCB, 2022b) and, as birth rates have dropped, the population is ageing. The proportion of individuals in Sweden aged 65 years and older was 20.3 per cent in 2020, an increase from 18.2 per cent in 2010. During recent years, however, the number of younger people in the population has increased due to foreign exchange students, refugees and labour immigration from Europe (Segendorf and Theobald, 2019).

About one in five adults (amounting to 1.3 million or 18 per cent of the adult population) in Sweden regularly provide help, support and/or care to a family member/significant other. Of these, about 900,000 are of working age. The average number of hours of care provision increased from 11 hours a week in 2012 to 13 hours a week in 2020 (NBHWS, 2012; Magnusson et al, 2022).

Any type of discrimination based on gender, transgendered identity or expressions, ethnicity, religion, disability, sexuality or age is strictly forbidden in Sweden according to the Swedish Discrimination Act (2008: 567). Discrimination due to social status, political beliefs and monetary status is also unlawful according to the EU Charter of Fundamental Rights (European Union, 2022). However, research has highlighted that some municipal decision makers have different expectations for women with an immigrant background and Swedish-born women, deriving from stereotypes of 'immigrants' care culture' affecting, for example, policy action plans for older and disabled people (Erlandsson, 2017).

Carer leave policies

The right to leave (unpaid and paid) to care for a family member or relative is regulated in national laws and in union agreements. However, carers' perspectives and needs have often been overlooked, although they are stronger for parents of children covered by LSS. In more recent years, however, some work to rectify the lack of a carer perspective has begun, as evidenced by the recent national carer strategy.

Short-term leave

In accordance with the Act (1998: 209) on the right to leave for urgent family reasons,[3] an employee is entitled to unpaid leave from employment for urgent family reasons that are related to illness or an accident that makes the employee's immediate presence absolutely necessary. The maximum length of the leave and possible compensations are mostly decided in collective agreements between national unions and employers. It is more common for larger employers to have a collective agreement. Thus, leave provisions vary across the country and range from part of a working day to several days.

Compensation for loss of earnings during the short-term leave is mostly decided in collective agreements between national unions and employers and ranges from no payment to 100 per cent of the normal pay. For example, some municipality and region employees have a maximum of ten days per year with full compensation in place. Employers without a central agreement decide if and what the compensation during a short-term leave is to be, although the right to a leave of absence remains. Thus, leave for urgent family reasons cannot be the sole grounds for dismissal, and employers are not allowed to alter working conditions for this reason. If the employee is nevertheless dismissed, the dismissal is annulled if the employee so requests, and if not, the employee can take their employer to court. Employers who break this law must pay compensation to the employee.

The Swedish Trade Union Confederation (LO) is one of the largest associations of trade unions in Sweden and is a central organisation with 14 affiliates. These affiliates organise workers from both the public and private sectors (LO, 2021). In a telephone interview conducted by the authors, Tina Nordling, who works at the Department for Collective Bargaining LO as an ombudsperson, explained that none of the 14 representatives for the affiliates are aware of an employer who does more than the bare minimum to support carers other than what is required by law.

The law does not specify any particular care-recipient characteristic/s but employers may request a medical certificate from their employee (Act [1998: 209] on the right to leave for urgent family reasons). Similarly, the law does not specify any carer-recipient characteristics, so the definition may vary depending on the authority, municipality and so on. However, it most often includes a partner/spouse, parent, child, grandparent and/or grandchild of an employee.

Temporary parental benefits (economic)

Two different areas within the law are applicable when a parent or relative needs to care for a child, depending on the child's illness: either the Social Insurance Code or the LSS. The Social Insurance Code relates to parents of children with a temporary non-life-threatening illness who are otherwise healthy. If the child is covered by the LSS, however, there are some additional regulations that are applicable.

If a child covered by the LSS or a child with a serious illness develops an additional illness, a parent has the right to temporary parental allowance for the care of the child up until the age of 21 years (with limitations) if the parent cannot work due to the illness. This is also valid if the carer has a temporary illness (child or carer) (Chp 13, Art 22, 27 Social Insurance Code). However, this is not applicable if the parent receives compassionate care leave for the same need of supervision and care. Additionally, if a child covered by LSS attends a special needs school, parents are entitled to temporary parental allowance until the spring of the year the child turns 23 years old (Chp 13 Art 27 Social Insurance Code). Likewise, if a child under 12 years old is seriously ill or has a disability and the parent needs to take time off work to visit the doctor, participate in the treatment of their child or learn to care for the child, the parent is entitled to temporary parental allowance (Chp 13 Art 20 Social Insurance Code). The maximum amount of days ranges from 10 to 120 days per child and per year, but for parents of children under the age of 16 the range is from 60 to 120 days per child and per year (Chp 13, Art 21, 25 of the Social Insurance Code).

Furthermore, if a child under the age of 18 is seriously ill, both parents have the right to temporary parental allowance (at the same time if they wish) when they need to take time off work or work fewer hours to care for the child. There is no limit on how long the temporary parental allowance in these types of cases can be paid, however, the parent can get benefits only for the time when they cannot work due to caring for their seriously ill child (Chp 13 Art 30–31 Social Insurance Code). Seriously sick or ill does not mean that the child's illness needs to be life-threatening, as during the whole period the parents can claim the temporary parental allowance. Benefits could be paid during, for example, an aftercare phase (Supreme Administrative Court, 2013).

Contact days

An employee with a disabled child under the age of 16 and covered by LSS is entitled to contact days, meaning time off work for reasons such as parent education, for instance, arranged by a non-governmental organisation, visits to the child's day care unit or school and participating in activities arranged by the school. The child themself does not need to participate in the training or activities. The aim is to increase the parents' knowledge of how to best support their child and the law covers all workplaces in Sweden.

The right for contact days is limited to a maximum of ten days per year and per child. Employers do not pay for the contact days, instead, compensation for loss of earnings during the contact days is applied for by the worker and approved by the Swedish Social Insurance Agency (national authority). The compensation is 80 per cent of lost pay per day.

To be eligible for contact days, the parent/s must have a Sickness Benefit Based Income (SGI), that is, earn a minimum annual income of SEK11,424 and work at least six months consecutively or have regular periods of paid work each year. Furthermore, the parent/s must also not undertake paid work or claim unemployment benefits during a contact day and must be insured in Sweden (SSIA, 2022a).

Long-term leaves

Compassionate Care Leave

In 1988, the Act (The Swedish Parliament, 1988: 1465) on the law providing leave for close relatives/next of kin gave employees the right to time off work to care for a family member, relative, friend or neighbour with a life-threatening illness that is administered with the Swedish Social Insurance Agency (SSIA). The law has been amended gradually, most recently by the Act 2010: 1241, but the right to time off work still applies, with a maximum length of leave of 100 days (or 240 days for a family member/significant other with HIV) in total. It is important to note here that care by the carer does not solely refer to medical care. Care provided can include emotional support to the care recipient. The days are attached to the care recipient and can be shared between family members or other people close to the care recipient without exceeding the maximum length of leave. It is also stated that employees have the right to get time off work even if the care recipient is being treated in a hospital or a long-term care facility. The law does not exempt any type of employer and clarifies that the employer cannot negotiate this right away. The compensation level is related to the income and the length of time away from work. Paid time off work is available for one quarter, half or three-quarters of a whole of a working day and the compensation is about 80 per cent of pay, although there is a maximum total amount (SEK543) a recipient can receive daily (SSIA, 2022d).

Compassionate Care Leave is available only to working carers who, through their caring activities, lose income from their paid work and are approved by the SSIA. Both the carer and the care recipient with a serious, life-threatening illness must be insured in Sweden. Consent from the care recipient with a life-threatening illness is necessary and the care should be given in Sweden or in an EU/ European Entry/Exit System (EES)-country. A medical certificate and treatment plan are required.

The number of people applying for and receiving Compassionate Care Leave is relatively low but has increased from around 8,000 people in 2000 to around 15,000 in 2019 (ISF, 2022; SSIA, 2022c). Many workers who take this form of leave are women (around 70 per cent), and in general under ten days per person are used. About half (47 per cent) of these carers use under five days and the most common reason for taking leave is to care for a parent who is seriously ill (ISF, 2022).

Reduced paid working hours for parents with eligible disabled children

The National Parental Leave Act (The Swedish Parliament, 1995: 584) covers all workplaces in Sweden, giving employees with disabled children covered by the law LSS, the right to shorten their weekly working hours up to a maximum of 25 per cent. Central collective agreements between employers and trade unions may allow minor changes to the law. The right to decreased working hours is present as long as the nursing allowance is approved by the SSIA, at most until June in the year the child turns 19. Thus, the employer does not compensate for the loss of income; however, employers may request a certificate from the SSIA.

Requirements are that the employee taking care of a child in need of special support and care due to a disability must provide care for at least six months. Both the carer and the child must be socially insured in Sweden and the employee must be the parent of the child or an adult with similar care responsibilities. Rules regulating this insurance are governed by the Swedish Social Insurance Code and international agreements and regulations. Additional requirements for reduced paid working hours are that the child must need more support and care than children of the same age without disabilities. Finally, the employee has a legal duty to inform their employer about the leave, but the employee should not be discriminated against in terms of pay and work tasks. Table 3.1 summarises the carer leave options available in Sweden as of November 2023.

Other support measures

In some instances, carers can be employed in a paid capacity to care for their family member if the supported person meets the criteria for one of the target groups of LSS. The legal basis for employing relatives as personal assistants varies depending on the extent of the individual's basic needs, which is shared by the municipality and the state. If the basic needs of the care receiver are assessed to be less than 20 hours per week, the decision is made by a municipal LSS or social welfare officer. If the needs are assessed to be over 20 hours per week, the Swedish Social Insurance Agency (SSIA) takes over the costs. The municipality can either provide the assistance directly or offer financial compensation if the individual wishes to employ their own assistant, who could be their informal carer. The same is applicable when the SSIA is responsible; however, SSIA then administers the pay to

Table 3.1: Carer leave schemes, Sweden (November 2023)

Leave details			Eligibility				
Leave name and introduced	Time period	Compensation	Worker/ employee status	Qualifying period	Person needing care	Evidence	Notice period and process
Temporary parental benefits, 1993/2010	10–120 days per annum	Paid	Employee	–	Children with disability/serious illness	Medical certificate, plus additional paperwork	–
Leave for urgent family reasons, 1998	Unspecified in the law but short-term (specified in collective agreements between national unions and employers)	Varies between 0% and 100% (an average) salary, depending on the company (specified in collective agreements). (Note: It is paid at many workplaces)	Employees	–	Unspecified	Employers can request a medical certificate	Notify employer ASAP
Contact days, 1993	10 days per annum	80% of pay	Employees	Earnings threshold, six months of work history/regular periods of paid work each year; no paid work or claim unemployment benefits during contact days	Children with disability/serious illness	–	–
Compassionate Care Leave, 1988	100 days (or 240 days for a family member/ significant other with HIV)	Approximately 80% of an average salary	Employees	–	Family member, relative, friend, neighbour with a life-threatening illness	Medical certificate required	Notify employer ASAP

either party depending on what is decided. The informal carer can then be employed through the municipality's home care services (or private home care service companies) as a personal assistant[4] (Sand, 2016).

Carers employed through municipal LSS often earn more than carers employed via the SSIA – up to approximately €35 per hour. Changes are, however, currently being investigated through SOU 2023: 9 'A State Principalship for Personal Assistance' with regards to the responsibility for investigating the need for assistance, proposing that it is all moved to more central administration via the SSIA rather than the municipality, which could in turn affect the frameworks of employment for informal carers.

In accordance with Chapter 4, Article 2, of the Social Insurance Act, a carer might also receive a Family Allowance/Home Care Allowance for providing services to the care recipient that the home care services otherwise would have provided. It is paid out to the *care recipient*, who is expected to pay the people/person taking care of them. This allowance is, however, not available in all municipalities, nor is it the same size or applicable to the same people in all municipalities. An example is the city of Stockholm, where a person caring for a relative once or twice a day in 2022 could receive around SEK1,200 per month. A person caring for someone 24 hours a day in 2022 could receive SEK4,830 per month. The sum is tax deductible if the carer/s lives with the care recipient. It is, however, up to the *care recipient* to decide how much, if any, of the money the carer will receive. The exact amount may vary slightly from year to year (City of Stockholm, 2022).

Furthermore, parents with a child covered by LSS are eligible to receive childcare allowance, which in 2023 ranges from SEK2,734 to SEK10,938 per month (SSIA, 2023a) and is not tax deductible. Additionally, compensation for additional costs for parents of a child with a disability lasts for more than six months, where they are insured in Sweden and where the additional costs exceed SEK13,125 per year (SSIA, 2023b).

Flexible working arrangements

In accordance with the EU Directive 2019/1159 on Work–life Balance for Parents and Carers (European Union 2019/1158, 2019), since August 2022 carers have the right to request flexible working arrangements (changes in work patterns via, for example, working from home, part-time and flexible working hours). It is up to the employer to decide whether to approve such a request; however, the employer is not allowed to discriminate or dismiss the worker due to the request or caring responsibilities. If the employer breaks these laws, the Equality Ombudsman can bring it to the Labour Court (The Swedish Parliament 2022: 1295 The Act amending the Act 1998: 209 on the right to leave for urgent family reasons, SFS, 2022).

In the Swedish ratification of the Directive (SOU, 2020: 81) the definition of carer is broad. It states that any person who wishes to take time off work to care for another person should be able to do so as they are then assumed to have a close enough relationship. By comparison, the definition provided by the EU Council in the EU Directive 2019/1159 on Work–life Balance for Parents and Carers (European Union 2019/1158, 2019) is more restrictive. Namely, family members and relatives include a worker's son, daughter, mother, father, spouse or, where such partnerships are recognised by national law, partner in a civil partnership.

It is important to note that in the EU Directive adopted by the European Council, it was agreed that workers providing personal care or support to a relative shall be entitled to five days of leave per year, but it did not stipulate if it should be paid leave or not. The Swedish ratification of the Directive states that the provision of leave is already covered within the existing Compassionate Care Leave, so further provision was deemed unnecessary (SOU, 2020: 81).

Adequacy of carer leave policies and programmes

In general, awareness of the existing support for working carers in Sweden among policy makers, decision makers and employers remains relatively low. A Swedish population study carried out in 2018 found that out of the ten different supports listed, only one (information and support) was either offered to or received by over 20 per cent of working carers (Vicente et al, 2022). This is rather surprising, given that the municipalities are obliged to offer support to carers, who are also entitled to an assessment of their needs. Possible explanations are that the support offered is not sufficiently flexible nor is it tailored to the needs of individual working carers (NBHWS, 2020).

Equity/inclusivity

Issues of inequity in Sweden's carer leave policies are mainly due to geography, such as the decentralised political system, differences in statutory supports and intersectional issues. One of the main sources of inequity derives from the decentralised political system, leading to differences between regions and municipalities. Different supports and provisions are available to varying extents and are applicable to different groups of people in different municipalities. One such example is local guidelines which might differ and so in some places may limit LSS support and activities, leading to families either having to move or pay out of their own pocket and time (NBHWS, 2020). This is also true for Family Allowance, which is not available in all municipalities, neither is the allowance the same amount or applicable to the same people in all municipalities. This means that this type of support is not accessible and available for all qualifying Swedish inhabitants. The same can be said about relevant national laws and local guidelines, as different groups of carers have varying degrees of accessibility to support.

Another source of inequity is whether the supported person is coved by LSS or not. Carers of a care recipient covered by LSS have a stronger and more extensive network of formal support, whereas working carers caring for people not covered by LSS may be unable to take paid time off work. Other examples are adolescents or adults with, for example, suicidal thoughts, eating disorders or other mental health conditions which may warrant supervision for longer or shorter periods, but for which compensation is not routinely granted. Thus, needs for care might still be present, but working carers might not be able to take paid or unpaid time off from work to care for a relative with mental health conditions, for example.

It is also important to note that LSS is available only for people with multiple and/or profound disabilities who apply before the age of 65 (note: an amendment to the Act concerning Support and Service for Persons with Certain Functional Impairments [1993: 387] went into effect as of 1 January 2023 and raised the age from 65 to 66. In 2026, the age limit will be raised to 67 years). Currently, for people aged 66 years and over with disabilities who are applying for support with their care needs, social services are responsible, and the supported person then receives care services for older people, which are less generous than LSS. This leads to inequity and unequal service provision among different groups of carers, leading to divisions, rather than seeing carers from a holistic and intersectional perspective.

Furthermore, the eligibility criteria for Compassionate Care Leave are quite narrow, as the care recipient's condition must be 'life-threatening', excluding a large group of carers who care for someone with a chronic, long-standing condition/s and/or disability/ies. As outlined earlier, the government at the time argued that the minimum of five days off required by the EU Directive 2019/1159 on work–life balance for carers (European Parliament, 2019) is fulfilled within existing Swedish legislation, referencing Compassionate Care Leave. However, many NGOs working with and for carers and people with long-term care needs and/or disabilities, together with Nationellt kompetenscentrum Anhöriga (Nka, the Swedish National Care Competency Centre), have argued that the interpretation is too narrow and thus does not live up to the intentions of the Directive, as it excludes, for example, care recipients who are living with long-term, chronic conditions and/or disabilities which might be fatal in the long term. Additionally, to receive Compassionate Care Leave, the employee must be the only available solution, meaning that if another person is available to care for the person in need, the employer does not need to give their employee time off work (Labour Court, 2016). Carers Sweden (2021) has argued that the focus should be on what care needs there are, as opposed to how seriously ill the person in need of care is.

Another source of inequity relates to both the decentralised system, as well as the differences between legal rights derived from employment practices. In Sweden, employers (for example, private actors, public actors, authorities and so on) have different collective agreements with different unions and have varying levels of awareness of carers' situations as well as the benefits of supporting them. As mentioned, a few basic rights are applicable across Sweden, for example, the right to unpaid leave from employment for a few days for urgent family reasons. Nevertheless, the details are set out in collective agreements between national unions and employers, including whether the leave is paid, resulting in regional and organisational variation in practice. In addition, this makes it difficult to secure a comprehensive overview of the support available to working carers across the country.

From a global perspective, Sweden ranks highly with regard to equality. Indeed, on the yearly ranking of 150 countries by the World Economic Forum, Sweden has not ranked lower than fifth place since 2006 (Swedish Institute, 2022). That said (see, for example, Sennemark et al, 2019; Vicente et al, 2022), female carers in Sweden still fare worse than male carers in terms of income, position on the labour market and pensions. Women in general provide more hours of care than men and are negatively affected to a greater extent by caring, for example, experiencing poorer mental health (Vicente et al, 2022). Even though the gap has been seen to close between the men and women in recent years, the extent of the care provided, and support received, remains unequal (SSIA, 2018; Sennemark et al, 2019). Women engage in more demanding care tasks than men, such as personal care and coordination of care (SOU, 2017: 21; Vicente et al, 2022). Additionally, women carry out more household chores and care for children to a greater extent than men (SCB, 2019). One explanation could be that it is difficult to leave household finances out of the equation when deciding who should stay home. The person with the lowest pay, often the woman, is thus often seen as the best choice for the household. Furthermore, it is more common for women to already work part time or reduce their paid work hours due to care activities, which further reinforces gender inequity. Clearly, there are limitations based on gender for carers to participate in paid work; however, they are not currently fully addressed in policies.

A further issue is those carers employed by municipalities to care for a family member/significant other who is not covered by LSS (Takter, 2019). Although there are positive aspects of carers being paid for their caring activities, it is in many ways a problematic form of employment from an intersectional standpoint, as it can be seen to reinforce traditional gender roles and cultural expectations (Magnusson, 2015; Erlandsson, 2017). In addition, a rather high proportion of female carers employed by the municipality and not covered by LSS have an immigrant background and generally have low wages, precarious employment conditions and a lack of collective agreements, which has led to many municipalities stopping any new appointments to this type of work. However, it is unclear what municipalities have done, if anything, to replace this type of appointment or if some carers continue to provide care without being paid (Brodin, 2018). More recently where staffing shortages in long-term care are particularly critical, municipalities can be seen to employ informal carers to attempt to cover the gap in service provision. This form of employment is traditionally seen to risk 'trapping' female carers, especially women from other cultures, at home, often caring in isolation for their care recipient (Sand, 2016). Thus, although many policies might not be directly discriminatory by mentioning certain sexes for example, the lack of an intersectional perspective in some policies can be argued to lead to discrimination. However, a positive signal is the follow-up to the launch of the national carers strategy, in which the government tasked the NBHWS to develop indicators for routinely following up the quality of carer support; part of this work specified that detailed gender analyses be carried out, which means that major gender differences and gaps will be clearly highlighted at municipal level.

Flexibility

There are several flexible features of the Compassionate Care Leave legislation which can make it easier for carers to reconcile paid work and care. For example, carers can share the days of leave between family members/ significant others, as the days are tied to the care *recipient*, and there is flexibility regarding the duration and timing of the leave. The circle of people who are included and defined as a carer is also relatively wide and includes both family members and other people close to the care recipient. In this way, it may enable family members/friends to share the care and the possible financial impact as well. It could mean that the people sharing the care might only have to slightly reduce their work hours, instead of one person having to take full-time leave from work and thus take on board larger financial and possibly negative health outcomes themselves. Similarly, parents with a child who is covered by LSS can share the paid role of being a personal assistant to their child.

The Swedish system also adopts a broader view of who is included in the circle of people who can get time off work to care for a person with care needs than, for example, the EU Council's Work–Life Balance Directive 2019/1158 (European Parliament, 2019; SOU, 2020: 81). Although there is no exact legal definition of an informal carer in Sweden, according to the NBHWS's database of terms (NBHWS, 2004), a carer is someone who cares for someone close to them who has a long-term illness, is older or has a disability. However, the lack of a definition of which people are included can and does lead to different outcomes (approval/denial), depending on which administrator handles the case (Abbas, 2016). Finally, the newly implemented right to ask for flexible working methods (arising from the EU Directive) could possibly have a positive impact on working carers and might allow them to better reconcile paid work and care, should their request be granted by their employer.

Job protection

In Sweden, an employer may not terminate employment based solely on the fact that their employee took time off work due to urgent family reasons or asked for flexible working arrangements. Likewise, an employer is not allowed to take away benefits or make working conditions worse for this reason. The dismissal can be annulled if the employee so requests, and the employee then has the right to seek compensation from their employer (Act 1998: 209 – the right to leave for urgent family matters). In court, the employee needs only to prove that there is a reasonable suspicion that they were treated differently due to exercising their legal rights. It is then up to the employer to prove otherwise.

Additionally, it is illegal to mistreat or dismiss employees based on their family situation. This means that working carers still have the right to engage in paid work if they wish to do so. That said, it is sometimes difficult for an employee to prove that they, for example, got laid off or had their hours reduced due to being a carer. If an employee's employment is terminated because their request for time off was denied but they took time off to provide care anyway, it is up to the employee to provide evidence to the court that it was necessary for them to be taking care of the care recipient and that no one else could do it. There are several court cases where employees have been dismissed, as they have been taking weeks or months off claiming urgent family matters, and the court has ruled in the employer's favour, as the employee was unable to provide evidence that they were the only person available to care for the care recipient (see, for example, Labour Court, 2016). There are, however, cases where the court has agreed with the employee (see, for example, Labour Court, 2003).

Income security

A national population study from 2018 which included 861 working carers aged 18–64 years revealed that 21.5 per cent of women and 5.5 per cent of men had reduced their working hours by half to care for a family member (aged parents, partners, children) (Magnusson et al, 2022). Reduced working hours have an immediate impact on a working carer's income but also long-term effects on carers' financial situation, as pensions are dependent on the person's income during their entire working life. This is one of many reasons why it is common for carers to use their vacation days or compensation time to provide care on certain days to try to limit the financial impact (Sand, 2016). Currently, no system of pension credits exists for the generally unpaid care activities carers provide to a family member/friend in Sweden, neither are there plans to explore this possible option, despite this form of income security being taken up within the recent European Care Strategy (Eurocarers, 2021). Additionally, Tina Nordling at LO explained in an interview with the first author that there have been proposals in Parliament about informal care, but that the consensus within LO is that the state, through taxpayers' money, should pay for this and not through abstaining wage increases (personal communication). She explained that prioritising paid leave for informal carers during the collective agreement negotiations would risk leaving workers with less room to increase their wages, highlighting the complexity of the issue.

As previously highlighted, the numbers of people using Compassionate Care Leave are relatively low. Possible reasons are a lack of information about it as well as the narrow rules of interpretation by physicians. Other types of financial compensation, as mentioned earlier, include employment to care for a family member through the Family Allowance[5] and via LSS, the childcare allowance and paid reduction of up to 25 per cent of working hours for parents of children covered by the LSS. However, in most cases, these compensation payments do not compensate for the entire loss of income for the carer. Additionally, there is a difference between securing financial compensation in the form of an allowance or through employment. Being employed as a carer for someone covered by LSS means the income is taxable and thus pensionable and provides access to the social security system, which is mostly not true for financial benefits (Sand, 2016).

Other support measures for carers

There have been few investigations of workplace practices for assisting carer employees in Sweden; however, some employers are aware of the challenges carers face and recognise that reconciling paid work and care is a workplace issue. One such employer is Swedish Radio, which has made efforts to create a more carer-friendly workplace by developing a policy that states that during yearly appraisals a discussion about the balance between work and leisure must be included, which opens up the possibility for informal caring to be raised.

Tina Nordling at LO explained in an interview with the authors that smaller or medium-sized companies can, in principle, do more for working carers but LO and its 14 affiliates are not aware of any employer who does anything extra for carers beyond what the law demands (personal communication). Clearly, it is important for employers and line managers to have an increased awareness of carers' needs and supports, including those at the workplace. A step in the right direction is to include employers as a key stakeholder group in NBHWS's commissioned work on supporting the implementation of Sweden's recent national carer strategy (MHSA, 2022).

COVID-19 pandemic response and implications for working carers

The MHSA granted Nka funding to identify the consequences for carers and carer support staff and to provide proposals for immediate and long-term measures to support carers during this and future pandemics/crises (Magnusson et al, 2021). Additionally, the NBHWS focused on the impact of the pandemic on people covered by LSS (Flyckt and Wallin, 2021).

The research resulted in two reports, which revealed that the pandemic significantly affected carers, contributing in particular to a decreased social network (80 per cent of respondents), a negative impact on carers' health (41 per cent of respondents) and financial situation, a worsening of overall quality of life and the risk for domestic violence increasing. There was an average increase of four hours of time per week spent caring for a care recipient during the pandemic, due to cancelled daily activities and subsequent isolation at home (Magnusson et al, 2021). Around one third of the municipalities cancelled daily activities such as day centre services and other external activities during the pandemic (Flyckt and Wallin, 2021).

Although there were no national policies directly aimed at helping carers during the pandemic, some temporary policies were implemented which might have affected carers. For example, temporary changes to requirements surrounding sick pay and compensation when having to stay at home were mandated by the government. The qualifying day (or waiting day) in relation to sickness benefits and other benefits was temporarily removed and people in high-risk groups received compensation. The requirement for a medical certificate when needing to be home from work to receive sick pay was also temporarily removed. Other examples were temporary exemption from paying off one's mortgage, temporary lower taxes for employers, possible redundancies and the possibility to work from home (42 per cent of adults of working age worked from home during the pandemic), which according to Nka's report (Magnusson et al, 2021), could help to explain why the financial situation of workers who were carers was not so badly affected as their health and social situation.

The maximum amount for compensation for sick pay, infection-risk monies, Compassionate Care Leave and rehabilitation was increased during the COVID-19 pandemic (SSIA, 2021). Up until 1 April 2022, someone who was not sick and could work, but was unable to do so because they might infect someone belonging to an at-risk group, could secure compensation. This meant that although they were not eligible for sick pay, the government instead paid them just under 80 per cent of their normal pay (maximum SEK1,027 per day) (SSIA, 2022b).

Other changes due to the pandemic that went into effect from early 2022 were increased flexibility for people on part-time sick leave, increased housing supplement for people with illnesses and other minor changes. If schools closed due to the pandemic, parent/s who were unable to work due to their child being home, even if the children were being taught online, had the right to parental leave pay (SSIA, 2021). This was applicable for a child aged under 12, or aged under 16 or 21 with special care needs or covered by LSS (SSIA, 2022c).

Additionally, many municipalities developed and/or changed their ways of working. For example, some swiftly set up ways for frail older people and their relatives to get help with, for example, grocery shopping. Also, digital support groups for carers were set up by municipal carer advocates, walk-and-talk small group meetings took place outdoors and individual meetings also took place over the phone (Magnusson et al, 2021).

It is also important to highlight the role of civil society and their efforts during the pandemic with, for example, digital funerals, one-to-one supportive phone calls and digital study circles. Several non-governmental organisations were able to reach carers who were usually out of their geographical reach via the internet. Magnusson et al (2021) argued for long-term planning and preparations for future crises to actively include carers. They suggested that this could be done by clarifying a carer perspective within the Social Services Act, the Health Care Act and the Patient Act and that carers should be included in the national COVID-19 strategy. Additionally, training staff members to take a carer perspective as well as develop digital knowledge was judged important (Flyckt and Wallin, 2021).

Conclusion

The Swedish state depends on carers to supplement its formal care systems. Indeed, one in five of the Swedish population is an informal carer (Magnusson et al, 2022). At the same time, the state also benefits from their participation in the labour market. This warrants support for the carer, but the reality in Sweden is that existing supports for working carers need to be more comprehensive and cover all groups of working carers. The state can be seen to ask a lot of working carers, but gives relatively little in return for carers as a whole, which risks putting a large strain on the system, care recipients and working carers themselves. Nevertheless, the launch of the first national carers strategy and subsequent commissioned work for the NBHWS, which includes targeted support for municipalities, regions and employers to implement the strategy, will hopefully lead to improvements. Additionally, the government's work commissioned from the NBHWS to propose a way forward for healthcare regions and municipalities regarding the systematic follow-up and evaluation of carer support will in time, hopefully, begin to help address the existing difficulties in obtaining a thorough national overview of the type, extent and take-up of carer support and its quality. These developments signal a political will and awareness that has not previously been witnessed. Furthermore, at the time of writing, the current government has initiated a further inquiry with the goal of further improving and strengthening individual support to carers (Dir, 2023: 77).

An ageing population, acute staff shortages and difficulties with retaining staff within health and social care, and more care delivered at home, makes the issue urgent. Sweden has a long way to go before carer support is as generous as its existing childcare policies. By international standards, Sweden enjoys generous parental leave policies. The leave can be split between the parents, taken at the same time by both parents or at different times. The Swedish Social Insurance Administration pays out for 480 days per child up until the child has finished Year 1 at compulsory school (around seven years old) and it is mainly income based.[6]

Compared to many other European countries, Sweden has a more generous support system for parents caring for children covered by LSS. However, different groups of carers do not have the same rights, which could be because carers are seldom the actual bearer of rights, with the exception of, for example, leave for urgent family matters. Instead, the rights bearer is the care recipient, as seen with the Compassionate Care Leave scheme, which leads to marginalising, and often hiding, the situation of working carers. LSS is an example of the strong individual focus that Swedish policies *can* have; people have a right to participate in society regardless of their disability or illness. However, carers still tend to be overlooked due to the belief that it is the state that provides most of the care, not carers. Labour market legislation and general support are not sufficiently adapted for working carers' caring situation and exclude a large proportion of carers from the leave and support available. If the state sees it as desirable for carers to keep participating in the labour force *and* care for relatives and others close to them, then carers' rights need to be fully met and improved. For the Swedish healthcare system to be sustainable, increased support for carers (through, for example, increased opportunities to take time off work applicable for *all* carers) is vital. This may require the Social Service Act to be as strong as the LSS legislation and more universal in its coverage across Sweden to avoid the current 'postcode lottery' of rights for carers.

The general invisibility of working carers means that employers are largely unaware of the struggles of many working carers, as well as of the benefits of supporting them, and are thus unlikely to make it possible for them to take more than a few (unpaid) days off work. Thus, national legislation and guidelines would benefit from being more direct. The NBHWS's government assignment to develop support aimed at employers, decision makers and managers in healthcare and social care, welfare officers and other health and social care personnel could possibly have a positive impact on the development of employers' occupational health practices for working carers. In sum, although some progress has been made, there is much work remaining to highlight working carers' situation, especially among the healthcare sector, industry and the general population.

As argued by Brodin (2018), the current individualised rhetoric no longer solely explains women taking on more care responsibilities than men due to their 'nature' and 'natural occurrences' and/or out of individual choice. Brodin (2018) explained that the idea of a free choice to engage in care hides a socialisation process and the lack of sufficient, quality public alternatives to care for relatives. This may reflect the lack of an intersectional perspective in policy discussions and debates. Granted, it could be argued that trying to improve the general situation for working carers through a national strategy could benefit female working carers. However, it is unlikely that it will 'by itself' change the gender, class and ethnicity related injustices that research shows exist (Katzin, 2014). Furthermore, the issue needs to be seen in the bigger picture: the issue with women providing more intensive care than men cannot solely be solved by support for carers; it is a systemic societal issue. The unproblematic view of the voluntary care of family members/relatives thus emerges from a lack of understanding of the structures linked to gender and other intersectional perspectives. Thus, care responsibility is presented as something neutral, despite research indicating that care responsibility is anything but evenly distributed between men and women (Katzin, 2014). Thus, strategic intersectional work needs to be further discussed and implemented. The gender analysis that the previous government included in the NBHWS's current assignments may be a step in the right direction and can be seen as a growing political awareness of the situation.

In conclusion, there is a greater political will to recognise the situation of carers in Sweden, as highlighted by the launch of the national carers strategy. However, there is still a long way to go before all working carers in Sweden receive the support they require to enable them to reconcile paid work with the care of a relative/loved one. Increased awareness of the situation of working carers in Sweden is needed, together with policies and practices sufficiently targeted at working carers, to help to empower and support them in their daily life and enable them to pursue their life goals.

Acknowledgements

We would like to thank the expert interviewees for their contributions to this chapter and their help in complementing and verifying the information and analysis. They include Tina Nordling, at the Department of Contractual Matters of the Swedish Trade Union Confederation; and Petra Ulmanen, Senior Lecturer and Professor Emeritus Marta Szebehely, both at the Department of Social Work, Stockholm University, Sweden.

Notes

[1] Carer advocates (*anhörigkonsulent*) provide direct individual and group support to carers and they also often have a strategic role in the development of carer support in their municipality, in collaboration with civil society.

[2] Eurostat calculates labour force participation among 20–64-year-olds whereas Statistics Sweden calculates the participation among citizens between the ages of 15 and 74.

[3] The law is based on the EG-directive 96/34/EG 3 July 1996.

[4] The first author discussed with an officer at the SSIA (date: 23 October 2023) in order to obtain the most current information on the subject.

[5] It is not available in all municipalities in Sweden.

[6] Parents mainly receive a percentage of their original pay.

References

Abbas, P.M. (2016) 'Municipalities' guidelines for employment of informal carers. A qualitative content analysis with a feminist theoretical approach'. Available from: http://www.diva-portal.org/smash/get/diva2:1044761/FULLTEXT01.pdf [Published in Swedish, accessed 20 November 2022].

Akademikernas A-kassa (Unemployment Insurance for University Graduates) (2021) 'The unemployment report'. Available from: https://arbetsloshetsrapporten.se/ [Published in Swedish, accessed 19 November 2022].

Brodin, H. (2018) 'At the intersection of marketisation, diversity and migration: reshaping the provision of paid family eldercare in Sweden?' *European Journal of Social Work*, 21(2): 222–34.

Carers Sweden (2021) 'Carers Sweden's response to the Government's Official Investigations of the Implementation of the Work Life Balance Directive'. Available from: https://www.regeringen.se/496a7a/contentassets/d7d957f021ea47cc9fa5e25bfb9d533b/anhorigas-riksforbund.pdf [Published in Swedish, accessed 20 November 2022].

City of Stockholm (2022) 'Home help services and home care allowance'. Available from: https://funktionsnedsattning.stockholm/olika-former-av-insatser/stod-i-hemmet/hemtjanst-hemvardsbidrag/ [Published in Swedish, accessed 20 November 2022].

Dir (2023: 77) 'Enhanced support for informal carers of individuals of long-term or seriously ill individuals'. Available from: https://www.regeringen.se/rattsliga-dokument/kommittedirektiv/2023/06/dir.-202377 [Published in Swedish, accessed 27 October 2023].

Ekonomifakta (Confederation of Swedish Enterprise – a Swedish employers' association). (2020) 'The State budget revenue'. Available from: https://www.ekonomifakta.se/fakta/offentlig-ekonomi/statsbudget/statsbudgetens-inkomster/ [Published in Swedish, accessed 19 November 2022].

Erlandsson, S. (2017) 'The value of gender and ethnicity in older people and disability policy', in E. Gunnarsson and M. Szebehely (eds), *Gender in everyday social care*, Stockholm: Gothia, pp 48–65. [Published in Swedish.]

Esping-Andersen, G. (1990) *The three worlds of welfare capitalism*, Cambridge: Polity Press.

EuroCarers (2021) 'The EU Strategy on Care: A new paradigm for carers across Europe?' Eurocarers position paper, EuroCarers. Available from: https://eurocarers.org/publications/the-eu-strategy-on-care/ [Accessed 19 November 2022].

European Parliament (2019) 'Directive (EU) 2019/1158 of the European Parliament and of the Council of 20 June 2019 on work–life balance for parents and carers and repealing Council Directive 2010/18/EU', Brussels: European Parliament. Available from: https://eur-lex.europa.eu/legal-content/EN/TXT/?uri=celex%3A32019L1158 [Accessed 30 June 2023].

European Union (2022) 'Charter of Fundamental Rights of the European Union'. Available from: https://eur-lex.europa.eu/legal-content/EN/TXT/?uri=CELEX:12012P/TXT [Accessed 22 November 2022].

Eurostat (2021) *'EU employment rate at 71.9 per cent in Q1 2021, Labour market slack at 14.8 per cent'*. Available from: https://ec.europa.eu/eurostat/web/products-eurostat-news/-/ddn-20210715-2 [Accessed 19 November 2022].

Finansinspektionen (Sweden's Financial Supervisory Authority) (2022) 'Stability in the Financial System. FI Ref. 22–14407'. Available from: https://fi.se/contentassets/41777fc48dca42a1beab132d38b160e1/stabiliteten-finansiella-systemet-22-1-eng.pdf [Accessed 20 November 2022].

Flyckt, K. and Wallin, E. (2021) 'The consequences of COVID-19 for people with special support according to LSS, Final Report'. The National Board of Health and Welfare Sweden (NBHWS). Available from: https://www.socialstyrelsen.se/globalassets/sharepoint-dokument/artikelkatalog/ovrigt/2021-8-7520.pdf [Published in Swedish, accessed 19 November 2022].

Hedström, K. (2020) 'They're breaking the circle', *Working Life*. Available from: https://www.prevent.se/arbetsliv/mer/20202/de-bryter-monstret/ [Published in Swedish, accessed 19 November 2022].

ISF (Inspection for Social Insurance) (2022) 'How is compassionate care leave used? An account of the financial support for care of next of kin/family members during the period 2000–2019'. Available from: https://isf.se/publikationer/rapporter/2022/2022-10-28-hur-anvands-narstaende penning [Published in Swedish, accessed 19 November 2022].

IVO (Inspection for Health and Social Care) (2021) 'The inspection of accessibility in the health care system, Final report of the government's mission to describe the risks of lack of accessibility and submit proposals for how supervision can be developed'. Available from: https://www.ivo.se/ [Published in Swedish, accessed 19 November 2022].

Johansson, L., Sundström, G. and Malberg, B. (2018) 'Half a century of Swedish elderly care – where do state and the family stand?' *Tidsskrift for omsorgsforskning*, 1(4): 62–68. [Published in Swedish.]

Katzin, M. (2014) 'The return to the family: private and public responsibility in the Swedish care for older people', *Retfærd: Nordisk Juridisktidsskrift*, 2: 37–53. [Published in Swedish.]

Labour Court (2003) 'Case Vårdförbundet vs Landstinget Västmanland i Västerås. AD 2003 nr 70'. Available from: https://lagen.nu/dom/ad/2003:70 [Published in Swedish, accessed 24 January 2024].

Labour Court (2016) 'Jusek v. state. Case nr 27/15 2016', Labour Court. Available from: https://lagen.nu/dom/ad/2016:24 [Published in Swedish, accessed 20 November 2022].

Liljeqvist, A. (2021) 'Final Report of The Board of Swedish Industry and Commerce for Better Regulations' (NNR) Municipal Review 2020 Survey of Swedish Municipalities, NNR'. Available from: https://www.kommungranskning.se/#rapporter [Published in Swedish, accessed 20 November 2022].

LO (The Swedish Trade Union Confederation) (2021) 'This is LO'. Available from: https://www.lo.se/english/this_is_lo [Accessed 20 November 2022].

Magnusson, F. (2015) 'Carers from other countries – an overview of the current knowledge', in M. Takter (ed), *Who shall pay for unpaid care? On social sustainable development*, Malmo: Holmbergs, pp 153–166. [Published in Swedish.]

Magnusson, L., Hanson, E., Larsson Skoglund, A., Ilett, R., Sennemark, E., Barbabella, F. and Gough, R. (2017) *Quality within care for older people from a carer perspective*, 2015:03. Available from: https://www.researchgate.net/publication/329338217_Kvalitet_i_aldreomsorg_ur_ett_anhorigperspektiv_The_quality_of_elder_care_from_a_family_carer_perspective#fullTextFile Content [Published in Swedish, accessed 24 January 2024].

Magnusson, L., Sennemark, E., Ekman, B., Johansson, P. and Hanson, E. (2021) *Consequences of the COVID-19 pandemic for informal carers who provide care, help and support for a person close to them*. 2021:3 Swedish Family Care Competence Centre (Nka). [Published in Swedish.]

Magnusson, L., McKee, K., Ekman, B., Vicenté, J. and Hanson, E. (2022) 'Informal caring, care and carers support, a national population survey 2018'. *Swedish Family Care Competence Centre (Nka)*. Available from the first author: lennart.magnusson@lnu.se [Published in Swedish].

MHSA (2022) 'Government bill for a closer and more accessible health care'. Available from: https://skr.se/skr/halsasjukvard/utvecklingavverksamhet/naravard/overenskommelseomengodochnaravard.28402.html [Published in Swedish, accessed 19 November 2022].

MHSA (2023) 'Agreement for closer and more accessible health care. Good and Accessible Health Care 2023. A transformation of health care with primary care as the hub. Agreement between the state and Sweden's Municipalities and Regions'. Available from: https://skr.se/skr/halsasjukvard/utvecklingavverksamhet/naravard/overenskommelseomengodochnaravard.28402.html ([Published in Swedish, accessed 27 October 2023]

Ministry of Finance (2023) 'High inflation continues to impact Swedish economy'. https://www.government.se/press-releases/2023/08/high-inflation-continues-to-impact-swedish-economy/ [Accessed 29 October 2023].

NBHWS (Socialstyrelsen) (2004) 'The National Board of Health and Welfare Sweden's term bank'. Available from: https://termbank.socialstyrelsen.se/?TermId=38&SrcLang=sv [Published in Swedish, accessed 20 November 2022].

NBHWS (National Board of Health and Welfare Sweden) (2012) 'Family members who provide care to someone close to them'. Available from: https://www.socialstyrelsen.se/globalassets/sharepoint-dokument/artikelkatalog/ovrigt/2012-8-15.pdf [Published in Swedish, accessed 24 January 2024].

NBHWS (National Board of Health and Welfare Sweden) (2020) 'Family members who care for or support older people close to them. Foundation Report to the National Carers Strategy'. Available from: https://www.socialstyrelsen.se/globalassets/sharepoint-dokument/artikelkatalog/ovrigt/2020-11-7045.pdf [Published in Swedish, accessed 20 November 2022].

OECD (2013) 'Long-term care in Sweden', in *OECD reviews of health care quality: Sweden 2013*. OECD Publishing. Available from: doi.org/10.1787/9789264204799-7-en [Accessed 20 November 2022].

SALAR (Swedish Association of Local Authorities and Regions – SKR) (2014) 'The State and the regional government bodies' assignments'. Available from: https://skr.se/skr/tjanster/rapporterochskrifter/publikationer/statenochderegionalasjalvstyrelseorganensuppgifter.30773.html [Published in Swedish, accessed 20 November 2022].

SALAR (2021) 'The European Union affects local Polices'. https://skr.se/skr/demokratiledningstyrning/euinternationellt/eukommunerochregioner.401.html [Published in Swedish, accessed 20 November 2022].

Sand, A.B. (2016) 'Informal carers who combine paid work with care of someone close to them, overview of the literature, updated version'. 2016:3. Available from: https://anhoriga.se/globalassets/media/dokument/publicerat/kunskapsoversikter/anhorigomsorg_sand_uppdat.pdf [Published in Swedish, accessed 20 November 2022].

SCB (Statistics Sweden) (2019) 'The division between paid and unpaid work'. Available from: https://www.scb.se/hitta-statistik/temaomraden/jamstalldhet/jamn-fordelning-av-det-obetalda-hem--och-omsorgsarbetet/fordelning-mellan-betalt-och-obetalt-arbete/#129904 [Published in Swedish, accessed 20 November 2022].

SCB (2020) 'Gainfully employed 16–64 years by profession, in 2020'. Available from: https://www.scb.se/hitta-statistik/statistik-efter-amne/arbetsmarknad/sysselsattning-forvarvsarbete-och-arbetstider/yrkesregistret-med-yrkesstatistik/pong/tabell-och-diagram/30-vanligaste-yrkena/ [Published in Swedish, accessed 20 November 2022].

SCB (2021) 'People born in other countries in Sweden'. Available from: https://www.scb.se/hitta-statistik/sverige-i-siffror/manniskorna-i-sverige/utrikes-fodda/ [Published in Swediah, accessed 20 November 2022]

SCB (2022a) 'Professions in Sweden'. Available from: https://www.scb.se/hitta-statistik/sverige-i-siffror/utbildning-jobb-och-pengar/yrken-i-sverige/ [Published in Swedish, accessed 20 November 2022].

SCB (2022b) 'Life expectancy in Sweden'. Available from: https://www.scb.se/hitta-statistik/sverige-i-siffror/manniskorna-i-sverige/medellivslangd-i-sverige/ [Published in Swedish, accessed 20 November 2022].

SCB (2023) 'Population statistics 2023'. Available from: https://www.scb.se/en/finding-statistics/statistics-by-subject-area/population/population-composition/population-statistics/pong/tables-and-graphs/population-statistics---month-quarter-half-year/population-statistics-2023/ [Accessed 29 October 2023].

Segendorf, O.Å. and Theobald, E. (2019) 'Can immigration solve the problem with an ageing population?' Swedish Riksbank. Available from: https://www.riksbank.se/globalassets/media/rapporter/pov/artiklar/engelska/2019/190613/er-2019_1-can-immigration-solve-the-problem-of-an-aging-population.pdf [Accessed 20 November 2022]

Sennemark, E., Andersson, J., Magnusson, L. and Hanson, E. (2019) 'Informal caring from a gender perspective, an overview of the literature'. 2019:3. *Nka*. https://anhoriga.se/globalassets/media/dokument/publicerat/rapporter/kunskapsoversikt_genus-webb.pdf [Published in Swedish, accessed 20 November 2022].

SFS (Svensk Författningssamling). (2008) Discrimination Act 2008:567. Available from: https://www.do.se/download/18.277ff225178022473141dda/1618941061391/discrimination-act-2018.pdf [Accessed 24 January 2024].

SFS (2022) 'Lag om ändring i lagen (1998:209) om rätt till ledighet av trängande familjeskäl' (*Act amending the Act (1998:209) on the right to leave for urgent family reasons*). Available from: https://svenskforfattningssamling.se/sites/default/files/sfs/2022-07/SFS2022-1295.pdf [Accessed 24 January 2024].

Skandia (2021) 'Equal work – different pension in 2021. This is how the pension is affected by part-time work after family formation'. Available from: https://www.skandia.se/globalassets/pdf/press-och-media/rappor ter-och-debatt/lika-arbete-olika-pension-2021.pdf [Published in Swedish, accessed 22 November 2022].

SOU (Statens Offentliga Utredingar) (The Government's Official Investigations) (2017: 21) 'Read me! The National Quality Plan for Health and Social Care of Older People, Part 1 and Part 2'. Available from: https://www.regeringen. se/4969b7/contentassets/9378aff4b35a427c99b772345af79539/sou-2017_2 1_webb_del1.pdf [Published in Swedish, accessed 20 November 2022].

SOU (2020: 81) 'Implementation of the balance directive – work–life balance for parents and informal carers'. Available from: https://www.regeringen. se/4af764/contentassets/07d6d56a63ba4ac1851ea632159fa940/genom forande-av-balansdirektivet--balans-mellan-arbete-och-privatliv-for-forald rar-och-anhorigvardare-sou-2020-81.pdf [Published in Swedish, accessed 20 November 2022].

SOU (2023: 9) 'A state principalship for personal assistance. Increased equality, long-term sustainability, and quality'. Available from: https:// www.regeringen.se/rattsliga-dokument/statens-offentliga-utredningar/ 2023/02/sou-20239/ [Published in Swedish, accessed 27 October 2023].

SSIA (Swedish Social Insurance Agency) (2018) 'Compassionate care leave amongst women and men. Less men than women provide care for a family member or loved one, short analyses', 2018:5. Available from: https://forsak ringskassan.se/statistik/sjuk/narstaendepenning [Published in Swedish, accessed 19 November 2022].

SSIA (2021) 'Changes in the Social Security Insurance law from 1 January 2022'. Available from: https://www.forsakringskassan.se/nyhetsarkiv/ nyheter-press/2021-12-20-forandringar-i-lagstiftning-for-socialforsakrin gen-arsskiftet-2022 [Published in Swedish, accessed 20 November 2022].

SSIA (2022a) 'Contact days'. Available from: https://www.forsakringskassan. se/privatpers/foralder/om_ditt_barn_har_en_funktionsnedsattning/konta ktdagar [Published in Swedish, accessed 19 November 2022].

SSIA (2022b) 'Disease carriers' allowance and reimbursement of travel expenses for employed persons'. Available from: https://www.forsak ringskassan.se/privatpers/sjuk/anstalld/smittbararpenning [Published in Swedish, accessed 19 November 2022].

SSIA (2022c) 'Statistics in the field of illness. Compassionate Care Allowance'. Available from: https://forsakringskassan.se/statistik/sjuk/narstaendepenn ing [Published in Swedish, accessed 19 November 2022].

SSIA (2022d) 'Family Care Allowance for job seekers'. Available from: https://www.forsakringskassan.se/privatperson/sjuk/arbetssokande/ narstaendepenning-for-arbetssokande [Published in Swedish, accessed 22 November 2022].

SSIA (2023a) 'Care allowance'. Available from: https://www.forsakring skassan.se/privatpers/funktionsnedsattning/om-ditt-barn-har-en-funkt ionsnedsattning/omvardnadsbidrag [Published in Swedish, accessed 29 October 2023].

SSIA (2023b) 'Additional cost compensation for children'. Available from: https://www.forsakringskassan.se/privatpers/funktionsnedsattning/om-ditt-barn-har-en-funktionsnedsattning/merkostnadsersattning-for-barn [Published in Swedish, accessed 20 October 2023].

Supreme Administrative Court (HFD – Högsta Förvaltningsdomstolen) (2013) 'Question on conditions for the right to temporary parents allowance for an unlimited time for care of a child who after completion of treatment for a serious illness needed intensive training etc. because of a remaining illness condition', HFD ref 76. Available from: https://www. domstol.se/globalassets/filer/domstol/hogstaforvaltningsdomstolen/avg oranden-2008-2018/2013/hfd-2013-ref.-76.pdf/ [Published in Swedish, accessed 20 November 2022].

Svallfors, S. and Tyllström, A. (2017) 'Lobbying for profits: private companies and the privatization of the welfare state in Sweden'. Working paper 2017:1, Institute for Future Studies. Available from: https://www.iffs.se/media/ 22171/2017_1.pdf [Accessed 20 November 2022].

Swedish Institute (SI) (2022) 'Equal power and influence for women and men – that's what Sweden is aiming for'. Available from: https://sweden. se/life/equality/gender-equality [Accessed 20 November 2022].

Takter, M. (2019) 'An Informal carer perspective – an opportunity for development? A national study of municipalities' support to carers', Carers Sweden, Nka. Available from: https://anhorigasriksforbund. se/site/wp-content/uploads/kartlapercentCCper cent88ggning_ 2019-reviderad-210518.pdf [Published in Swedish, accessed 20 November 2022].

The Swedish Parliament (1949: 381) 'The Act concerning The Parental Code'. Available from: https://www.riksdagen.se/sv/dokument-lagar/ dokument/svensk-forfattningssamling/foraldrabalk-1949381_sfs-1949-381 [Published in Swedish, accessed 24 January 2024].

The Swedish Parliament (1987: 230) 'The Marriage Code'. Available from: https://www.riksdagen.se/sv/dokument-lagar/dokument/svensk-forfattningssamling/aktenskapsbalk-1987230_sfs-1987-230 [Published in Swedish, accessed 24 January 2024].

The Swedish Parliament (1988: 1465) 'The Act concerning leave for close relatives/next of kin'. Available from: https://www.riksdagen.se/sv/dokum ent-lagar/dokument/svensk-forfattningssamling/lag-19881465-om-ledig het-for-narstaendevard_sfs-1988-1465 [Published in Swedish, accessed 24 November 2022].

The Swedish Parliament (1993: 387) 'The Act concerning Support and Service for Persons with Certain Functional Impairments'. Available from: https://www.riksdagen.se/sv/dokument-lagar/dokument/svensk-forfattningssamling/lag-1993387-om-stod-och-service-till-vissa_sfs-1993-387 [Published in Swedish, accessed 21 November 2022].

The Swedish Parliament (1995: 584) 'The Parental Leave Act'. Available from: https://www.riksdagen.se/sv/dokument-lagar/dokument/svensk-forfattningssamling/foraldraledighetslag-1995584_sfs-1995-584 [Published in Swedish, accessed 24 November 2022].

The Swedish Parliament (1998: 209) 'The Act on the Right to Leave for Urgent Family Reasons'. Available from: https://www.riksdagen.se/sv/dokument-lagar/dokument/svensk-forfattningssamling/lag-1998209-om-ratt-till-ledighet-av-trangande_sfs-1998-209 [Published in Swedish, accessed 24 November 2022].

The Swedish Parliament (2001: 453) 'The Act concerning Social Services Act 2001: 453 (2009: 549)' Available from: https://www.lagboken.se/Lagboken/start/socialratt/socialtjanstlag-2001453/d_361777-sfs-2009_549-lag-om-andring-i-socialtjanstlagen-2001_453 [Published in Swedish, accessed 24 November 2022].

The Swedish Parliament (2010: 110) 'The Act concerning Social Insurance Code'. Available from: https://www.riksdagen.se/sv/dokument-lagar/dokument/svensk-forfattningssamling/socialforsakringsbalk-2010110_sfs-2010-110 [Published in Swedish, accessed 24 November 2022].

The Swedish Parliament (2010: 1241) 'The Act amending the Act (1988:1465) on compensation and leave for family care'. Available from: https://www.lagboken.se/Lagboken/start/arbetsratt-och-arbetsmiljoratt/lag-19881465-om-ledighet-for-narstaendevard/d_693846-sfs-2010_1241-lag-om-andring-i-lagen-1988_1465-om-ersattning-och-ledighet-for-narstaendevard [Published in Swedish, accessed 22 November 2022].

Ulmanen, P. (2015) 'The price of care in times of austerity. Informal care for Older people from a Gender perspective', Report in Social Work, no. 150. Stockholm University, Department for Social Work. Holmbergs tryckeri. Available from: https://su.diva-portal.org/smash/get/diva2:858835/FULLTEXT01.pdf [Published in Swedish, accessed 20 November 2022].

Vicente, J., McKee, K., Magnusson, L., Johansson, P., Ekman, B. and Hanson, E. (2022) 'Informal care provision among male and female working carers: findings from a Swedish national survey', PLoS ONE, 17(3): e0263396.

4

Australia

Kate O'Loughlin and Alison Williams

Introduction

Australia has a national Carer Recognition Act 2010 (Commonwealth of Australia, 2010) and states and territories also have legislation and strategies in place to recognise and support unpaid carers. Such legislation is intended to recognise the social and economic contribution of family carers and supports needed to ensure carers have rights and choices related to paid work, income security, health and well-being (Chomik, Williams and Baird, 2019). Central to the introduction of legislation and policies recognising and supporting carers is the influence of carers' organisations (Yeandle, 2016). A carer movement emerged in Australia in the 1970s with the Carers Association of New South Wales (NSW) established in 1980 as the first independent advocacy organisation (Carers Australia, nd). Australia now has a national carers' organisation as well as state- and territory-based associations, whose lobbying role has been instrumental in gaining recognition and forms of support (carer payments, access to services, flexible work arrangements) for unpaid family/friend carers (Yeandle, Kröger and Cass, 2012).

While this recognition is significant, a gap remains between the legislative and policy framework intended to recognise and support carers and what translates into practice with carer leave entitlements for employees under the Fair Work Act 2009 and National Employment Standards (NES) (Cheng, Jepsen and Wang, 2020).

This chapter provides an overview of the political, economic and social contexts influencing policy making in Australia, before outlining carer leave policies available to Australian workers. A critical assessment of the adequacy of the policies follows, with specific reference to the implications for employed carers in the context of the COVID-19 pandemic and its legacy.

National context

Political context

Australia has a federated government system comprised of one national, six state and two territory governments, with municipal governments at the local level. Australia's constitution represents an 'integrated federation' (Fenna, 2012), outlining the relationship and power-sharing arrangements between the national parliament and the states/territories. Each level of government has jurisdiction over policy domains; however, there are areas of overlap. Should any conflict arise between the national provisions and state/territory provisions, the national law overrides the state/territory law. For example, an area of overlap relevant to carers is anti-discrimination legislation.

The national government has centralised fiscal powers as it controls the taxation base, thus shaping its key policy-making role in socioeconomic life (for example, health, aged care, disability, childcare, income support). The states take on a service-delivery role (for example, hospitals, schools, transport, policing) and rely on transfers from the national government for approximately half of their funding needs (Koutsogeorgopoulou and Tuske, 2015). Carer leave policies are covered by national legislation through the NES, with some employees covered by state-based legislation as detailed later.

Historically, Australia has been considered a liberal welfare state based on collectivist values and commitment to equity and inclusion. This is reflected in legislative and policy provisions, providing universal benefits (for example, health, education) as well as support for people with specific needs (for example, unemployment, low-income families, aged care, disability). However, there has been a shift towards more individual responsibility and marketised systems in many public policy areas, including aged and disability care services, with the introduction of a consumer-directed funding model as a means of relieving fiscal pressures on government but, at the same time, putting pressure on family/friend carers to fill the gap when formal care services are not available (Fine and Davidson, 2018).

Economic and labour market context

Australia has a mixed market economy with almost half of the country's economic output derived from key industries including health and education (13.2 per cent); mining (14.6 per cent); finance (7.6 per cent); construction (7.3 per cent); manufacturing (6 per cent) with export share related to resources (63.3 per cent), services (16.5 per cent), rural (10.8 per cent) and manufactured (7.2 per cent) (Reserve Bank of Australia, 2023). While the COVID-19 pandemic impacted the economy, in 2020–21 Australia fared better among Organisation for Economic Co-operation and Development (OECD) countries through initially using a suppression approach to limit transmission (for example, lockdowns, border closures) and then a containment approach (for example, vaccinations, co-existing with the virus). Gross domestic product (GDP) has recovered to pre-pandemic levels, with unemployment falling from 7.4 per cent in 2020 to 4.6 per cent in 2021 (OECD, 2021a).

Changes in Australia's labour market over the last 50 years show increased participation rates for women, while men's rates have remained relatively stable (Australian Institute of Family Studies, 2023). There is a high incidence of part-time work among women (Sila and Dugain, 2019). Women make up 38.4 per cent of all full-time employees and 68.5 per cent of all part-time employees (Australian Bureau of Statistics [ABS], 2022; Workplace Gender Equality Agency [WGEA], 2022). An important point of distinction in Australia's industrial relations provisions is defining an 'employee' and a 'worker'. The Fair Work Act 2009 predicates its provisions on the employment relationship established between employer and employee (working hours, pay rates, leave entitlements); however, due to increasing casualisation there are now many Australian workers (for example, working under a contract, or as part of the gig economy) not classified as employees under the Act (Stanford, 2021) and, as casual workers, without paid leave entitlements.

Labour force data indicate Australia's participation rate is 66.4 per cent, unemployment rate 4 per cent and underemployment rate 6.6 per cent (ABS, 2022). Women's participation in paid work continues to be shaped by sociocultural and economic issues associated with gender roles, including industrial and occupational segregation, interrupted work histories and expectations of providing care at various life stages (Foley and Cooper, 2021; WGEA, 2021). The gender pay gap and women's under-representation in senior executive/management roles remain barriers to equal participation in paid employment (WGEA, 2022). The national gender pay gap is 13.8 per cent between women and men, with the gap highest for women employed in professional, scientific and technical services (WGEA, 2022).

The Australian Bureau of Statistics (ABS) Survey of Disability, Ageing and Carers (2018) reported that 10.8 per cent of all Australians are carers[1] and, overall, more likely to be women (12.3 per cent of all females, 9.3 per cent of all males), with 56.1 per cent aged between 45 and 74 years (ABS, 2018). Women also are more likely to take on a primary carer role (Figure 4.1). The impact of a carer role on paid employment is evident, with carers in the usual working age range of 15–64 years having a lower employment rate (66 per cent) than non-carers (77.4 per cent). Male carers were more likely to be employed (71.8 per cent) than female carers (63.2 per cent). The participation rate for primary carers (58.8 per cent) was significantly lower than for non-carers (81.5 per cent) (ABS, 2018). For primary carers aged 15–64 years, 55.5 per cent were employed, with employment status influenced by the hours of care provided per week: 28.6 per cent of primary carers providing 40+ hours of care per week were employed, as compared to 52.8 per cent of those providing up to 20 hours of care per week (ABS, 2018).

Figure 4.1: Primary carers by age and sex

■ Number of primary carers, by age and sex, 2018 Male ('000)

▨ Number of primary carers, by age and sex, 2018 Female ('000)

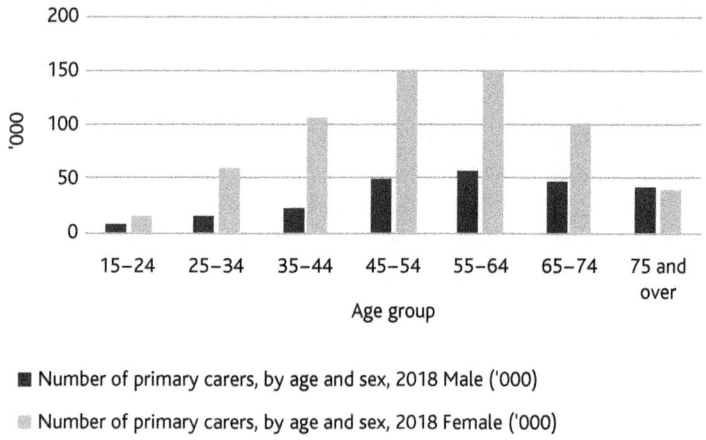

Source: ABS (2018)

Social context

As Kendig and Lucas note (2014: 212): 'Australia is growing older, with a predominantly Western heritage and an increasingly Asian future'. The current population of ~25.5 million is concentrated in the large coastal cities, with few people living in the interior. Australia has a relatively small Indigenous population (2 to 3 per cent) that, in general, experiences severe disadvantage and lower life expectancy (Australian Institute of Health and Welfare, 2020). Population growth has been driven by successive waves of immigration starting with 19th-century British colonisation, followed by post-World War II migration from Europe and, more recently, from many parts of Asia. Australia had a major, sustained baby boom from the late 1940s to the mid-1960s. The people born in this period are now entering mid-to-later life, with many becoming multigenerational carers (O'Loughlin, Barrie and Kendig, 2018).

With population ageing, the Australian population aged 65 years and over is projected to double to approximately 8.9 million in the period 2019–20 to 2060–61, to represent 23 per cent of an expected population of 38.3 million. The ratio of the working age population to those aged 65+ is projected to decrease from 4 to 2.7 in the same time frame (Commonwealth of Australia, 2021). According to OECD data, overall life expectancy in Australia is 83.2 years; for men 81.2 years and women 85.3 years (OECD, 2021b, OECD, 2022).

Carer leave policies

Australian employees can access several paid and unpaid forms of leave to enable them to care for dependents/household members. In the national sphere, the policies are known as Personal/Carer's Leave (paid), Compassionate Leave (paid) and Carer's Leave (unpaid), noting that they may be known by alternative names in state and territory legislation and in workplace-based collective agreements. The availability of these forms of leave was developed during the 1990s through a number of decisions by federal and state industrial relations tribunals prompted by Australia's ratification of the International Labour Organization (ILO) Workers with Family Responsibilities Convention (#156), and introduced for the first time the concept that an employee's sick leave entitlement could be used to care for family or household members (Chapman, 2009: 457). Several 'test cases' brought before industrial relations tribunals between 1994 and 2005 sought to broaden the range of employees who were entitled to this benefit, but coverage remained uneven. However, in 2006 a suite of employee minimum standards was created at the federal level, including personal/carer's leave and compassionate leave, and in 2010 these were incorporated into the current NES, which provide minimum entitlements/standards under the Fair Work Act. The Fair Work Act applies to all Australian employees covered by the national workplace relations system (approximately 87 per cent of employees) (ABS, 2018).

Prior to the introduction by the federal government of a national workplace relations system in 1996, each state had its own industrial relations system, with great variation in employee entitlements. Most states (NSW, Queensland, South Australia, Tasmania) have retained industrial relations powers over their public service and local government sector. Western Australia has retained more of its industrial relations powers than the other states and has a small number of employees not covered by the national system as well as state public servants. All Victorian employees are covered by the national Fair Work Act, as are employees in the Northern Territory and the Australian Capital Territory.

Another important feature of the Australian system is that employees may have their pay, leaves and other entitlements determined by several interconnected means. As well as the Fair Work Act and other employment-related legislation such as health and safety and workers compensation, there is also a system of 'modern awards' and 'enterprise agreements'. A modern award is a uniquely Australian instrument providing a set of minimum conditions for a particular industry or occupation that is determined by the Fair Work Commission as the national industrial relations tribunal. Currently there are 122 modern awards covering a wide range of industries, occupations and employment conditions. An enterprise agreement is a collectively negotiated instrument between an employer and employees, or their representatives, that provides conditions of employment that are above the award minimum. There are also employees, such as managers and professionals, who are outside the industrial relations system and who have their conditions of employment determined by common law contracts.

While this does lend a complexity to the Australian system, essentially most Australian employees are covered by the Fair Work Act, with the modern award and/or enterprise agreements providing additional entitlements.

Longer-term leave

Paid Personal/Carer's Leave is part of the NES and therefore available to permanent full-time and part-time employees of employers covered by the Fair Work Act; however, casual employees are not entitled to this leave. Eligible employees are entitled to ten days' leave per year to care for or support an immediate family or household member because of illness, injury or emergency.

Immediate family is defined by the Fair Work Act (s.12) as: (a) a spouse/ former spouse, de facto partner/former de facto partner, child, parent, grandparent, grandchild or sibling of the employee; or (b) a child, parent, grandparent, grandchild or sibling of a spouse or de facto partner of the employee. The definition includes step-relations and adoptive relations, and 'child' includes adult children.

Public sector employees in most states are entitled to the same amount of paid personal/carer leave as provided by the NES. The following pieces of legislation provide carer's leave to employees not covered by the Fair Work Act, including state public sector employees:

- NSW Crown Employees (Public Service Conditions of Employment) Reviewed Award 2009, providing leave to care for a family member;
- Queensland Employment Standards, made under Chapter 2 Part 3 of the Industrial Relations Act 2016;
- Western Australian Minimum Conditions of Employment Act 1993;
- South Australian Fair Work Act 1994;
- Tasmanian Industrial Relations Act 1984.

While ten days' leave per annum is the minimum entitlement, formal industrial instruments and individual common law contracts can set out different entitlements, but these cannot be less than this minimum. Many public sector employees receive more than the minimum ten days; for example, Commonwealth public servants receive 18 days per annum (APSC, 2018), NSW public servants receive 15 days per annum (see: Crown Employees (Public Service Conditions of Employment) Reviewed Award 2009 [NSW]), South Australian public servants receive 12 days per annum (South Australian Office of the Commissioner for Public Sector Employment, 2022) and Western Australian public servants receive 13 days per annum (Government Services (Miscellaneous) General Agreement 2021, cl.47). Employees are paid at their base rate of pay for their ordinary hours of work in the period, not including penalty rates or overtime (Fair Work Act, s.99).

Short-term leaves

Unpaid Carer's Leave is also provided by the NES and provides two consecutive full days or four consecutive half days for each caring episode if an employee's immediate family or household requires care or support because of personal illness, injury, death or an emergency. Importantly, full-time and part-time employees must have exhausted any paid personal/carer's leave entitlement before being eligible to take unpaid carer's leave. Casual employees are eligible immediately, as they have no paid entitlement.

State government employees in NSW, Queensland, South Australia, Tasmania and Western Australia, including temporary or casual employees, are also entitled to this leave. State government employees in NSW are additionally entitled to 1–2.5 days of Family Leave, which is paid leave for unplanned and emergency family responsibilities or other emergencies (not related to sickness).

Paid Compassionate Leave is also provided by the NES and comprises two consecutive full days or separate periods of one day each time an immediate family or household member suffers a life-threatening illness or injury, or death. It is available for full-time and part-time employees for each occasion, as needed. Casual employees are entitled to the same amount of Compassionate Leave, but it is unpaid.

Most state government employees are also entitled to an equivalent form of Paid Compassionate Leave; however, Western Australian employees not covered by the Fair Work Act do not have an entitlement to compassionate leave for caring but are entitled to Bereavement Leave on the death of a family or household member.

Table 4.1 summarises the carer leave options available in Australia as of November 2023.

Other legislated carer supports

Flexible working arrangements

Flexible working arrangements assist workers to manage their care responsibilities (Fair Work Ombudsman, 2019). The Fair Work Act (s.65) provides employees with the right to request flexible working arrangements. A right to request, however, does not guarantee that the request will be granted or that it will be implemented consistently across workplaces (O'Loughlin et al, 2019). While a right to request was initially associated with childcare, in 2013 the Fair Work Act Amendment Act 2013 extended the 'right to request' to mature-age workers over 55 and workers with added

Table 4.1: Carer leave schemes, Australia (November 2023)

Leave details			Eligibility					
Leave name and introduced	Time period	Compensation	Worker/employee status	Qualifying period	Person needing care	Evidence	Notice period and process
Unpaid Personal/ Carer's Leave, 2009	2 days/4 half days per annum	Unpaid	Employees, including casual workers	–	Family	Employer can ask for medical certification	Have to have exhausted paid carers' leave entitlement
Compassionate Leave, 2009	2 days per annum	Paid, but not for casual workers	All, but not paid for casual workers	–	Family/ household member	Employer can ask for medical certification	Notify employer ASAP
Personal/Carer's Leave, 2005	10 days per annum but accrues	Yes, at base salary	Full-time/part-time employees, not casual workers	Accrues from day one	Family/ household member	Employer can ask for medical certification	Notify employer ASAP

caring responsibilities (Williamson and Pearce, 2022). Further, in 2018 the Fair Work Commission issued a decision that all modern awards should contain a term that facilitated employees to make a request for flexible working arrangements. The award term requires employers to provide written reasons for any refusal of a request and to consider alternatives to the request that could provide a compromise (Fair Work Commission, 2018). The employer is allowed to refuse on 'reasonable business grounds' essentially related to cost and inconvenience such as the impact on efficiency, productivity and customer service, and/or the impact on, or employer's capacity to change, other workers' working arrangements (Fair Work Act s.65(5A); Williamson and Pearce, 2022).

The Act also allows employers and employees to agree to a formal Individual Flexibility Arrangement (IFA); these are variations of awards and enterprise agreements agreed to by both the employer and an individual employee to provide more flexibility in working conditions. For example, an IFA could stipulate that a carer is allowed a longer break in the middle of the day to assist with taking a family member to medical appointments, combined with an earlier start time or later finishing time. Note that because the NES and modern awards provide the minimum (safety net) conditions for workers, an IFA cannot be used to disadvantage the employee compared to the award, or their enterprise agreement if they have one. Instead, the worker must be 'better off overall'. There is no oversight of IFAs by the Fair Work Commission, so little data is available on whether IFAs in practice provide flexible working arrangements that benefit workers rather than employers. However, recent research shows that while the overall prevalence of IFAs is low, they are more common in certain industries such as healthcare and social assistance, financial and insurance services and retail trade, and used slightly more by women than men (Fair Work Commission, 2021a).

Financial support for carers

In addition to leave provisions available to employees, a number of forms of direct public payments are available to eligible Australian carers. There has been some form of 'carer' pension since the 1940s; initially this was called a 'wife's allowance/wife pension' (for caring for an invalid/age pensioner) and in 1983 became the 'Spouse Carer's Pension' to cover men caring for a spouse. Reflecting social change and, as outlined previously, the influence of emerging carer advocacy groups, in 1997 it was renamed as a 'Carer Payment' to cover anyone meeting specified criteria in taking on a carer role.

Additional government payments include:

- Carer payment: means–tested, including an assets test (principal residence exempt) to provide fortnightly income support, paid at the same rate as other social security pensions (for example, age pension). The carer must provide constant care in a private home for a person with a severe disability/illness, or frail aged person, and cannot be away from the recipient for more than 25 hours a week for paid work.

- Carer's allowance: means-tested extra fortnightly payment for daily care provided for person with disability/serious illness or frail aged person where care will be needed for at least 12 months or remainder of recipient's life.
- Carer supplement: an additional payment of AU$600 per year automatically paid to those receiving a carer allowance/payment, and can be paid for each eligible payment (for example, receiving carer allowance for more than one person).

Social assistance benefits

Carers, if they are receiving a Carer Payment/Carer Allowance, automatically receive a Health Care/Pensioner Concession Card to assist with medication costs and other personal costs (for example, electricity, public transport). They may also qualify for further payments such as a remote area allowance and rent assistance in the private rental market. Carers are also eligible for certain tax deductions or credits with means-tested eligibility. For example, there is a tax offset payment available if the carer receives a carer payment/allowance and has been wholly engaged in providing care to a person in receipt of a disability support pension (for example, spouse, child/adult with a disability). While care recipients are able to self-manage their nationally funded personal budgets for Aged Care and National Disability Insurance Scheme care packages, these funds cannot be used to pay a family member(s) to provide care.

Services for carers

The national government provides free services and supports for carers through a recently reformed (2019–20) initiative called Carer Gateway. These are provided online, by phone or in person. Supports include support planning, counselling, coaching, educational resources, peer support, financial support, emergency respite and assistance with accessing local government and non-government funded services (Carer Gateway, nd).

Analysis and discussion of the adequacy of carer leave policies and programmes

The national legislative and policy framework intended to protect industrial rights and important aspects of diversity and inclusion in Australian workplaces, including recognition and support for carers, does not always translate into equitable practices in all workplaces. This section reviews the effectiveness of short- and long-term carer leaves and other support measures for carers in Australia. It draws on research into the operation of the provisions of the Fair Work Act that allow flexible working arrangements; equity issues related to the use of flexible work; and income security.

Equity/inclusivity

Two sources of inequity related to working carers will be considered here: employment status and gender. Fundamentally, employment status determines who has access to paid leave entitlements including carer leave. Workers employed on a casual basis do not have access to paid leave, but their hourly pay rate includes an additional 15–25 per cent as acknowledgement and recompense for this (Gilfillan, 2021). However, evidence indicates that the median wage for casual workers is 26 per cent lower than that of permanent employees, reflecting the variable hours of work and low hourly rates of pay associated with this form of work (Stanford, 2021). From a carer perspective, those employed under these conditions likely cannot afford to take time away from paid work to provide care for a family/ household member.

In 2021 Australia had 2.4 million casual employees (~19 per cent of all employed) (ABS, 2021). The increase in non-standard and insecure forms of employment essentially advantages employers, as it provides flexible employment options particularly in service-based industries such as health and social care, though the case is also made that it provides opportunities for those wanting temporary work (for example, women, students) and as a 'foot in the door' for those with low skill levels, including migrant workers (Gilfillan, 2021). Effectively this move towards casual and insecure work has eroded Australia's long-held form of permanent full-time employment that provided basic protections and entitlements, including paid leave, through industrial awards (Stanford, 2021). What we have now is legislated changes to the Fair Work Act introduced by the conservative Liberal-National coalition government in power from 2013 to 2022 that facilitate the continuation of casual and insecure work by allowing employers to determine the ways in which they employ casual workers and limiting previous provisions around turning casual appointments into permanent positions (Stanford, 2021).

As outlined previously, Australia's 2.65 million carers are more likely to be women, older and with a lower employment rate than non-carers (ABS, 2020), and women also have higher rates of casual and insecure employment than men (Stanford, 2021). About half (50.2 per cent) of all carers, as compared to a quarter (25.6 per cent) of non-carers, live in a household in the lowest two equivalised gross income quintiles (ABS, 2020). However, this demographic profile is not necessarily reflected in carer leave entitlements, particularly in the case of those in a primary carer role, where 28.6 per cent provide 40+ hours of care per week while also being employed (ABS, 2020). A study of Australia's baby boomers aged 60–64 years found that the experiences of older working carers is mediated by socioeconomic position, age and gender; carers were more likely to be women, employed part-time or not in paid work, and dependent on government income support such as the Age Pension or Carer Payment (O'Loughlin, Loh and Kendig, 2017).

The legal right to request flexible work arrangements to accommodate carer responsibilities is discussed in detail in the next section; however, the issue of equity arises in considering who has access and how/when such access is granted. Data from a Carers NSW survey indicate that not all working carers are fully aware of their right to request and, for those who are, barriers remain, including limited paid carer leave options and negotiating flexible work arrangements with often unsupportive managers and co-workers (O'Loughlin et al, 2019).

Flexibility

There are several features of the Australian system that provide flexibility in the accrual and banking of leaves and granting and taking leaves. These will be discussed along with the increasing use of formal flexible working arrangements.

Flexibility is built into Personal/Carer's Leave in several ways. The leave accrues progressively during a year of service from the first day of employment, with the effect that new employees gradually build up leave and do not have to wait for an eligibility period to pass. Additionally, a bank of available paid leave accumulates from year to year. This means that there is no minimum or maximum amount of paid Personal/Carer's Leave that can be taken at a time – it is dependent on how much leave has accrued. Arguably, one of the most flexible aspects of the Australian system is that 'personal' leave is interchangeable with 'carer' leave; that is, an individual can use the leave for their own personal needs (such as sickness) or for their caring activities.

The Fair Work Act does not place restrictions on the taking of Personal/Carer's Leave, so in practice employees can take it in smaller blocks of time (for example, one or two days, or part days), to provide short-term care. This leave also can be used to care for a family member(s) who is living overseas.

Personal Carer's Leave may be taken in the form of cash (paid out) only if provided for in a formally registered award or enterprise agreement. There are no official records kept of this practice, however, anecdotally such 'cashing out' is considered rare, mainly because the conversion of leave to cash is seen as a way of eroding and potentially removing leave entitlements and commoditises an entitlement meant to assist workers (Henderson, 2016).

These arguments were made in relation to annual leave but can also be applied to Personal/Carers' Leave. As there is little research into cashing out Personal/Carer's Leave it is unclear whether this does or could potentially disadvantage workers.

The Australian system has very limited flexibility when it comes to sharing of carer leave, as both short-term and longer-term leaves are attached to the individual worker. In most circumstances the leaves therefore cannot be shared with the worker's partner or other family member(s). It is possible, with the agreement of the employer, for an employee to 'gift' leave entitlements to another employee; however, this can only be done legally via a registered collective or individual agreement that is ratified by the Fair Work Commission. An example might be where a group of employees decide to assist a work colleague caring for a family member with a serious illness by each 'donating' some of their unused personal leave to their colleague, providing them with more time off to care.

Employees are given a degree of flexibility in providing evidence of their need to take paid Personal/Carer's Leave. The evidence must 'satisfy a reasonable person' and usually takes the form of a medical certificate or statutory declaration (s.107). Certificates are commonly provided by medical doctors but may also be provided by allied health practitioners such as pharmacists, physiotherapists and dentists. However, this is a grey area, as it is up to the employer as a 'reasonable person' to decide whether to accept, for example, a certificate from an allied health professional. Evidentiary requirements are set out in the award or enterprise agreement and an employee can challenge their employer's decision about a medical certificate under its dispute resolution procedure. Nonetheless, the Fair Work Commission has taken the view that the crucial feature of a medical certificate is that it should enable the employer to make an informed decision about the employee's fitness for work (see, for example, *Tawanda Gadzikwa v Australian Government Department of Human Services* [2018] FWC 4878).

Employees are unable to accrue unpaid Carer's Leave or paid/unpaid Compassionate Leave from year to year, but arguably there is no need, as the entitlement is attached to each caring episode, and these are unlimited. While this gives the impression of greater flexibility, in practice there is the possibility that employees with multiple short-term leaves for caring could be seen as less committed by the employer (Productivity Commission, 2015). Given that a permanent employee may only access unpaid Carer's Leave after their ten days of paid Carer's Leave has been exhausted, there is the possibility of increased employer intervention in managing performance if the amount of time spent caring increases.

Part-time employees are catered for in the Fair Work Act, as it specifies the amount of leave in 'days'. They are entitled to the same number of 'days' of leave as full-time employees, equivalent to the number of hours worked in a day or week. Women are the main beneficiaries of this policy, as 68.5 per cent of part-time Australian workers are women (WGEA, 2022) and, as mentioned previously, women are more likely to be carers (ABS, 2020). Additionally, unpaid Carer's Leave is specified as two (2) full days or four (4) part days, enshrining flexibility in its definition. In practice, employers could grant the leave in even smaller amounts (for example, hours), should they so choose, and while this level of detail is not formally recorded, anecdotal evidence indicates this does occur.

As the Fair Work Act provides other avenues for flexibility for carers apart from leaves, it is important to consider how effective these are in operation. A recent study involving a survey and interviews with key stakeholders in the industrial relations system such as trade unions, employers, lawyers and employer representatives provided an assessment of how the system was working from their perspectives (Fair Work Commission, 2021b). The researchers found that the use of the right to request flexibility remains gendered, with mainly women making these requests and very few requests from men in male-dominated industries (Fair Work Commission, 2021b: 8).

While the Act gives the right to request flexible working arrangements to statutorily specified groups, including people with a disability, carers and older workers, it is mainly parents seeking to care for school-age or younger children who make use of the right to request (Fair Work Commission, 2021b: 8). The most requested flexibility arrangement was for reduced working hours, mostly from full-time to part-time, followed by changes to the pattern of hours, for example starting and finishing early. Most respondents had encountered requests for flexible working arrangements by mature workers to care for spouses, older family members and grandchildren, indicating the uptake of these flexibility provisions in the context of population ageing and the need for multi-generation care.

As reported by 83 per cent of survey respondents (Fair Work Commission, 2021b), most requests for flexibility were being acceded to by employers and, where a request was refused, it was common for it to ultimately be granted in some way after negotiation. It appears that flexible work is becoming accepted, with the caveat that it is still seen as 'something for women'.

The report further found that IFAs are not commonly used, although there is evidence of a slight increase in some industries. Where IFAs are used, the evidence indicates that women who seek out an IFA are doing so to meet care responsibilities (for example, by reducing their working hours), in contrast with higher skilled employees, usually men, who are using IFAs to achieve higher wages (Fair Work Commission, 2021a).

Job protection

Employees are protected when taking leave for personal or caring needs by the industrial relations legislation and by national and state anti-discrimination laws. The Fair Work Act prohibits employers from taking adverse action against an employee because of their family or carer responsibilities, age, sex, physical and mental disability, plus some other protected grounds (s.351(1)). Adverse action includes dismissing the employee, changing or 'injuring' their employment and discriminating between that employee and other employees. Penalties of up to AU$66,600 apply for a corporation and AU$13,320 for an individual; for example, an employer was ordered to pay AU$32,131 to an employee denied Personal/Carer's Leave to pick up their child from primary school (Fair Work Commission, 2022).

Two pieces of Commonwealth legislation seek to prevent employers from discriminating against carers either directly or indirectly. The Sex Discrimination Act 1984 (s.7A) makes it illegal for an employer to discriminate based on an employee's family responsibilities and the Disability Discrimination Act 1992 (s.7) makes it illegal for an employer to discriminate against an employee because of their association with someone with a disability. Formal complaints are rare: in 2020–21 only 5 per cent of 479 complaints made to the Australian Human Rights Commission (AHRC) under the Sex Discrimination Act related to family responsibilities, and 2 per cent of 1,006 complaints made under the Disability Discrimination Act related to being a carer or associated with a carer (AHRC, 2020). While this could be taken as evidence that the legislation is working as intended, it is more likely that discrimination occurs in an indirect way. It is well supported in the literature (Adams, 2005; Broderick, 2012) that women are discriminated against based on their carer responsibilities, and this often occurs in an indirect way; for example, requiring all workers to work full time, or be office-based, could indirectly discriminate against carers who need to be at home more because of their caring roles.

State-based provisions such as Victoria's Equal Opportunity Act 2010 (s.19) make it illegal to discriminate against a person because of their carer status. However, discrimination legislation in most states and territories (NSW, Northern Territory, Queensland, South Australia, Tasmania and Western Australia) only confers protection to carers of family members or dependents, or based on family responsibilities, rather than the broader provisions of the Fair Work Act that also recognise care of household (non-family) members.

Income security

Working carers in Australia are eligible for paid leave to provide care for a family/household member but, as noted earlier, it depends on one's employment status. However, evidence at a national and international level indicates that there are income and career penalties for carers (Loretto and Vickerstaff, 2015; Austen and Mavisakalyan, 2018), and that where carer leave provisions or flexible working arrangements are available, they are not always adequate if the care required is ongoing (O'Loughlin, Triandafilidis and Judd-Lam, 2019; Austin and Heyes, 2020).

Income security is of concern for older working carers in Australia, particularly women, as they are more likely to take extended leave or leave paid work to care for a family member(s) (Temple, Dow and Baird, 2019). Additionally, there can be significant out-of-pocket expenses for carers (Duncan et al, 2020), with an Australian survey reporting that financial responsibility for adult children/grandchildren and ageing parents was a major consideration in retirement planning (National Australia Bank, 2014). A study of Australia's baby boomers aged 60–64 years found that the experiences of older working carers are influenced by a person's socioeconomic position, age and gender. Those with caring responsibilities were more likely to be women, in part-time work or not in paid work, and dependent on government income support such as the Age Pension or Carer Payment (O'Loughlin, Loh and Kendig, 2017).

Australian government financial support and other benefits to carers are means tested and available only to those providing 'constant care'. Constant care is defined as personally providing care on a daily basis for a 'significant period' during each day; a significant period is deemed to be at least equivalent to a normal working day (Commonwealth of Australia, 2022). While the statutory rate of carer payments is equivalent to other government pensions, leaving paid employment, whether full-time or part-time, will result in a significant loss of income and in no way compensates for the hours of unpaid care provided. At the structural and policy level, a compelling statistic for Australia is the estimated AU$77.9 billion replacement cost if unpaid care provided by families were to be done by the formal paid care workforce (Deloitte Access Economics, 2020). The same report also calculated the opportunity cost of lost productivity and earnings associated with workers leaving paid work to provide care at an estimated AU$15.2 billion.

COVID-19 pandemic response and implications for employed carers

Australian governments at both national and state level provided significant financial support to businesses and the community during the COVID-19 pandemic (Ramia and Perrone, 2021), with many of the programmes assisting carers. The national government subsidised up to AU$1,500 per fortnight as wage replacement for many employees under the Job Keeper programme that ran from March 2020 to March 2021, tapering off by September 2021 (The Treasury, nd). Childcare centres remained open during the pandemic, particularly for children of essential workers, with the national government subsidising the full cost. Up to AU$750 per week was paid as Pandemic Leave Disaster Payment to workers without sick leave entitlements and those unable to work due to caring for a household member with COVID-19, children, people with a disability and close contacts of persons with COVID-19 (Services Australia, 2022). This leave payment remains, although rules around eligibility have changed with the 'living with the virus' approach.

During the lockdown period (March 2020–November 2021), approximately 40 per cent of workers worked from home (Productivity Commission, 2021). Few workers used the formal right to request flexible work arrangements in the Fair Work Act, relying instead on informal arrangements (Baird et al, 2021). Interviews with employers during this time indicate that the suddenness and necessity of shifting operations to remote working meant many had to act, and worry about the formalities later (Fair Work Commission, 2021b). At the same time, the Fair Work Commission proactively made temporary changes to many modern awards to support flexibility. These changes allowed remote working, unpaid pandemic leave, extended ordinary hours of work and doubled annual leave at half pay. A survey of employer groups and unions indicated that working at a different location was most common, followed by flexible start and finish times (Baird et al, 2021). However, all these formal changes were temporary, and now most awards have reverted to their previous provisions, except for allowing employees with COVID-19 to take unpaid pandemic sick leave.

People working from home and living with care recipients bore the brunt of the pandemic, as not only did they have to deal with additional care responsibilities as schools and care facilities closed, but they also had to contend with employer expectations that productivity would continue at the pre-pandemic level (Craig and Churchill, 2021). Beyond this, carer responsibilities were unequal, as women did most of the care during the pandemic (Johnston et al, 2020), although men did increase carer time (Craig and Churchill 2021). Women were also disproportionately affected by the pandemic itself, as they made up 78 per cent of those employed in caring professions such as nursing and aged care and 55 per cent of workers in the service industries (for example, hospitality, retail).

While flexibility was available, the pandemic exposed the impact of casual and insecure employment in the labour force. During lockdown periods many casual workers lost jobs and income, particularly in industries where working from home was impossible (for example, hospitality, health/social care). While the Job Keeper scheme provided income support, qualifying conditions for casual workers to receive this support differed from permanent employees (for example, only those who had been with an employer for at least 12 months). Data show that in 2021 those employed in part-time, casual positions made up to three-quarters of job losses in the Australian labour force (Stanford, 2021).

Casual workers in service sectors such as aged and disability care were placed under considerable personal and financial stress. These low-paid workers were deemed 'essential workers' during lockdown; however, it came to public attention that the casual and insecure nature of their employment required them to work across multiple care sites for one employer or for multiple employers (Macdonald and Charlesworth, 2021). Because of this, they were considered as spreading the virus both to clients and within their own families (Bessant and Watts, 2021), but without paid leave entitlements they could not afford the time away from work (O'Neil, 2021; Stanford, 2021).

Conclusion

It remains unclear whether the flexibilities obtained both formally and informally during the COVID-19 pandemic will become enshrined in working arrangements. Encouragingly, in interviews conducted with employers and unions in 2021, both groups indicated that they would seek formal changes to retain greater flexibility in working hours (Baird et al, 2021: 54). Productivity reportedly was unaffected by working from home during lockdown (Beck and Hensher, 2022), so employers may be inclined to retain flexible working options. However, an important point is that employers retain the right to direct their employees to return to pre-pandemic working conditions (Baird et al, 2021). While working carers in permanent full-time and part-time employment may have benefited from working from home, particularly in reduced travel time and potentially improved work–life balance, challenges associated with working while providing care remain. Carer support services were severely interrupted during the pandemic, and it is unclear whether these have returned to pre-pandemic levels, particularly with ongoing staff shortages among community and personal care workers (National Skills Commission, 2021).

Moving beyond COVID-19, strengthening carer entitlements from the formal right to *request* flexible working arrangements to the right to be *granted* flexible work arrangements may be what is required to fully normalise combining caring and work. That employers pre-COVID may have refused the very flexible arrangements that suddenly were implemented en masse suggests that refusal of requests may be more about managerial prerogative than business needs. Giving employees the right to challenge the employer's business grounds for refusal (Dayaram et al, 2020) or giving the Fair Work Commission powers to order an employer to agree to their employee's flexibility requests (Temple et al, 2019) have both been suggested as means to provide employees with more control over their flexibility needs.

A further theme in this chapter has been the unequal experiences of men and women with care responsibilities, particularly during the pandemic. Australia has persistent gender norms around unpaid care work which are unlikely to be resolved just by increasing access to flexible working arrangements (Foley and Cooper, 2021). Wider influences are at play; free childcare, available during the pandemic, is once again the responsibility of individual families and women have further to recover from higher COVID-induced unemployment rates in feminised industries (Craig and Churchill, 2021). Policy makers will need to carefully unpick these strands of influence so as not to further entrench gendered paid and unpaid carer roles.

While the pandemic exposed inequities and pressures on casual and insecure workers with care responsibilities, the duality of the Australian labour market for these workers and other employees covered by the industrial relations system is unlikely to change without government intervention. The centre-left Australian Labor Party, elected in 2022, introduced key amendments to the Fair Work Act that strengthen the right to request flexible working arrangements to assist eligible employees to negotiate workplace flexibilities that suit both them and their employer (Commonwealth of Australia, 2023a). These amendments came into effect on 6 June 2023.

The current national government also established a Senate (Upper House) Select Committee on Work and Care to inquire into the impact combining work and care responsibilities has on the well-being of workers, carers and those they care for. The Committee's Report (Commonwealth of Australia, 2023b) was released in March 2023 and addressed all forms of care required across the lifecourse and the work undertaken by carers (unpaid, paid). It contained a total of 33 recommendations and while it is too early to consider how these recommendations may translate to policy reforms, the report clearly stated that the government needs to take a comprehensive and integrated approach to addressing the challenges of work and care. Some of the recommendations of relevance to the issues covered in this chapter include: recognising the social and economic value of care and carers and reviewing the level of Carer Payment and Carer Allowance; requesting the Fair Work Commission to review access to and compensation for paid, sick and annual leave for casual and part-time workers; and introducing an updated social contract around work and care that enshrines a right to care alongside a right to paid work (Commonwealth of Australia, 2023b).

Note
[1] The definition of a carer used in the Survey of Disability, Ageing and Carers: 'A carer is defined as a person who provides any informal assistance, in terms of help or supervision, to people with disability or older people (aged 65 years and over). Assistance must be ongoing, or likely to be ongoing, for at least six months.'

References
Adams, K.L. (2005) 'Indirect discrimination and the worker-carer: it's just not working', *Law in Context*, 23(1): 23–44.

Austen, S. and Mavisakalyan, A. (2018) 'Gender gaps in long-term earnings and retirement wealth: the effects of education and parenthood', *Journal of Industrial Relations*, 60(4): 492–516.

Austin, A. and Heyes, J. (2020) *Supporting working carers: How employers and employees can benefit*, Research report CIPD/University of Sheffield.

Australian Bureau of Statistics (ABS) (2018) 'Disability, ageing and carers, Australia: summary of findings'. Available from: https://www.abs.gov.au/statistics/health/disability/disability-ageing-and-carers-australia-summary-findings/latest-release [Accessed 26 January 2024].

ABS (2020) 'Disability, ageing and carers, Australia: summary of findings'. Available from: https://www.abs.gov.au/statistics/health/disability/disability-ageing-and-carers-australia-summary-findings/latest-release [Accessed 17 November 2023].

ABS (2021) 'Characteristics of employment, Australia'. Available from: https://www.abs.gov.au/statistics/labour/earnings-and-working-conditions/characteristics-employment-australia/latest-release [Accessed 26 January 2024].

ABS (2022) 'Labour force, Australia: February 2022'. Available from: https://www.abs.gov.au/statistics/labour/employment-and-unemployment/labour-force-australia/latest-release [Accessed 23 March 2022].

Australian Human Rights Commission (AHRC) (2020) '2019–20 Complaint statistics'. Available from: https://humanrights.gov.au/sites/default/files/2020-10/AHRC_AR_2019-20_Complaint_Stats_FINAL.pdf [Accessed 18 April 2022].

Australian Institute of Family Studies (May 2023) 'Employment of men and women across the lifecourse'. Available from: https://aifs.gov.au/research/facts-and-figures/employment-men-and-women-across-life-course [Accessed 20 October 2023].

Australian Institute of Health and Welfare (2020) 'Profile of Indigenous Australians'. Australia's health 2020 snapshots. Australia's Health Series No. 17. AIHW, Canberra. Available from: https://www.aihw.gov.au/reports/australias-health/profile-of-indigenous-australians [Accessed 24 July 2020].

Australian Public Service Commission [APSC] (2018) 'APSC enterprise agreement 2018–21'.

Baird, M., Hamilton, M., Gulesserian, L., Williams, A. and Parker, S. (2021) *An employer lens on COVID-19: Adapting to change in Australian workplaces*, Sydney: Centre of Excellence on Population & Ageing Research.

Beck, M.J. and Hensher, D.A. (2022) 'Australia 6 months after COVID-19 restrictions part 2: The impact of working from home', *Transport Policy*, 128: 274–85.

Bessant, J. and Watts, R. (2021) 'COVID, capital, and the future of work in Australia', *AQ: Australian Quarterly*, 92(1): 20–8.

Broderick, E. (2012) 'Women in the workforce', *Australian Economic Review*, 45(2): 204–10.

Carers Australia (n.d.) 'Our History'. Available from: https://www.carersaustralia.com.au/about-us/our-history/ [Accessed 26 January 2024].

Carer Gateway (n.d.) Available from: https://www.carergateway.gov.au [Accessed 1 October 2022].

Chapman, A. (2009) 'Employment entitlements to carer's leave domesticating diverse subjectivities', *Griffith Law Review*, 18(2): 453–74.

Cheng, Z., Jepsen, D.M. and Wang, B.Z. (2020) 'A dynamic analysis of informal elder caregiving and employee wellbeing', *Journal of Business and Psychology*, 35: 85–98

Chomik, R., Williams, A. and Baird, M. (2019) *Legal protections for mature workers*. Available from: https://cepar.edu.au/sites/default/files/cepar-fact-sheet-legal-protections-for-mature-workers.pdf [Accessed 26 January 2024].

Commonwealth of Australia (2010) 'Carer Recognition Act 2010'. Canberra: Australian Government.

Commonwealth of Australia (2021) '2021 Intergenerational Report – Australia over the next 40 years'. Canberra: Australian Government.

Commonwealth of Australia (2022) 'Social Security Guide Version 1.299'. Australian Government, Canberra. Available from: https://guides.dss.gov.au/social-security-guide/1/1/c/310 [Accessed 1 October 2022].

Commonwealth of Australia (2023a) 'The Fair Work Legislation Amendment (Secure Jobs, Better Pay) Act 2022'. Department of Employment and Workplace Relations, Canberra.

Commonwealth of Australia (2023b) 'The Senate Select Committee on Work and Care Final Report'. Available from: https://parlinfo.aph.gov.au/parlInfo/download/committees/reportsen/024994/toc_pdf/FinalReport.pdf;fileType=application%2Fpdf [Accessed 26 January 2024].

Craig, L. and Churchill, B. (2021) 'Working and caring at home: gender differences in the effects of Covid-19 on paid and unpaid labor in Australia', *Feminist Economics*, 27(1–2): 310–26.

Dayaram, K., Fitzgerald, S. and McKenna, S. (2020) 'Working from home remains a select privilege: it's time to fix our national employment standards', *The Conversation*. Available from: https://theconversation.com/working-from-home-remains-a-select-privilege-its-time-to-fix-our-national-employment-standards-139472 [Accessed 26 January 2024].

Deloitte Access Economics (2020) 'The value of informal care in 2020', report commissioned by Carers Australia. Available from: https://www2.deloitte.com/au/en/pages/economics/articles/value-of-informal-care-2020.html [Accessed 26 January 2024].

Duncan, K., Shooshtari, S., Kerstin, R., Fast, J. and Han, J. (2020) 'The cost of caring: out-of-pocket expenditures and financial hardship among Canadian carers', *International Journal of Care and Caring*, 4(2): 141–66.

Fair Work Act (2009: 28) Available at: https://www.legislation.gov.au/
C2009A00028/2017-09-20/text [accessed 3 April 2024].

Fair Work Commission (2018) 'Family Friendly Working Arrangements
[2018] FWCFB 5753', Canberra: Commonwealth of Australia.

Fair Work Commission (2021a) 'General Manager's report into individual
flexibility arrangements under s.653 of the Fair Work Act 2009 (Cth): 2015–
18', Canberra: Commonwealth of Australia.

Fair Work Commission (2021b) 'General Manager's report into the
operation of the provisions of the National Employment Standards relating
to requests for flexible working arrangements and extensions of unpaid
parental leave under s.653 of the Fair Work Act 2009 (Cth): 2015–18',
Canberra: Commonwealth of Australia.

Fair Work Commission (2022) 'General protections benchbook',
Canberra: Commonwealth of Australia.

Fair Work Ombudsman (2019) 'Flexible working arrangements',
Canberra: Fair Work Ombudsman.

Fenna, A. (2012) 'The character of Australian nationalism', *eJournal of Tax
Research*, 10(1): 12–20.

Fine, M. and Davidson, B. (2018) 'The marketization of care: Global challenges
and national responses in Australia', *Current Sociology*, 66(4): 503–16.

Foley, M. and Cooper, R. (2021) 'Workplace gender equality in the post-
pandemic era: Where to next?' *Journal of Industrial Relations*, 63(4): 463–76.

Gilfillan, G. (2021) 'Recent and long-term trends in the use of casual
employment', *Parliamentary Library*, Canberra. Available from: https://
www.aph.gov.au/About_Parliament/Parliamentary_Departments/Parlia
mentary_Library/pubs/rp/rp2122/TrendsCasualEmployment [Accessed
26 January 2024].

Henderson, T. (2016) *Hard to get away. Is the paid holiday under threat in
Australia?* Briefing Paper, Centre for Future Work at The Australia Institute.

Johnston, R.M., Mohammed, A. and Van Der Linden, C. (2020) 'Evidence
of exacerbated gender inequality in child care obligations in Canada
and Australia during the COVID-19 pandemic', *Politics & Gender*,
16(4): 1131–41.

International Labour Organization (1985) *ILO's Convention on Workers with
Family Responsibilities Convention, 1981 (C156).* Available from: https://
www.ilo.org/century/history/iloandyou/WCMS_213324/lang--en/
index.htm [Accessed 29 November 2023].

Kendig, H. and Lucas, N. (2014) 'Individuals, families and the state: changing
responsibilities in an aging Australia', in A. Torres and L. Samson (eds), *Aging
in Asia-Pacific: Balancing the state and the family*, Quezon City: Philippine
Social Science Center, pp 211–24.

Koutsogeorgopoulou, V. and Tuske, A. (2015) *National-state relations in Australia*, OECD Economics Department Working Papers, No. 1198, OECD Publishing, Paris.

Liberal Party of Australia (2020) *Greater certainty for casuals and small business.* Available from: https://www.liberal.org.au/latest-news/2021/03/18/grea ter-certainty-casuals-and-small-business [Accessed 11 May 2022].

Loretto, W. and Vickerstaff, S. (2015) 'Gender, age and flexible working in later life', *Work, Employment and Society*, 29(2): 1–17.

Macdonald, F. and Charlesworth, S. (2021) 'Regulating for gender-equitable decent work in social and community services: bringing the state back in', *Journal of Industrial Relations*, 63(4): 477–500.

National Australia Bank (2014) 'MLC quarterly Australian wealth sentiment survey, Q2 2014'. Available from: http://business.nab.com.au/wp-cont ent/uploads/2014/08/MLC-Quarterly-Australian-Wealth-Sentiment-Sur vey-Q2-2014-PDF-301KB.pdf [Accessed 1 October 2022].

National Skills Commission (2021) 'Skills priority list'. Available from: https://labourmarketinsights.gov.au/our-research/skills-priority-list/ [Accessed 11 May 2022].

O'Loughlin, K., Barrie, H. and Kendig, H. (2018) 'Australia's baby boomers as the future older generation', in M. Higo, N. Dhirathi and T. Klassen (eds), *Ageing and old-age in Asia-Pacific,* Routledge, chapter 14.

O'Loughlin, K., Loh, V. and Kendig, H. (2017) 'Carer characteristics and health, wellbeing and employment outcomes of older Australian baby boomers', *Journal of Cross-Cultural Gerontology*, 32(3): 339–56.

O'Loughlin, K., Triandafilidis, Z. and Judd-Lam, S. (2019) 'How flexible is flexible? Australia's flexible work policies to support working carers', Paper presented in symposium 'Innovation for sustainable care: International perspectives from industry and practice', Transforming Care Conference, Copenhagen, 24–26 June. Available from: http://www.transforming-care. net/symposium-2-innovation-for-sustainable-care-international-perspecti ves-from-industry-and-practice/ [Accessed 26 January 2024].

O'Neil, M. (2021) 'The Australian industrial system in the era of COVID-19', *Journal of Industrial Relations*, 63(3): 422–31.

Organisation for Economic Co-operation and Development (OECD) (2021a) 'Economic Survey of Australia (September 2021)', Paris: OECD Publishing. Available from: https://www.oecd.org/economy/australia-economic-snapshot/ [Accessed 25 March 2022].

OECD (2021b) 'Health at a GLANCE 2021: OECD indicators', Paris: OECD Publishing. Available from: https://www.oecd-ilibrary.org/ social-issues-migration-health/health-at-a-glance-2021_ae3016b9-en [Accessed 30 March 2022].

OECD (2022) 'Life expectancy at birth (indicator)', Paris: OECD Publishing. Available from: https://www.oecd-ilibrary.org/social-issues-migration-health/life-expectancy-at-birth/indicator/english_27e0fc9d-en [Accessed 30 March 2022].

Productivity Commission (2015) 'Review of the workplace relations system', Vol. 1, p 519.

Productivity Commission (2021) 'Working from home', Research Paper, Canberra.

Ramia, G. and Perrone, L. (2021) 'Crisis management, policy reform, and institutions: the social policy response to COVID-19 in Australia', *Social Policy and Society*, THEMED SECTION: Social Policy Responses and Institutional Reforms in the Pandemic, 22(3): 562–76.

Reserve Bank of Australia (2023) 'Composition of the Australian Economy 5 October 2023'. Available from: https://www.rba.gov.au/snapshots/economy-composition-snapshot/pdf/economy-composition-snapshot.pdf?v=2023-10-29-15-19-26 [Accessed 20 October 2023].

Services Australia (2022) 'Pandemic leave disaster payment.' Available from: https://www.servicesaustralia.gov.au/pandemic-leave-disaster-payment [Accessed 2 May 2022].

Sila, U. and Dugain, V. (2019) 'Income, wealth and earnings inequality in Australia: evidence from the HILDA survey', OECD Economics Department Working Papers, No. 1538, Paris: OECD Publishing. Available from: https://www.oecd-ilibrary.org/economics/income-wealth-and-earnings-inequality-in-australia_cab6789d-en [Accessed 26 January 2024].

South Australian Office of the Commissioner for Public Sector Employment (2022) 'Determination 3.1: Employment Conditions – Hours of Work, Overtime and Leave'. Available from: https://www.publicsector.sa.gov.au/hr-and-policy/Determinations,-Premiers-Directions-and-Guidelines/Determinations/Source/20230426-Determination-3.1-Employment-Conditions-Hours-of-Work,-Overtime-and-Leave.pdf [Accessed 24 January 2024].

Stanford, J. (2021) *Shock troops of the pandemic: Casual and insecure work in COVID and beyond*, Centre for Future Work, The Australia Institute. Available from: https://australiainstitute.org.au/wp-content/uploads/2021/10/Shock-Troops-of-the-Pandemic.pdf [Accessed 26 January 2024].

Temple, J., Dow, B. and Baird, M. (2019) 'Special working arrangements to allow for care responsibilities in Australia: availability, usage and barriers', *Australian Population Studies*, 3(1): 13–29.

The Treasury (undated) 'JobKeeper payment'. Available from: https://treasury.gov.au/coronavirus/jobkeeper [Accessed 20 May 2022].

Victorian Equal Opportunity and Human Rights Commission (undated) 'Parent and carer status.' Available from: https://www.humanrights.vic.gov.au/for-individuals/parent-and-carer-status/ [Accessed 18 April 2022].

Williamson, S. and Pearce, A. (2022) 'COVID-normal workplaces: should working from home be a "collective flexibility"?' *Journal of Industrial Relations*, 64(3): 461–73.

Workplace Gender Equality Agency (2021) 'Flexible work post-COVID', Canberra: Australian Government. Available from: https://www.wgea.gov.au/publications/flexible-work-post-covid [Accessed 28 March 2022].

Workplace Gender Equality Agency (2022) 'Gender equality workplace statistics at a glance 2022', Canberra: Australian Government. Available from: https://www.wgea.gov.au/publications/gender-equality-workplace-statistics-at-a-glance-2022 [Accessed 28 March 2022].

Yeandle, S. (2016) 'Caring for our carers: an international perspective on policy developments in the UK', *Juncture*, 23: 57–62.

Yeandle, S., Kröger, T. and Cass, B. (2012) 'Voice and choice for users and carers? Developments in patterns of care for older people in Australia, England and Finland', *Journal of European Social Policy*, 22(4): 432–45.

5

United Kingdom

Kate Hamblin, Jason Heyes and Camille Allard

Introduction

Managing paid work and care has become an increasingly prominent policy issue in the United Kingdom (UK) and the importance of providing adequate forms of support for working carers has been highlighted as being of critical importance in this regard. Since the 1980s, carers' organisations, trade unions and some employers have sought to build support for interventions to assist working carers (Yeandle and Buckner, 2017). The UK's policy approach to supporting work–care reconciliation has largely focused on flexible work practices, in addition to some rights related to unpaid time off for care emergencies. However, carers' organisations, such as Carers UK,[1] have emphasised that provision of publicly funded care services has been rolled back and families have come under increased pressure to '"fill the care gap", either providing care themselves or sourcing and coordinating care for their relative, often at a distance' (Starr and Szebehely, 2017: 116). Indeed, Lloyd (2023) highlights that social care is on the periphery in terms of policy prioritisation in the UK and therefore most susceptible to neglect and cuts in investment.

The pressures and stress associated with attempting to combine paid employment and care provision can lead to working carers reducing their hours of paid work or leaving employment altogether. Carers UK reports that, on average, 600 people a day leave their jobs to care (Carers UK, 2019), and that three-quarters of carers in employment worry about their ability to continue balancing work and care (Carers UK, 2022). These issues have been the focus of political attention, with inquiries such as the recent House of Lords Adult Social Care Committee inquiry highlighting that the UK 'lags behind established practice in other comparable economies' (Yeandle, in House of Lords Adult Social Care Committee, 2022: 109) with regards to carers leave specifically (although, as will be explained, this situation has very recently changed). This chapter examines the extent and impact of measures to support working carers in the UK, situating the policy approach within the wider political, economic and social policy context. The chapter is organised as follows. The next section provides an overview of the national context within which demands for support for working carers have been articulated. This is followed by a section charting the development of policies and employer practices to support working carers, focusing on the period following the election of the New Labour government in 1997. The adequacy of the support available to working carers, and the impact of the COVID-19 pandemic, are then discussed in the two following sections. The chapter concludes with an assessment of progress to date and some thoughts regarding prospects for strengthening support.

National context

This section outlines the political, economic and social context in the UK, which provides a backdrop to the leave and associated policies for carers currently in place.

Political context

In exploring issues related to carers leave, we examine the intersection between employment legislation and statutory care entitlements, as the former governs the protection and support carers receive in work while the latter influence the level of care provided by family members, friends and neighbours. To reflect on the policy context in terms of statutory care provision, in the UK 'adult social care' (ASC) as a distinct field of social policy was created relatively recently in 2005, when children's and adult's services were formally separated within local government (Gray and Birrell, 2013; Hall et al, 2020). Statutory responsibility for ASC policy is 'devolved' to the national administrations of the four UK nations and, in turn, the delivery of ASC services themselves is the responsibility of individual local authorities (152 in England and 22 Wales), councils (32 in Scotland) or 'health and social care trusts' (five in Northern Ireland) (Gray and Birrell, 2013). The UK nations operate different ASC assessment systems, but all use a financial means and a needs test, with those who have assets and savings above set thresholds paying for all or some of their care.

The financial sustainability of ASC in the four nations has been a topic of debate, and the sector is often described as being in 'crisis' (Dayan and Heenan, 2019; Clifton, 2021; Glasby, 2021; Needham and Hall, 2023). The demographic changes described later and the reduction in spending in real terms on ASC have resulted in systems across the four nations where care and support are 'rationed ... [and] quality and consistency of services has suffered acutely as local authorities have raised the threshold to receive support' (House of Lords Adult Social Care Committee, 2022: 15).

The lack of state care entitlements has been argued to have 'forced other solutions on UK families. Among middle-income families there is now extensive use of private and often informal solutions to the burden of housework' (Yeandle, 1999: 102). In the literature on 'care regimes', the UK has been treated as an example of a liberal model of care (O'Connor, Orloff and Shaver, 1999), with a familialistic approach that exhibits minimal state intervention and extensive privatisation and marketisation of care provision services. Estimates indicate the value of care provided by carers in England and Wales exceeds the annual expenditure on the National Health Service (£162 billion versus £156 billion, Petrillo and Bennett, 2023). For Yeandle (1999), the absence of state-provided care meant that the UK became a 'dual-earner/marketised-female-domestic-economy' model, where families are polarised according to whether they can afford to purchase care services and assistance. In addition, the onus on purchasing care in the market results in an increasing demand for female domestic workers, whose jobs tend to be poorly paid and insecure (International Labour Organization [ILO], 2021).

While care as a policy area is devolved to the four nations of the UK in terms of legislation and administration, employment law is not, and Parliament is the main legislative body with jurisdiction over this area (the exception being Northern Ireland). Various stakeholder groups have sought to influence policy and practice related to working carers, through research, policy papers, lobbying members of both the House of Commons and the House of Lords and contributing to public inquiries or consultations. The carers' movement in the UK has been highly important in drawing the attention of policy makers to the needs of carers. Carers' representative organisations have provided a 'collective voice' for carers for many years (Yeandle et al, 2012) and have been described as 'instrumental in demanding and shaping' (Larkin and Milne, 2014: 29) policies such as the Carers (Recognition and Services) Act (HM Government, 1995) and cross-government Carers Strategies (see later). The UK carers' movement began with the creation of the National Council for the Single Woman and her Dependents in 1965, later shifting in focus to include a diverse range of caring experiences and situations. This organisation became today's Carers UK, which continues to have a key role in lobbying government regarding issues related to carers, as well as offering practical support and advice. Alongside other national carers' organisations (Crossroads Caring for Carers and the Princess Royal Trust for Carers [merged into the Carers Trust], Contact a Family), Carers UK has raised the profile of care and caring, and pressed for the 'right to a life outside caring', including paid employment (Yeandle and Buckner, 2017: 8).[2] Trade unions have also engaged with policy debates related to unpaid carers and employment, including recent discussions regarding legislated leave arrangements (NASUWT, 2020; TUC, 2020), as well as shaping enterprise-level arrangements (UNISON, 2021).

Economic context

The economy of the UK – the sixth-largest in the world – is dominated by the service sector, comprising 82 per cent of its gross domestic product (GDP) (Booth, 2021). Its model of economic growth is highly reliant on finance capital and private consumption fuelled by household debt (Heyes, Lewis and Clark, 2012; Reisenbichler and Wiedemann, 2022). The UK has also experienced persistently weak productivity growth relative to other advanced economies (Van Ark and Venables, 2020).

The UK's employment and welfare models have variously been described as an example of a 'market regime' (Gallie, 2009), a 'liberal welfare state' (Esping-Andersen, 1990, 1999) or a 'liberal market economy' (Hall and Soskice, 2001). These labels highlight essential features of the UK's labour market institutions and approach to employment rights and social protections. They denote a system in which trade unions have relatively little labour market power or involvement in decision making within enterprises, opportunities for social dialogue are extremely restricted and policy makers' concerns with preserving labour market 'flexibility' restrict the progress of employment rights. In addition, social protections are relatively weak, particularly for vulnerable groups, with modest and often means-tested state benefits and strict eligibility rules.

Price (2006) argues that the UK also adheres to a 'male breadwinner/female part-time care' model of welfare, with women combining paid part-time work and care in practice because policy reinforces this division. Thirty-eight per cent of women in employment worked part-time, as compared to 13 per cent of men, in 2022 (Irvine et al, 2023). Women's disproportionate involvement in part-time employment relative to men reflects the domestic division of labour, in which women typically continue to perform a larger amount of unpaid domestic work than men, even when both men and women living in the same household work full time (Zamberlan et al, 2021). Gender differences in this regard became even more pronounced during the COVID-19 pandemic (Zamberlan et al, 2021; Andrew et al, 2022). A lack of affordable childcare provision also serves to restrict the options of mothers when it comes to decisions relating to their labour market participation.

Women are most commonly employed in health and social care (21 per cent of all jobs held by women), wholesale and retail (13 per cent) and education (12 per cent in 2022) (Irvine et al, 2023). The gender pay gap between men and women was 14.9 per cent in 2022 for all employees, but when part- and full-time work are considered, women were paid 2.8 per cent more than men in part-time work and 8.3 per cent less in full-time work.[3] The gap in employment rates between the genders is closing, with 79 per cent of men employed in 2022, as compared to 72.3 per cent of women (Irvine et al, 2023).

Social context

In 2020, there were 67 million people living in the UK (56.5 million in England, 3.1 million in Wales, 5.5 million in Scotland and 1.9 million in Northern Ireland) (Office for National Statistics [ONS], 2022). The UK's population is increasing, its growth driven by migration and increased longevity (ONS, 2021). Though migration levels have remained stable since 2016, there has been a change in migration patterns as net migration from European Union (EU) countries has decreased since 2015, while non-EU net migration has increased since 2013 (ONS, 2021).

Population ageing has implications for the supply of, and demand for, care. In the UK, people aged 65 years and over are the fastest-growing age group in the population; over the next 50 years, it is projected that there will be an additional 7.5 million people in this age category (ONS, 2021). Though life expectancy at birth has increased in recent years, progress related to healthy and disability-free life expectancy has been more modest (Jagger, 2015). This has implications for the demand for care, as when increases in HLE do not rise at the same rate as life expectancy, periods of ill-health at the end of life are extended. Older people are also more likely than younger age groups to experience certain long-term conditions and disabilities (for example, diabetes, arthritis, congestive heart failure, dementia) (Guzman-Castillo et al, 2017).

Coinciding with these changes in demand for care and support, the total fertility rate per woman in 2021 was 1.63, below the population replacement rate of 2.1 children per female (ONS, 2021). This creates an imbalance between older and younger populations which has significant implications for care provision and demand. The 2021 Census indicated there are five million people in England and Wales providing unpaid care (Petrillo and Bennett, 2023). There is significant churn in the population that are unpaid carers: every year in the period 2010–20, 4.3 million people moved into an unpaid caring role in the UK – 12,000 people a day (Petrillo et al, 2022). During this period, more than 1.9 million people in paid employment became unpaid carers every year (Petrillo et al, 2022).

Carer leave policies

Short-term leave

Care leave policy entered the UK policy discourse in the mid-1990s due to its relevance to the balance between paid work and family life, a key concern for the Labour government that came to power in 1997. This 'family-friendly' agenda – highlighted in Tony Blair's first speech as Prime Minister and in the 1998 White Paper 'Fairness at Work' (Department of Trade and Industry, 1998) – focused on parents and involved the introduction of parental leave and an expansion of childcare provision. At this point, the policy focus did not include those caring for other family members. In response, the UK carers' movement launched a series of media campaigns, as well as lobbying policy makers to raise the profile of carers (Bytheway and Johnson, 1998).

Their lobbying and campaigning for a national carers' strategy met with some success when, in 1999, *Caring about Carers: A National Strategy for Carers* (Department of Health [DH], 1999) was launched (Yeandle, 2016). This strategy was argued to embody 'the principles of choice, consumer control, access to paid work and social inclusion, the hallmarks of the New Labour approach to welfare' (Lloyd, 2000: 136–7). Organisations representing carers were actively involved in the consultation process leading up to the strategy and 'their influence is evident in the range of issues addressed and the strategic response proposed' (Lloyd, 2000: 136). The strategy outlined the 'business case' for policies to support people to combine work and care, citing reduced absence and employee turnover and better staff morale. Equivalent strategies were introduced in Scotland (1999) and Wales (2000), reflecting the increased awareness on the part of the UK Government and devolved administrations of the importance of carers and their needs (Yeandle and Buckner, 2007). According to Lloyd (2000: 148), the introduction of these strategies also provided a 'major boost to carers' organisations whose position in the policy process [was] reinforced, expanded and increasingly influential.'

Also introduced in 1999, the Employment Relations Act provided employees with the right to a 'reasonable' (but unspecified) amount of unpaid leave to take 'necessary' action to deal with emergency situations involving their dependents (not limited to children). This Act states that:

> [a]n employee is entitled to be permitted by his employer to take a reasonable amount of time off during the employee's working hours, where it is reasonable for him to do so, in order to deal with a domestic incident, with 'domestic incident' referring to an event which (a) occurs in the home of the employee, or (b) affects a member of the employee's family or a person who relies on the employee for assistance. (Employment Relations Act 1999, Part II, Schedule 4, section 57A)

The unpaid time off can be:

a. 'to provide assistance on an occasion when a dependent falls ill, gives birth or is injured or assaulted,
b. to make arrangements for the provision of care for a dependent who is ill or injured,
c. in consequence of the death of a dependent,
d. because of the unexpected disruption or termination of arrangements for the care of a dependent, or

e. to deal with an incident which involves a child of the employee and which occurs unexpectedly in a period during which an educational establishment which the child attends is responsible for him'.

'A dependent' refers to 'a spouse, a child, a parent, a person who lives in the same household as the employee, otherwise than by reason of being his employee, tenant, lodger or boarder' (Employment Relations Act, Part II, Schedule 4, section 57). The Act also includes provisions to protect employees from dismissal for responding to an emergency related to someone they care for.

The carers' movement continued to campaign for a right to paid care leave and Carers UK gave evidence on this subject to the government's Cross-Government Action Plan on Carers (Department of Health and Social Care, 2018), the Independent Review of the State Pension Age (Cridland, 2017), the government's Industrial Strategy (BEIS, Department of Business, Energy and Industrial Strategy, 2017) and a Select Committee inquiry into support for working carers (House of Commons Work and Pensions Committee, 2008). Reform related to care leave was attempted in 2016 with a Private Members' Bill (introduced by Baroness Tyler of Enfield, Liberal Democrat), 'the Carers (Leave entitlement) Bill',[4] which had its first reading in the House of Lords.[5] This Bill aimed to amend the Employment Rights Act 1996 to provide more specificity around the duration of leave (including a maximum period and allowances for a single period or a series of leave periods), what constitutes caring activities and to make the leave paid. The Bill did not, however, progress beyond the House of Lords.

A subsequent opportunity to secure a specified period of care leave for working carers in the UK was missed due to the country's exit from the European Union (EU). Through membership of Eurocarers, Carers UK played a role in shaping the EU Work–life Balance Directive (2019/1158), approved on 4 April 2019 (European Parliament, 2019), which included the right for all carers to take five days of leave per year. Opposition from several EU member states resulted in the removal of a proposal that the leave period be paid at the level of national statutory sickness benefits. With the UK's Brexit from the EU, this Directive was not applicable to the UK. However, former Prime Minister Theresa May, who had been Minister of Women and Equalities from 2010 to 2012, stated that, as part of the EU-UK Withdrawal Agreement, she planned to implement parallel UK legislation. Her successor as Prime Minister, Boris Johnson, subsequently stated that mirroring newer EU directives was not a priority (de la Porte, Larsen and Szelewa, 2020).

Current and previous Conservative governments, however, stated that they aimed to introduce five days unpaid carers leave, including it as a manifesto pledge in the 2019 election (The Conservative Party, 2019), and this commitment was also included in the Queen's Speech of that year. In March 2020, the government initiated a consultation on carers leave, which was extended due to the COVID-19 pandemic (BEIS, 2020), with scope for leave entitlement to be included in an anticipated Employment Bill. The consultation was welcomed by both Carers UK (2020a) and trade unions, although they expressed concern that the UK might fall behind other European countries if legislation did not introduce more generous care leave policy in line with the EU Work–life Balance Directive (TUC, 2021). Both Carers UK (2020b) and the UK Trades Union Congress (TUC, 2020) responded to the consultation, indicating their support for paid care leave.

In May 2021, Conservative MP Jack Brereton introduced a Private Member's Bill, the Employment (Caring Leave) Bill, which included the right to five days' unpaid leave for carers. This Bill did not receive a second reading. In September of the same year, the Conservative government restated its intention to introduce an entitlement to one week of unpaid care leave, which could be used flexibly (BEIS, 2021), but the Employment Bill was not included in the 2022 Queen's Speech announcing Parliament's new legislative programme.

In June 2022, Scottish Liberal Democrat MP Wendy Chamberlain announced her intention to introduce a Private Member's Bill which would include leave for carers to be debated in November 2022 (Redpath, 2022). This Bill, the Carers Leave Bill, had its first reading on 15 June 2022 and passed its second reading on 21 October that year. On 2 November 2022, it completed its committee stage with no amendments, with MPs from both sides of the House speaking in favour and no opposition raised. The Bill included carers leave as a 'day one' right for all employees with no qualifying period and applicable to 'anyone caring for a spouse, civil partner, child, parent or other dependent who needs care because of a disability, old age or any illness or injury likely to require at least three months of care' (Brione, 2023: 5). The proposal was that the leave would be unpaid and the duration would be set by regulations, with a minimum of one week per year (that is, five working days for full-time employees and pro rata for part-time employees). The Bill would be applicable to England, Scotland and Wales but not Northern Ireland, where employment law is devolved. On 19 May 2023, the Bill was successful at its third reading in the Lords, thereby finishing its passage through the UK Parliament. It received Royal Assent on 24 May 2023, alongside other Acts related to issues of care – the Neonatal Care (Leave and Pay) Act and Protection from Redundancy (Pregnancy and Family Leave) Act. Acts either come into operation within a set period after Royal Assent (typically two months later) or at a time fixed by the government. It is anticipated the Carer's Leave Act will come into effect in 2024.

Table 5.1 summarises the carer leaves available in the UK.

Table 5.1: Carer leave schemes, UK (November 2023)

Leave details				Eligibility		Person needing care	Evidence	Notice period and process
Leave name and introduced	Time period	Compensation		Worker/employee status	Qualifying period			
Emergency leave, 1999	Unspecified but short term	Unpaid		Employees, not casual workers	–	A 'dependant' (spouse, partner, child, grandchild, parent, or someone who depends on person for care)	Not required	Not required – cannot be applied for in advance
Carers' Leave, 2023[a]	5 days	Unpaid		Employees, not causal workers	None – 'day one' right	Family member, a loved one or anyone if they 'reasonably rely on the employee to provide or arrange care'[b]	Not required	Twice the length of time being requested as leave + one day

Notes: [a] Not enacted as of November 2023.

[b] Carer's Leave Act 2023, chapter 18.

Other support measures

Flexible working

From 2000, the policy discourse shifted away from 'family-friendly' policies to the promotion of 'work–life balance' (Lewis and Campbell, 2007) with the launch of the Department for Education and Employment's (DfEE) policy document *Work Life Balance: Changing Patterns in a Changing World* (DfEE, 2000). The conception of policies for the reconciliation of work and life as simply a concern of families, and therefore primarily women, was expanded to include men and leisure time (Lewis and Campbell, 2007). The emphasis was on persuading employers of the business case for introducing or improving policies that would allow employees to reconcile work and family life. The DfEE outlined changes to working patterns that could support work–life balance, including changes in when employees worked (such as part-time, job sharing, V-time [working part time for certain periods then moving back to regular hours, DfEE, 2000: 15], term-time working, flexitime, compressed working hours, shift-swapping, self-rostering); where they worked (home working) and complete breaks from work (sabbaticals, carers leave, career breaks).

The change in terminology from 'family-friendly' to 'policies for work–life balance' was, as Lewis and Campbell (2007) suggest, connected to New Labour's third major policy initiative in the area: the right for individuals to request flexible working hours, led by the Department of Trade and Industry (DTI). The Flexible Working (Eligibility, Complaints and Remedies) Regulations were introduced in 2002 for people with children under five years of age (or under 18 if the child was disabled) and amended to include carers of dependent adults in the Work and Families Act 2006 (implemented in 2007). The Children and Families Act 2014 extended the request for flexible working to all employees[6] (distinct from workers) who had worked for their employer for at least 26 weeks. The regulations entitled them to make only one request per year (ACAS, 2014)[7] and employers were permitted to refuse their request if they were able to demonstrate a reasonable business case for doing so. The implication of the latter provision was that 'the *expectation* that employers will respond positively to requests for flexible employment patterns does not secure rights for employees' (Lloyd, 2006: 951, original emphasis). The Employment Rights Act (1996) outlined eight grounds upon which the employer could refuse requests:

- Burden of additional costs.
- Detrimental effect on ability to meet customer demand.
- Inability to reorganise work among existing staff.
- Inability to recruit additional staff.
- Detrimental impact on quality.
- Detrimental impact on performance.

- Insufficiency of work during the periods the employee proposes to work.
- Planned structural changes. (Employment Rights Act, 1996, Section 80[G][1][b])

In June 2022, the Employment Relations (Flexible Working) Bill, another private member's Bill, originated in the House of Commons. It then passed through its first, second and third readings and the committee stage, receiving Royal Assent on 20 July 2023. The Act amends the sections of the Employment Rights Act (1996) related to flexible working and will require employers to consult with employees before rejecting any flexible working requests, increase the number of requests that can be made annually from one to two and curtail the time employers have to consider requests from three months to two. The Act itself does not include the right to request flexible working from day one but it is anticipated this will be introduced as secondary legislation alongside the implementation of the Act in 2024. It is also slightly opaque as to whether the Act will include workers as well as employees; the preamble states it is 'An Act to make provision in relation to the right of employees and other workers to request variations to particular terms and conditions of employment, including working hours, times and locations', but the Act and the Employment Rights Act (1996) which the new legislation amends refer only to the former (House of Commons, 2023).

Equality and anti-discrimination legislation

Progress in terms of protection from discrimination in the workplace was made when the Equality Act 2010 expanded the scope of protection to include carers (in England, Scotland and Wales) through a requirement to 'have due regard' to promoting equality of opportunity for carers. Carers UK (2015), however, has expressed concerns that carers are protected from 'discrimination by association', that is, when a person is treated less favourably because they are linked or associated with a protected characteristic under *the Equality Act 2010*. This means that while carers are protected from direct discrimination and harassment in the UK, they are not protected from indirect discrimination or entitled to 'reasonable adjustment' (House of Lords, 2016).[8] Carers UK proposes the status of carer should become a protected characteristic in its own right, thereby protecting carers from indirect discrimination and enabling them to require 'reasonable adjustment' in the workplace (Carers UK, 2020e).

Carers Allowance

The UK has one benefit provided to carers in the UK which can be combined with a limited amount of paid work (Fry, Price and Yeandle,

2009; Kennedy and Gheera, 2018). Carers Allowance is paid at a lower rate than all other income-replacement benefits in the UK system. This is a reflection of its origins in 1976 as a benefit for those who lacked a social insurance contribution record (House of Commons, 2008, 2022). It was originally referred to as the 'Invalid Care Allowance' and is now called the Carers Allowance, providing a benefit (£69.70 a week for 2022/23) for those caring for at least 35 hours a week for a person in receipt of a disability benefit. Those in work can earn up to £132 a week[9] alongside this benefit after tax, National Insurance and up to 50 per cent of any private or occupational pension contributions and expenses, which can include some of the costs of caring while the claimant is at work. Carers in receipt of certain benefits do not receive a Carers Allowance payment if they receive more than the amount of Carers Allowance from any other benefits, but can still have an 'underlying entitlement', should that benefit be paid at a lower rate than Carers Allowance for any period. In November 2021, 1.3 million people in Great Britain were in receipt of Carers Allowance, of whom 69 per cent were women. Of the 1.3 million Carers Allowance claimants, only 70 per cent were receiving a payment, with 386,600 people barred due to the 'overlapping benefits' rule (including pensions) or other income. Between 2003 and 2021 the number of Carers Allowance claimants more than doubled, from 632,000 to just over 1.3 million (DWP, 2022).

In addition to its very low rate, Carers Allowance has been criticised for having an abrupt employment earnings cut-off, rather than a tapered threshold. For claimants, earning any amount over £132 per week results in withdrawal of the entire allowance (House of Commons, 2008; Fry, Price and Yeandle, 2009; Kennedy and Gheera, 2018; House of Lords Adult Social Care Committee, 2022). The combination of a low level of state support for carers via Carers Allowance and 'the assumption, held by our society and policy makers, that social care happens first and foremost in the family circle' has prompted those engaged in policy making, campaigning groups and sections of the media to draw the conclusion that in the UK, 'the work of unpaid carers is largely invisible, unrecognised and unsupported' (House of Lords Adult Social Care Committee, 2022: 4; see also various discussions in the UK media: Fox-Leonard, 2020; Shereen, 2020; Carers UK, 2020a, 2020b, 2020c, 2020d, 2020e; Dalton, 2022).

Carers Assessment

The Care Act 2014 introduced a new legal entitlement to assessment and public support for carers in England, including support to enable them to remain in or re-enter work, independent of whether or not the person they provide care for has been assessed as having eligible needs. However, in practice local authorities in England have found implementing the Care Act challenging, due to a lack of resources, and data indicate that the number of Carers Assessments and associated provision have declined. In addition, carer-related expenditure following the Care Act has also declined by 6 per cent in cash terms, versus an overall increase for adult social care by 3 per cent by 2017 (Fernandez et al, 2021). Following a Carers Assessment, it is possible for carers to receive a Direct Payment to meet their own assessed needs, but due to modest local authority budgets impacted by austerity cuts (Burstow, 2016), a relatively small number of carers receive this support. In 2021–22, 380,725 carers in England were supported by local authorities or were/had their needs assessed or reviewed, and of that total, 18.8 per cent (71,710 carers) received Direct Payments (NHS Digital, 2022).

Employer-provided carers leave

Improving the working lives of carers has continued to be the focus of the UK carers' movement's lobbying and campaigning. Carers' organisations participated in the task force which shaped the 2008 National Carers Strategy and contributed evidence to a parliamentary enquiry on carers in the same year (House of Commons Work and Pensions Committee, 2008; Clements, 2010; Yeandle et al, 2012). In 2009, Carers UK launched Employers for Carers (EfC), a membership organisation to develop and share good practice among employers, building on an EU-funded project, Action for Carers and Employment (ACE National, 2002–2007). EfC's current (2021) membership of 215 organisations includes large public and private organisations as well as small businesses (Yeandle, 2017: 22). EfC provides its members with forms of support that include advice for employers seeking to develop carer-friendly policies in their workplace, including care leave. An EfC survey (2020)[10] showed that half of employers surveyed said their organisations offered care leave or special leave to carers within their workforce. More than four out of ten employers said that they had introduced additional leave arrangements for carers because of the COVID-19 pandemic. Employer-provided support, such as paid care leave, can be very valuable for working carers' mental and physical health. For example, findings from a survey of working carers in England and Wales[11] showed that mental well-being is higher among organisations that provide support for their employees with care responsibilities (Austin and Heyes, 2020). Implementing support for carers also has benefits for employers. The same survey findings showed, for example, that carers who received support were less likely to consider reducing their hours or quitting their job.

Trade unions are a further potential influence on employers' practices relating to working carers. Women now form the majority of trade union members in the UK (TUC, 2021), and growing membership diversity has also led to enhanced representation of different groups' interests in union governance structures (Parker, 2006: 423). For example, the trade union for public sector workers, UNISON, has been a pioneer in improving the representation of women trade union members' interests. UNISON has published a guideline for its branches on collective bargaining on carers' policies (UNISON, 2019) such as care leave. This guideline was published with the aim of reducing the number of 'cases' requiring union representation, recruiting more members as well as increasing branches' activist base. The guideline on negotiating a paid carer's leave policy included the following points:

(5) 'development of the carer policy in consultation with the trade unions; commitment from the employers;
(ii) clear definition of carer;
(iii) review of the policy on a regular basis and data confidentiality'.

Other trades union initiatives have also been taken to promote the interests of carers at work. For example, as a result of the increase of care responsibilities due to the pandemic, Wales TUC has been calling on employers to do more to support workers with caring responsibilities. It launched a survey of working carers in Wales, with the aim to influence the Welsh Government's actions to support carers and to work directly with employers to improve workplace support (Wales Trade Union Congress Cymru, 2022).

Employer-led policies such as care leave may also be implemented as part of a Diversity and Inclusion (D&I) strategy in workplaces. For some, a D&I approach holds the promise of transformative organisational opportunity, with disadvantage tackled by acknowledging individual differences between employees (Williams, 2014: 124). The D&I perspective has, however, been criticised, as it can result in managers preferring to deal with individual differences on a case-by-case basis, rather than implementing changes in a more standardised way, especially if those changes bear a cost to the business (Williams, 2014; Kirton and Greene, 2015). Hoque and Noon (2004) observe that these practices and policies implemented as part of a D&I approach can become 'empty shells' or 'box ticking' measures. These measures are not always supported in practice or might be restricted to certain groups of employees. In addition, as noted by Williams (2014: 125), there may be limited opportunities for employees to have a say in the development and implementation of such policies and, as a result, policies and practices may not adequately address employees' needs in relation to combining paid work and care.

Despite inclusion in enterprises' D&I strategies, access to support and leave policies is not, however, available to all working carers even when they are employed by an organisation that provides support to carers. Austin and

Figure 5.1: Steps taken to manage care responsibilities and paid work over the past 12 months (per cent)

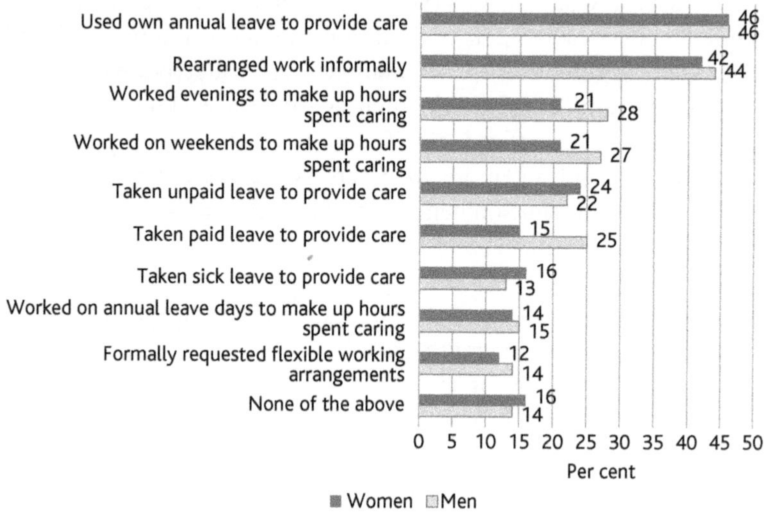

Source: Authors' presentation of data from Austin and Heyes (2020)

Heyes (2020) found that a lack of knowledge about support was a problem affecting 14 per cent of working carers who had not made use of employer-provided support, and there was a difference between men and women, with women being less likely to take paid care leave. Figure 5.1 outlines the differences between the types of support used by men and women from a representative survey of 970 working carers (Austin and Heyes, 2020).

In addition, there are disparities in union membership which in turn have implications for the support available in different sectors for working carers. Although a union agenda focused on care is important, union representation in the UK is far more widespread in the public sector than the private sector. Where private sector collective bargaining does occur, it is predominantly at the level of enterprises and workplaces, as opposed to the sectoral or national levels (Gregory and Milner, 2009). This imbalance in terms of trade union representation might be a factor influencing inequalities in the support available to working carers in the private and public sectors. According to Carers UK (2019), private sector employees are less likely than those in the public and third or voluntary sectors to have options available to them that enable them to reconcile paid work and care responsibilities.

Adequacy of carer leave policies

The UK lacks data on the number and nature of flexible working requests or requests for emergency, unpaid leave as legislated by the Employment

Relations Act; the Carer Leave Act has yet to come into law at the time of writing (November 2023), so its effectiveness remains to be seen. Employers are not required to report formally the use of either flexible working requests or the unpaid care leave introduced by the Employment Rights Act 1996, and again the amendment through the Employment Relations (Flexible Working) Act 2023 has yet to be enacted. However, a survey conducted in England and Wales found that 23 per cent of working carers had taken unpaid leave and 19 per cent had taken paid leave (Austin and Heyes, 2020). Another survey conducted by Carers UK (2014) found that only 12 per cent of working carers had accessed any form of leave for carers and 7 per cent had used 'dependents' leave'. In contrast, 38 per cent had used up annual leave and 22 per cent had used sick leave to provide care.

With regards to flexible working, the Employment Rights Act 1996 has been criticised for introducing a 'weak' right to request flexible work, with employers able to decline for several reasons. A survey by the Trades Union Congress found that one in three requests were turned down (TUC, 2019), with requests more likely to be declined for those in routine or semi-routine occupations, prompting them to state that 'the current law isn't working' (TUC, 2021). A survey of working carers in England conducted more than ten years ago found that only 13 per cent had submitted a flexible working request (Family Friendly Working Hours Taskforce, 2010). At the same time, flexible work can attract carers back into the labour force (Family Friendly Working Hours Taskforce, 2010). One survey found that 21 per cent of working carers had left the labour market because they could not access flexible working arrangements or because of their line manager's attitude (Carers UK, 2014). Carers UK's later research has highlighted that the forms of support that working carers regard as most important in enabling them to remain in employment are flexible working, care leave and a supportive line manager (Carers UK, 2019). Other studies have pointed to the importance of the option to reduce hours of work from full time to part time, job sharing, working from home or tele-work, compressed working weeks and carers' networks/support services (Budd and Mumford, 2006; Hamblin and Hoff, 2011; Schneider et al, 2013; Ireson et al, 2018).

COVID-19 pandemic response and implications for employed carers

The COVID-19 pandemic created significant change, both in terms of the demands upon working carers and the increased prevalence of flexible working arrangements in the UK and across Europe (Phillips et al, 2022). Data indicate that, as care services were paused or overstretched, increasing numbers of people combined work and care in the UK (Carers UK, 2020a, 2020c, 2020d; Muldrew et al, 2022), with women over-represented in the growing population of carers (King et al, 2020; Power, 2020). Carers UK reported that 81 per cent of carers in 2020 were providing more care than before the national 'lockdowns' which they calculated saved the UK state £530 million in care costs per day (Carers UK, 2020c, 2020d). Initially, the UK's policy response to the pandemic centred on the message 'Stay at home. Stay safe. Save lives'. Subsequently it evolved to 'Stay at home. Save the NHS. Save lives', resulting in the closure of day and respite services, the support of which many carers relied on to facilitate their paid employment, with repercussions for their well-being (Giebel et al, 2021a, 2021b; Akafekwa, Dalgarno and Verma, 2021).

The UK Government created the Coronavirus Job Retention Scheme, which included 'furlough'[12] payments from March 2020 until 30 September 2021, which allowed employers to claim the cost of 80 per cent of their employees' wages. Explicit reference in the guidance was made to offering this option to employees who 'have caring responsibilities resulting from coronavirus, such as caring for children who are at home as a result of school and childcare facilities closing or caring for a vulnerable individual in their household'.[13] There are, however no, data on the number of people who were furloughed due to caring responsibilities, or who identified as carers.

While flexible working increased during the pandemic, the extent to which unpaid carers were able to access these arrangements, and whether they were formalised as part of flexible working requests, is as yet unclear (Chartered Institute of Professional Development [CIPD], 2020). A recent paper observed: 'carers have had the chance to "road-test" a range of flexible working arrangements. Attributable to the pandemic, the flexibility of remote working for some has resulted in greater autonomy and increased time with family, which may have alleviated some strains associated with reconciling work with care' (Phillips et al, 2022: 291–2). However, while flexible working arrangements have been reported to be beneficial for carers (Eurocarers, 2017), it is important to examine which specific types have the greatest impact. For example, research in Wales found that the flexibility offered by working from home during the pandemic was welcomed by some carers but was felt to be at the expense of their ability to take time away from caring while at their place of work (Burrows et al, 2021). Phillips et al (2020) highlight that flexibility in terms of working location may not protect working carers from additional strain.

The increase in flexible working during the pandemic was not evenly spread across all sectors or regions of the UK. The CIPD, for example, mapped flexible working 'notspots' across the UK using Labour Force Survey data, where employers were less likely to offer flexibility in terms of working hours and/or location, with the south-east of England assessed as offering the most opportunities for flexible work (CIPD, 2021). ONS data highlight that flexibility regarding working location is occupationally segmented, with only 10 per cent of those employed in the transportation and storage sector and accommodation and food services sector reporting that they had ever been able to work from home, in contrast to half of those working in the telecommunications sector (ONS, 2020). These findings underscore the importance of nuance in considering whether some people are more likely to be excluded from flexibility around working arrangements, and the extent to which working carers are disproportionately affected. While there have been arguments made by trades unions and carers' organisations (BEIS, 2022) for the strengthening of the rights around flexible working, a government consultation concluded that 'legislation should remain a "right to request", not a "right to have"' flexible working arrangements (BEIS, 2021).

Conclusion

This chapter has explored an increasingly pressing issue in the context of population ageing in the UK: the provision of carers leave. The UK has been described as 'lagging behind' other comparable nations in this area (House of Lords Adult Social Care Committee, 2022), despite the campaigning and lobbying efforts of carers' organisations and trades unions. More broadly, the UK's position as a 'liberal' nation in the care regime literature reflects its relatively limited statutory care entitlements for older and disabled adults. In turn, the provision of support for working carers is also modest, reflecting a long-standing assumption that families should, first and foremost, be the providers of care.

Currently (November 2023), the UK legislation covers emergency unpaid leave for carers for an unspecified period and the 'weak' right to request flexible working arrangements which is available to qualifying employees ('workers' do not have access to this right[14]), but the latter may change when the Employment Relations (Flexible Working) Act 2023 becomes law in 2024. The pandemic certainly resulted in renewed calls for a strengthening of the right to flexible work, and while some of the secondary details of the Act have yet to be confirmed, in December 2022 the UK Government announced that the right to request flexible working, which was previously subject to a 26-week qualifying period, would become a day one right. However, they also announced that employers will continue to have the right to decline requests on business grounds. There is, however, evidence that employee expectations have increased in relation to flexible work, with half of employers surveyed by Advisory, Conciliation and Arbitration Service (ACAS) indicating that they anticipated that the increase in working from home witnessed during the pandemic would lead to a growth in the number of formal requests for flexible working arrangements (ACAS, 2021).

Advances on the issue of paid and unpaid care leave have been stymied by the UK's exit from the EU, the COVID-19 pandemic and significant political upheaval. The UK's exit from the EU meant it was no longer obliged to introduce legislation in line with the EU Work–life Balance Directive (2019/1158; European Parliament, 2019). Following significant efforts from the carers' movement and the efforts of individual politicians, the imminent introduction in early 2024 of a right for carers to take five days' unpaid care leave following the Carer's Leave Act 2023 represents a further important development. However, is too early to judge what impact it will have. It is possible that the unpaid nature of the leave will limit uptake among lower-paid employees.

The adequacy of existing measures to support carers – emergency leave and flexible working requests – is hard to assess, due to a lack of robust, national data on the use of these policies. Employers in the UK also have discretion over their own policies that go beyond the statutory requirements, but again, data on the intricacies, uptake and impact of these policies is limited. Nevertheless, the evidence that is available strongly indicates that those employers that do provide support to carers can experience significant benefits in relation to issues such as staff turnover and absence rates, and that support for carers results in improvements in their work–life balance and well-being (Carers UK and HM Government, 2013; Carers UK, 2019; Austin and Heyes 2020).

Notes

[1] Carers UK includes Carers Cymru, Carers Scotland and Carers NI.

[2] Carers' organisations also play a role in the delivery of services for carers, including via contracts with local authorities and councils (Lloyd, 2023), and are therefore a key part of the UK's 'care diamond' (Razavi, 2007).

[3] The higher gender pay gap for all employees than for full- and part-time work reflects the higher share of women than men working part time, where part-time employees generally earn less.

[4] The Carers (Recognition and Services) Act 1995, the Carers and Disabled Children Act 2000 and the Carers (Equal Opportunities) Act 2004 were all initiated as Private Members' (rather than government) Bills. Private Members' Bills are public Bills introduced by MPs and Lords who are not government ministers and most fail to become law, making the success of these somewhat remarkable. Where they do not become law, they can indirectly affect policy by bringing attention and publicity to particular issues.

[5] There are two chambers to the Houses of Parliament through which legislation must be passed before it becomes law: the House of Commons (made of up elected Members of Parliament [MPs]) and the House of Lords (made up of appointed members). Policy often begins as a 'Green Paper' or consultation, aimed to invite discussion and comments from the opposition, stakeholder groups and the public. A White Paper might follow, with more detail, and then may be followed by a Bill which is submitted to either House (or government can omit the Green and White Papers and produce a Bill immediately). When passed through both Houses, a Bill receives Royal Assent, after which it becomes an Act of Parliament and law.

[6] Workers (and employees if they have already made a statutory request in the last 12 months) can make non-statutory requests for flexible working, but as these are not covered by legislation, there is no set procedure for applicants or employers. This is an

important distinction: as has been highlighted by the Taylor Review (2017) and the TUC (2014), the casualisation of employment, and in particular the casualisation of employment for certain groups such as women, has repercussions for their employment rights. The TUC found that women in particular did not consider their contract type problematic until they needed access to rights such as flexible working and could have it because they were workers, not employees. Some employees are also not eligible to make a statutory request (members of the armed forces and agency workers, unless returning from parental leave).

[7] https://www.gov.uk/flexible-working [Accessed 20 October 2020].

[8] As an example of the distinction between direct and indirect discrimination: a carer would be protected from being dismissed because they are caring for someone with a protected characteristic (for example, age or disability), but if an employer introduced a new working time pattern that applied to all staff but was not possible for a carer due to their caring responsibilities, this would be indirect discrimination. A carer in this scenario could ask for flexible working arrangements. As being a carer is currently not a protected characteristic – unlike having a disability – carers are not entitled to 'reasonable adjustment' and the flexible working right is only a 'right to request' – therefore an employer can decline this request and it would not be classed as discrimination in the law as it stands. There is, however, one example of a case where, at tribunal, a carer's claim of indirect discrimination was upheld (*Follows v Nationwide Building Society*, HM Courts and Tribunals Service and Employment Tribunal, 2021) as they followed a European Court of Justice case from 2015 (*Chez Razpredelenie Bulgaria*), a law retained post-Brexit (HM Courts and Tribunals Service and Employment Tribunal, 2021). In the UK, the Supreme Court and the Court of Appeal may depart from EU case law 'when it appears right to do so', so it remains to be seen whether future indirect discrimination cases may be successful (Rollin, 2021).

[9] By comparison, the UK average regular weekly pay in September 2023 was £617 (ONS, 2023).

[10] Based on responses from 114 member organisations.

[11] The achieved sample size was 970 unpaid carers in employment (excluding the self-employed).

[12] During the pandemic, companies unable to operate were able to 'furlough' their workers, that is, place them on temporary leave, and they then received 80 per cent of their wages while their employer received Government subsidies.

[13] https://www.gov.uk/guidance/check-which-employees-you-can-put-on-furlough-to-use-the-coronavirus-job-retention-scheme

[14] In UK employment law, 'worker' is an intermediate category that relates to people in work who are judged to be neither employees nor independently self-employed. The employment rights available to 'workers' are more restricted than those available to employees.

References

ACAS (2014) *The right to request flexible working: an ACAS guide (including guidance on handling requests in a reasonable manner to work flexibly)*. Available from: http://m.acas.org.uk/media/pdf/1/7/The-right-to-request-flexible-working-the-Acas-guide.pdf [Accessed 13 May 2019].

ACAS (2021) *'New study reveals half of employers expect more flexible working requests from staff after the pandemic is over'*. Available from: https://www.acas.org.uk/new-study-reveals-half-of-employers-expect-more-flexible-working-after-pandemic [Accessed 31 January 2023].

Akafekwa, T., Dalgarno, E. and Verma, A. (2021) 'The impact on the mental health and well-being of unpaid carers affected by social distancing, self-isolation and shielding during the COVID 19 pandemic in England – a systematic review', *medRxiv*, 2021. 08.20.21262375

Andrew, A., Cattan, C., Costa Dias, M., Farquharson, C., Kraftman, L., Krutikova, S., et al (2022) 'The gendered division of paid and domestic work under lockdown', *Fiscal Studies: The Journal of Applied Public Economics*, 43(4): 325–40.

Austin, A. and Heyes, J. (2020) 'Supporting working carers: how employers and employees can benefit', CIPD/University of Sheffield.

BEIS (Department of Business, Energy and Industrial Strategy) (2017) 'Industrial Strategy: building a Britain fit for the future'. Available from: https://www.gov.uk/government/publications/industrial-strategy-building-a-britain-fit-for-the-future [Accessed 31 May 2023].

BEIS (2020) 'Consultation on Carer's Leave'. Available from: https://www.gov.uk/government/consultations/carers-leave [Accessed 3 September 2021].

BEIS (2021) 'Consultation outcome: making flexible working the default', London: BEIS. Available from: https://www.gov.uk/government/consultations/making-flexible-working-the-default [Accessed 31 January 2023].

BEIS (2022) 'Consultation on making flexible working the default: government response'. Available from: https://assets.publishing.service.gov.uk/government/uploads/system/uploads/attachment_data/file/1121682/flexible-working-consultation-government-response.pdf [Accessed 31 January 2023].

Booth, L. (2021) 'Components of GDP: key economic indicators. House of Commons Library', London: HMSO. Available from: https://commonslibrary.parliament.uk/research-briefings/sn02787/ [Accessed 31 January 2023].

Brione, B. (2023) 'Carer's Leave Bill 2022–23: Progress of the Bill, Research Briefing', London: House of Commons Library.

Budd, J.W. and Mumford, K.A. (2006) 'Family-friendly work practices in Britain: availability and perceived accessibility', *Human Resource Management*, 45: 23–42.

Burrows, D., Lyttleton-Smith, J., Sheehan, L. and Jones, S. (2021) 'Voices of carers during the COVID-19 pandemic: messages for the future of unpaid caring in Wales'. Cardiff University Report.

Burstow, P. (2016) 'The Care Act: one year on – lessons learned, next steps', Carers Trust. Available from: https://carers.org/downloads/resources-pdfs/care-act/care-act-for-carers-one-year-on.pdf [Accessed 23 June 2023].

Bytheway, B. and Johnson, J. (1998) 'The social construction of carers', in A. Symonds and A. Kelly (eds), *The social construction of community care*, Basingstoke: Palgrave Macmillan, pp 241–53.

Carers UK (2014) *Caring and family finances inquiry: UK report*, London: Carers UK. Available from: https://www.carersuk.org/for-professionals/policy/policy-library/caring-family-finances-inquiry [Accessed 30 April 2019].

Carers UK (2015) 'Evidence on the Equality Act 2010 and Disability, consultation report'. Available from: Evidence on the Equality Act 2010 and Disability – Carers UK.

Carers UK (2019) 'Juggling work and unpaid care: a growing issue, policy report', London: Carers UK. Available from: https://www.employersforcar ers.org/resources/research/item/1460-juggling-work-and-unpaid-care-a-growing-issue [Accessed 31 January 2023].

Carers UK (2020a) 'Carers Week 2020 research report', London: Carers UK. Available from: www.Carersuk.org/for-professionals/policy/policy-library/carers-week-2020-research-report [Accessed 30 January 2023].

Carers UK (2020b) 'Unseen and undervalued: The value of unpaid care provided to date during the COVID-19 pandemic', London: Carers UK. Available from: https://www.carersuk.org/media/gi1b4oup/unseenand undervalued.pdf [Accessed 7 January 2021].

Carers UK (2020c) 'Caring behind closed doors: forgotten families in the coronavirus outbreak', London: Carers UK. Available from: https:// www.carersuk.org/media/a5dpp3ng/caring-behind-closed-doors-forgot ten-families-in-the-coronavirus-outbreak.pdf [Accessed 30 January 2023].

Carers UK (2020d) 'Caring behind closed doors: six months on'. Available from: https://www.carersuk.org/media/cptbrdal/caring-behind-closed-doors-six-months-on.pdf [Accessed 7 January 2021].

Carers UK (2020e) 'Vision 2025: our five year direction of travel', London: Carers UK. Available from: https://www.carersuk.org/media/0caka4bn/carers-uk-direction-of-travel-vision-2025.pdf [Accessed 24 January 2024].

Carers UK (2022) 'State of caring report', London: Carers UK. Available from: https://www.carersuk.org/reports/state-of-caring-2022-report/ [Accessed 31 January 2023].

Carers UK and HM Government (2013) 'Supporting working carers: the benefits to families, business and the economy'. [Available from: https:// www.gov.uk/government/publications/supporting-working-carers-the-benefits-to-families-business-and-the-economy [Accessed 30 May 2023].

CIPD (Chartered Institute of Personnel and Development) (2020) 'Coronavirus (COVID-19): flexible working during the pandemic and beyond', London: CIPD. Available from: www.cipd.co.uk/knowledge/ fundamentals/relations/flexible-working/ during-COVID-19-and-beyond [Accessed 30 January 2023].

CIPD (2021) ' "Employers must do more to address flexible working inequality" says CIPD, as new analysis highlights "flexible working notspots" across the UK'. Available from: https://www.cipd.co.uk/about/media/ press/flexible-working-inequality#gref [Accessed 31 January 2023].

Clements, L. (2010) Carers and their rights, London: Carers UK.

Clifton, A. (2021) 'Social care: a system at breaking point?' in E. Henderson and H. Johnson (eds), *What's next? Key issues for the Sixth Senedd*, Cardiff: Welsh Parliament Senedd Research, pp 34–39.

Cridland, J. (2017) 'Independent review of the state pension age: smoothing the transition'. Available from: https://www.gov.uk/government/publications/state-pension-age-independent-review-final-report [Accessed 31 May 2023].

Dalton, J. (2022) '"We're invisible": the hidden lives of the UK's unpaid carers', *The Independent*, 14 January. Available from: https://www.independent.co.uk/independentpremium/long-reads/unpaid-carers-social-care-cost-benefits-b1982970.html [Accessed 31 January 2023].

Dayan, M. and Heenan, D. (2019) *Change or collapse: lessons from the drive to reform health and social care in Northern Ireland*, London: The Nuffield Trust.

De la Porte, C., Larsen, T. and Szelewa, D. (2020) 'The EU's work–life balance directive: a lost opportunity for the UK in gender equality?' in M. Donoghue and M. Kuisma (eds), *Whither social rights in (post-) Brexit Europe? Opportunities and challenges*, Berlin and London: Social Europe Publishing and the Friedrich Ebert Stiftung, pp 96–99.

Department for Education and Employment (DfEE) (2000) *Work–life balance: changing patterns in a changing world*, London: DfEE.

Department of Health (1999) *Caring about carers: a national strategy for carers*, London: HMSO.

DHSC (Department of Health and Social Care) (2018) *'Carers action plan 2018 to 2020: supporting carers today'*. Available from: https://assets.publishing.service.gov.uk/government/uploads/system/uploads/attachment_data/file/713781/carers-action-plan-2018-2020.pdf [Accessed 31 May 2023].

Department of Trade and Industry (1998) 'Fairness at work', London: HMSO.

Department of Work and Pensions (DWP) (2022) DWP benefits statistics: August 2022. Available from: https://www.gov.uk/government/statistics/dwp-benefits-statistics-august-2022/dwp-benefits-statistics-august-2022 [Accessed 11 November 2023].

Esping-Andersen, G. (1990) *The three worlds of welfare capitalism*, New York: Princeton University Press.

Esping-Andersen, G. (1999) *Social foundations of postindustrial economies*, Oxford: Oxford University Press.

Eurocarers (2017) *Reconciling work and care: The need to support informal carers,* Brussels: Eurocarers. Available from: https://www.eurocarers.org/userfiles/files/factsheets/Eurocarers%20-%20Work%20Life%20balance_final.pdf [Accessed 13 April 2019].

European Parliament (2019) 'Directive (EU) 2019/1158 of the European Parliament and of the Council of 20 June 2019 on work–life balance for parents and carers and repealing Council Directive 2010/18/EU', Brussels: European Parliament. Available from: https://eur-lex.europa.eu/legal-content/EN/TXT/?uri=celex%3A32019L1158 [Accessed 30 June 2023].

Family Friendly Working Hours Taskforce (2010) *Flexible working: Working for families, working for business*. Available from: https://webarchive.natio nalarchives.gov.uk/20130701172411/http://www.dwp.gov.uk/docs/fam ily-friendly-task-force-report.pdf [Accessed 12 March 2019].

Fernandez, J.-L., Marczak, J., Snell, T., Brimblecombe, N., Moriarty, J., Damant, J., et al (2021) 'Supporting carers following the implementation of the Care Act 2014: eligibility, support and prevention: The Carers in Adult Social Care (CASC) study', Care Policy and Evaluation Centre, London School of Economics and Political Science and NIHR Policy Research Unit in Health and Social Care Workforce.

Fox-Leonard, B. (2022) 'Our second NHS: Britain's invisible army of unpaid carers need your help', *The Telegraph*, 8 November. Available from: https:// www.telegraph.co.uk/hristmas/2020/11/08/second-nhs-britains-invisi ble-army-unpaid-carers-need-help/ [Accessed 31 January 2023].

Fry, G., Price, C. and Yeandle, S. (2009) 'Local authorities' use of Carers Grant. A report prepared for the Department of Health', London: Department of Health.

Gallie, D. (2009) 'Institutional regimes and employee influence at work: a European comparison', *Cambridge Journal of Regions, Economy and Society*, 2(3): 379–393.

Giebel, C., Lord, K., Cooper, C., Shenton, J., Cannon, J., Pulford, D. et al (2021a) A UK survey of COVID-19 related social support closures and their effects on older people, people with dementia, and carers, *International Journal of Geriatric Psychiatry*, 36(3): 393–402.

Giebel, C., Pulford, D., Cooper, C., Lord, K., Shenton, J., Cannon, J. et al (2021b) 'COVID-19-related social support service closures and mental well-being in older adults and those affected by dementia: a UK longitudinal survey', *British Medical Journal Open*, 11(1): e045889.

Glasby, J. (2021) 'Adult social care in England: more disappointment, delay, and distraction', *BMJ*, 374: n2242.

Gray, A.M. and Birrell, D. (2013) *Transforming adult social care*, Bristol: Policy Press.

Gregory, A. and Milner, S. (2009) Editorial: Work–life balance: a matter of choice? *Gender, Work & Organization*, 16(1): 1–13.

Guzman-Castillo, M., Ahmadi-Abhari, S., Bandosz, P., Capewell, S., Steptoe, A., Singh-Manoux, A., et al (2017) 'Forecasted trends in disability and life expectancy in England and Wales up to 2025: a modelling study', *The Lancet Public Health*, 2(7): e307–e313.

Hall, P.A. and Soskice, D. (eds) (2001) *Varieties of capitalism: The institutional foundations of comparative advantage*, Oxford: OUP Oxford.

Hall, P., Needham, C. and Hamblin, K. (2020) 'Social care', in N. Ellison and T. Haux (eds), *Handbook of society and social policy: Social care*, Cheltenham: Edward Elgar, pp 321–32.

Hamblin, K.A. and Hoff, A. (2011) Carers@ Work. *Carers between work and care-Conflict or chance? Results of interviews with working carers in the United Kingdom*, Oxford: Oxford Institute of Population Ageing. Available from: https://www.ageing.ox.ac.uk/publications/view/22 [Accessed 23 November 2023].

Heyes, J., Lewis, P. and Clark, I. (2012) 'Varieties of capitalism, neo-liberalism and the economic crisis of 2008', *Industrial Relations Journal*, 43(3): 222–41.

HM Courts and Tribunals Service and Employment Tribunal (2021) 'Mrs J Follows v Nationwide Building Society: 2201937/2018'. Available from: https://www.gov.uk/employment-tribunal-decisions/mrs-j-follows-v-nationwide-building-society-2201937-slash-2018 [Accessed 30 June 2023].

HM Government (1995) *Carers (Recognition and Services) Act*, London: HMSO.

Hoque, K. and Noon, M. (2004) 'Equal opportunities policy and practice in Britain: evaluating the "empty shell" hypothesis', *Work, Employment and Society*, 18(3): 481–506.

House of Commons (2023) *Employment Relations (Flexible Working) Act 2023*. Available from: https://www.legislation.gov.uk/ukpga/2023/33/enacted [Accessed 23 November 2023].

House of Commons Work and Pensions Committee (2008) *Valuing and supporting carers*, volume 1, London: The Stationery Office.

House of Lords (2016) 'The Equality Act 2010: the impact on disabled people Select Committee on the Equality Act 2010 and Disability Report of Session 2015–16'. Available from: https://lordslibrary.parliament.uk/the-equality-act-2010-impact-on-disabled-people/ [Accessed 19 June 2023].

House of Lords Adult Social Care Committee (2022) 'A "gloriously ordinary life": spotlight on adult social care', London: HMSO.

International Labour Organization (ILO) (2021) 'Making decent work a reality for domestic workers: progress and prospects ten years after the adoption of the Domestic Workers Convention, 2011 (No. 189)' Geneva: ILO.

Ireson, R., Sethi, B. and Williams, A. (2018) 'Availability of caregiver-friendly workplace policies (CFWPs): an international scoping review', *Health & Social Care in the Community*, 26(1): e1–e14.

Irvine, S., Clark, H., Ward, M. and Francis-Devine, B. (2023) 'Women and the UK economy', research briefing, House of Commons Library, London: HSMO.

Jagger, C. (2015) *Trends in life expectancy and healthy life expectancy*, London: Government Office for Science.

Kennedy, S. and Gheera, M. (2018) 'Carer's Allowance, briefing paper number 00846', 19 July 2018, London: House of Commons.

King, T., Hewitt, B., Crammond, B., Sutherland, G., Maheen, H. and Kavanagh, A. (2020) 'Reordering gender systems: can COVID-19 lead to improved gender equality and health?' *The Lancet*, 396(10244): 80–1.

Kirton, G. and Greene, A. (2015) *The dynamics of managing diversity: A critical approach*, 4th edn, Abingdon: Routledge.

Larkin, M. and Milne, A. (2014) 'Carers and empowerment in the UK: a critical reflection', *Social Policy and Society*, 13(1): 25–38.

Lewis, J. and Campbell, M. (2007) 'Work/family balance policies in the UK since 1997: a new departure?' *Journal of Social Policy*, 36(3): 365–81.

Lloyd, L. (2000) 'Caring about carers: only half the picture?' *Critical Social Policy*, 20(1): 136–50.

Lloyd, L. (2006) 'Call us carers: limitations and risks in campaigning for recognition and exclusivity', *Critical Social Policy*, 26(4): 945–60.

Lloyd, L. (2023) *Unpaid care policies in the UK: Rights, resources and relationships*, Bristol: Policy Press.

Muldrew, D.H., Fee, A. and Coates, V. (2022) 'Impact of the COVID-19 pandemic on family carers in the community: a scoping review', *Health & Social Care in the Community*, 30(4): 1275–85.

NASUWT (2020) 'Department for Business, Energy and Industrial Strategy (BEIS) Carer's Leave Consultation, NASUWT submission'. Available from: https://www.nasuwt.org.uk/asset/84BE73B5-1651-4451-BBA0D 67DA184F1E8/ [Accessed 31 January 2023].

Needham, C. and Hall, P. (2023) *Social care in the UK's four nations: Between two paradigms*, Policy Press: Bristol.

NHS Digital (2022) 'Adult social care activity and finance report, England, 2021–22'. Available from: https://digital.nhs.uk/data-and-information/ publications/statistical/adult-social-care-activity-and-finance-report/2021- 22/carers [Accessed 23 June 2023].

O'Connor, J., Orloff, A. and Shaver, S. (1999) *States, markets, families: Gender, liberalism and social policy in Australia, Canada, Great Britain and the United States*, Cambridge: Cambridge University Press

ONS (2020) 'Coronavirus and homeworking in the UK labour market: 2019'. Available from: https://www.ons.gov.uk/employmentandlabourmarket/ peopleinwork/employmentandemployeetypes/articles/coronavirusandhom eworkingintheuklabourmarket/2019#occupations-of-homeworkers per cent20 [Accessed 31 January 2023].

ONS (2021) 'Overview of the UK population: January 2021'. Available from: https://www.ons.gov.uk/peoplepopulationandcommunity/populat ionandmigration/populationestimates/articles/overviewoftheukpopulat ion/january2021 [Accessed 31 August 2021].

ONS (2022) 'Population estimates for the UK, England, Wales, Scotland and Northern Ireland: mid-2021'. Available from: https://www.ons.gov.uk/peopl epopulationandcommunity/populationandmigration/populationestimates/ bulletins/annualmidyearpopulationestimates/mid2021 [Accessed 21 June 2023].

ONS (2023) 'Average weekly earnings in Great Britain: September 2023'. Available from: https://www.ons.gov.uk/employmentandlabourmarket/ peopleinwork/employmentandemployeetypes/bulletins/averageweeklyear ningsingreatbritain/september2023 [Accessed 3 November 2023].

Parker, J. (2006) 'Trade union women's groups and their effects on union goals and strategies', *Human Resource Management Journal*, 16(4): 411–31.

Petrillo, M. and Bennett, M. (2023) 'Valuing Carers 2021: England and Wales', London: Carers UK.

Petrillo, M., Bennett, M.R. and Pryce, G. (2022) 'Cycles of caring: transitions in and out of unpaid care', London: Carers UK.

Phillips, D., Paul, G., Fahy, M., Dowling-Hetherington, L., Kroll, T., Moloney, B. et al (2020) 'The invisible workforce during the COVID-19 pandemic: carers at the frontline', *HRB Open Research*, 3: 24.

Phillips, D., Duffy, C., Fahy, M., Dowling-Hetherington, L., Paul, G., Moloney, B. et al (2022) 'Beyond the COVID-19 pandemic for working carers across the European Union: work, policy and gender considerations', *International Journal of Care and Caring*, 6(1–2): 289–98.

Price, D. (2006) 'Gender and generational continuity: breadwinners, caregivers and pension provision in the UK', *International Journal of Ageing and Later Life*, 1(2): 31–66.

Power, K. (2020) 'The COVID-19 pandemic has increased the care burden of women and families', *Sustainability: Science, Practice and Policy*, 16(1): 67–73.

Razavi, S. (2007) 'The political and social economy of care in a development context: conceptual issues, research questions and policy options', #Gender and Development Programme Paper No. 3, United Nations Research Institute for Social Development, Geneva: UNRISD.

Redpath, E. (2022) 'Chamberlain to present "landmark" unpaid carers leave Bill'. Available from: https://www.northeastfifelibdems.org.uk/chamberlain_to_present_landmark_unpaid_carers_leave_bill [Accessed 9 August 2022].

Reisenbichler, A. and Wiedemann, A. (2022) 'Credit-driven and consumption-led growth models in the United States and United Kingdom', in L. Baccaro, M. Blyth and J. Pontusson (eds), *Diminishing returns: The new politics of growth and stagnation*, Oxford: Oxford University Press, pp 213–37.

Rollin, F. (2021) 'A carer had the right to bring indirect discrimination claims based on her association with a disabled person'. Available from: https://www.stevens-bolton.com/site/insights/articles/indirect-associative-discrimination-claimaints-association [Accessed 30 June 2023].

Schneider, U., Trukeschitz, B., Mühlmann, R. and Ponocny, I. (2013) '"Do I stay or do I go?" Job change and labor market exit intentions of employees providing informal care to older adults', *Health Economics*, 22(10): 1230–49.

Shereen (2020) 'Unpaid carers were isolated even before lockdown – now we're invisible', *The Guardian*, 12 May. Available from: https://www.theguardian.com/society/2020/may/12/unpaid-carers-isolated-lockdown-invisible [Accessed 31 January 2023].

Starr, M. and Szebehely, M. (2017) 'Working longer, caring harder – the impact of "ageing-in-place" policies on working carers in the UK and Sweden', *International Journal of Care and Caring*, 1(1): 115–19.

Taylor, M., Marsh, G., Nicol, D. and Broadbent, P. (2017) *Good work: The Taylor review of modern working practices* (Vol 116), London: Department for Business, Energy & Industrial Strategy.

The Conservative Party (2019) *Get Brexit done, unleash Britain's potential: The Conservative and Unionist Party Manifesto 2019*, London: Paragon.

Trades Union Congress (TUC) (2014) 'Women and casualisation: Women's experiences of job insecurity'. Available from: https://www.tuc.org.uk/sites/default/files/Women_and_casualisation.pdf [Accessed 30 April 2019].

Trades Union Congress (TUC) (2019) 'One in three flexible working requests turned down, TUC poll reveals'. Available from: https://www.tuc.org.uk/news/one-three-flexible-working-requests-turned-down-tuc-poll-reveals [Accessed 31 January 2023].

Trades Union Congress (TUC) (2020) 'BEIS Carer's leave consultation response', London: TUC. Available from: https://www.tuc.org.uk/research-analysis/reports/beis-carers-leave-consultation-response [Accessed 30 January 2023].

Trades Union Congress (TUC) (2021) 'Good news, bad news, and the same challenges'. Available from: https://www.tuc.org.uk/blogs/good-news-bad-news-and-same-challenges-trade-union-membership-statistics [Accessed 30 January 2023].

UNISON (2019) '"Carer policies": How branches can benefit from bargaining on carers' rights at work', London: UNISON.

UNISON (2021) 'Carers' policies: a bargaining guide and model policy'. Available from: https://www.unison.org.uk/content/uploads/2021/12/Model-carers-policy.docx [Accessed 31 January 2023].

van Ark, B. and Venables, A. (2020) 'A concerted effort to tackle the UK productivity puzzle', *International Productivity Monitor*, 39: 3–15. Available from: https://research.manchester.ac.uk/en/publications/a-concerted-effort-to-tackle-the-uk-productivity-puzzle [Accessed 24 January 2024].

Wales Trade Union Congress Cymru (2022) 'Working and looking after others: new survey'. Available from: https://www.tuc.org.uk/news/working-and-looking-after-others-new-survey [Accessed 24 January 2024].

Williams, S. (2014) *Introducing employment relations: A critical approach*, Oxford: Oxford University Press.

Yeandle, S. (1999) 'Women, men, and non-standard employment: breadwinning and caregiving in Germany, Italy, and the UK, in R. Crompton, *Restructuring gender relations and employment: The decline of the male breadwinner*, Oxford: Oxford University Press, pp 80–105.

Yeandle, S. (2016) 'Caring for our carers: an international perspective on policy developments in the UK', *Juncture*, 23(1): 57–62.

Yeandle, S. (2017) 'Work–care reconciliation policy: legislation in policy context in eight countries.' Report prepared for the German Bundesministeriumfür Familie, Senioren, Frauen und Jugend. Available from: https://drive.google.com/file/d/1ZSErSTrCgUek4AxM1SkWV 0nJ2FW6AXoM/view [Accessed 24 January 2024].

Yeandle, S. and Buckner, L. (2007) *Carers, Employment and Services: time for a new social contract?* Carers UK. Available from: https://essl.leeds.ac.uk/ download/downloads/id/218/carers_uk_report_6.pdf [Accessed 24 January 2024].

Yeandle, S. and Buckner, L. (2017) 'Older workers and care-giving in England: the policy context for older workers' employment patterns', *Journal of Cross-Cultural Gerontology*, 32(3): 303–21.

Yeandle, S., Kröger, T. and Cass, B. (2012) 'Voice and choice for users and carers? Developments in patterns of care for older people in Australia, England and Finland', *Journal of European Social Policy*, 22(4): 432–45.

Zamberlan, A., Gioachin, F. and Gritti, D. (2021) 'Work less, help out more? The persistence of gender inequality in housework and childcare during UK COVID-19', *Research in Social Stratification and Mobility*, 73: 100583.

6

Canada

Janet Fast and Jacquie Eales

Introduction

In many respects, support for carers in Canada is underdeveloped compared to its Organisation for Economic Co-operation and Development (OECD) counterparts. There is no publicly endorsed carer strategy, no national carer recognition legislation, nor a national carer allowance scheme, despite repeated calls for a more systematic approach to carer support (see, for example, Canadian Centre for Caregiving Excellence, 2022; The Petro-Canada CareMakers Foundation, 2021/2022). Yet the care that carers provide is estimated to be worth three times the national expenditures on home, community and long-term care (Fast et al, 2023). Some progress has been made since 2000, especially where policy reform is consistent with prevailing policy-maker values favouring labour force participation; indeed, addressing employment challenges for carers has become a mainstay of Canadian government responses.

In this chapter, we describe the political, economic and social contexts underpinning Canada's policy initiatives around supporting employed carers. We then describe Canada's legislated carer leave programmes in some detail, and offer a critical reflection on their adequacy in terms of equity, flexibility, job protection and income security. We briefly report on the impact of the COVID-19 pandemic on employed carers and Canada's response to this impact. Finally, we set the carer leave provisions in the context of other (limited) carers support measures.

National context

Policy and policy instruments are not developed, implemented or enforced in a vacuum. The political, social, economic and cultural contexts within which policy is made create barriers and enablers that influence policy analysis and design and explain policy success and failure (Lohman et al, 2009). In this section, we describe the political, economic and social contexts that influence policy making in Canada.

Political context

A key characteristic of Canada's political context is its federated government system. Canada comprises one federal, ten provincial and three territorial governments; municipal governments (cities, towns, villages) also play a role. Canada's constitution sets out which level(s) of government have jurisdiction over which policy domains, but there is significant overlap such that multiple levels of government have some jurisdiction over some of the same policy domains, including health, labour, income security and family policy. This results in considerable regional variability in eligibility criteria, coverage, specific provisions, delivery and enforcement of policy instruments. This is certainly true of carer leave policies.

Canada is considered to be a liberal welfare state, with more collectivist values than some developed countries (for example, US) but less collectivist than others (for example, Nordic countries) (Olsen, 2007). Further, within the Canadian federation, the province of Quebec is more collectivist and socially liberal than the rest of Canada. It also operates under a different legal system (the Napoleonic code) than the rest of Canada (common law). Social values of collectivism but with a trend toward more individual responsibility, and stated commitment to equity, diversity and inclusion, underpin public policy making in Canada.

Despite this collectivist inclination, there has always been an expectation that individuals will be responsible for meeting their own day-to-day needs as and when they can. In addition, and with specific relevance to care, filial responsibility legislation has existed in all Canadian jurisdictions since the Great Depression of the 1920s–30s (though the province of Alberta repealed the parental support provisions of its Family Law Act in 2005) (Moore, 2016). The original legislation, requiring adult children to support parents who may be dependent due to age, illness or financial status, was motivated largely by a desire to contain government expenditures. It has been enforced rarely (Gardiner, 2011), but there is now active debate about whether population ageing, renewed public expenditure concerns and a re-emergence of familialist ideology will (or should) result in more vigorous enforcement or more widespread rejection of the legislation (BCLI, 2007). More recent directives from governments, such as those to improve 'carer preparedness', are strengthening an individual responsibility expectation, similarly motivated by fiscal considerations.

Yet Canada's history with respect to seizing opportunities to support carers is not encouraging. In 2004, the then Liberal government appointed a Minister of State for Families and Caregivers, who promised a national carer strategy to guide federal policy. Before such a strategy could be developed, an election saw a change in government that eliminated the Minister of State for Families and Caregivers portfolio. In 2009, a Special Senate Committee on

Aging also recommended the development of a National Caregiver Strategy, but 13 years later, this remains unfulfilled. In 2015, the federal government established an Employers for Caregivers Panel as part of its economic action plan. The Panel's mandate was to consult with Canadian employers with a view to helping employees balance paid work with their care responsibilities to decrease cost to employers and the Canadian economy by reducing the impact of employees' caregiving responsibilities on job performance, absenteeism, turnover and productivity. The Panel was disbanded once its final report, highlighting some best practices for supporting working carers, was tabled, and no further government action has been taken. Even as recently as 2022, the Petro-Canada CareMakers Foundation (The Petro-Canada CareMakers Foundation, 2021/22) and the Canadian Centre on Caregiving Excellence (Canadian Centre for Caregiving Excellence, 2022), in separate reports, recommended enhanced financial supports for carers, more supportive labour policies and a national carer strategy.

Economic and labour market context

The nature and health of the national economy profoundly influence policy choices and options. Canada is considered to have a developed economy, though it is more dependent on natural resource industries than most others (Natural Resources Canada, 2020). This, and the fact that the US is by far Canada's largest trading partner (accounting for 75 per cent of all Canadian exports), makes Canada's public policy process highly susceptible to US influence (Dymond and Hart, 2004).

Like in most developed countries, women comprise an increasing share of the Canadian labour market, facilitated by evolving social gender norms, smaller families, educational gains, new household technologies, service sector employment opportunities and related labour and family policies (pay equity, maternity and parental leave, non-parental childcare services) (Statistics Canada, 2015). Yet women's labour force participation (LFP) continues to be affected by family care responsibilities to a greater extent than men's (Moyser, 2017): marriage and presence of young children still depress LFP and increase incidence of part-time work for women (though this relationship is weakening), while family responsibilities are associated with higher LFP for men.

Pre-COVID, Canadian employment rates were strong and unemployment rates shrinking: the unemployment rate stood at 5 per cent in February 2020; rose to a high of 13.7 per cent in May 2020; and by December 2022 had returned to 5 per cent (Statistics Canada, 2022a). In stark contrast to previous economic downturns when women were less disadvantaged than men, women were more likely to drop out of the labour force due to COVID, with women's LFP rates reaching their lowest level in 30 years (Desjardin et al, 2020). Women also accounted for 45 per cent of the reduction in work hours and have not regained employment as quickly as men since COVID-19 containment measures were relaxed. As of December 2022, employment losses have recovered somewhat, with 81 per cent of women in peak employment years (age 25–54) participating in the paid labour force (Statistics Canada, 2023a).

Social context

Canada's population is relatively small and sparse, reaching 40 million Canadians living in the second-largest land mass in the world in 2023 (Statistics Canada, 2023a). Its population is projected to grow to 47.7 million by 2036 (Sheets and Gallagher, 2013). Most are urban dwellers living within 100 miles of the US border. Its population is increasingly ethnically diverse, as much of its population growth comes from immigration. Official bilingualism (English and French) is a distinguishing feature of Canadian society.

Canada's population is ageing, but at a more moderate pace than other countries. In 2015, there were more older adults (aged 65 and older) than youth (aged 15 and younger) for the first time in Canadian history (Statistics Canada, 2017). Canadians aged 65 and older are expected to rise from 18.5 per cent of the population in 2021 to 23.1 per cent in 2043 and 25.9 per cent in 2068 (Statistics Canada, 2022b). By 2056, it is projected that one in ten Canadians will be aged 80 or older (Bélanger et al, 2005). Canadians' life expectancy at birth is currently 82 years (OECD, 2023).

Estimates of the proportion of the Canadian population that provides care to a family member or friend with a long-term health condition, a physical or mental disability, or problems related to ageing tend to be higher than for comparable developed countries: one in four Canadians aged 15+ living in the ten provinces (7.8 million people) in 2018 (Hango, 2020). The majority of these caregivers are employed (26 per cent of Canadians of employment age, 5.2 million in 2018) and most of these are employed full time (Magnaye et al, 2022).

Carer leave policies

Discrimination based on gender, ethnicity/race, age, disability, family status and other biasing personal characteristics is officially prohibited in Canada by its Charter of Rights and Freedoms and provincial equivalents, and employment and pay equity legislation. In September 2019, the Canada Labour Code was amended to provide workers in federally regulated industries with the right to request flexible working arrangements. The Canada Labour Code applies to about 10 per cent of all Canadian employees, but provincial human rights codes have been interpreted as requiring employers to accommodate employees' family responsibilities, so long as this does not create undue hardship for the employer (Canadian Human Rights Commission, 2014). Yet gender differences persist in employment, social and care contexts. In 2018, only a slight majority (54 per cent) of Canadian carers were women (Hango, 2020). Women are also more disadvantaged by their carer status than men, reporting social, health, employment and financial consequences in higher proportions in each of the five nationally representative surveys on care conducted since 1998.

There are several legislated leave programmes that support carers' abilities to balance paid work and care responsibilities by providing them with job-protected time off work. These include (mostly unpaid) short leaves of a few days per year, commonly referred to as family responsibility leave, and three more extended leaves of absence, accompanied by partial income replacement through the Employment Insurance programme: Compassionate Care Leave, Critical Illness Leave for Children and Critical Illness Leave for Adults (Table 6.1). We start with a description of Family Responsibility Leave – the only short-term leave available in Canada – including its intent, eligibility criteria and benefits, followed by similar descriptions of the longer carer leaves.

Short-term leaves

Family Responsibility Leave (FRL) was first introduced in 1995 as part of a consolidation of the federal Employment Standards Act, which, as already noted, applies only to workers in federally regulated industries. Provincial governments subsequently enacted FRLs that apply to other workers, while the northern territories (Yukon, Northwest Territories and Nunavut) have not followed suit. FRL is an employee entitlement that enables workers to meet responsibilities for the care, health or education of a child or other immediate family members. The definition of immediate family varies somewhat across jurisdictions, but most have a broad and liberal interpretation that includes at least partner/spouse, child, parent, guardian, sibling, grandchild or grandparent of an employee, and any person who lives with an employee as a member of the employee's family. The province of Manitoba also includes extended family members like aunts, uncles, nieces and nephews.

In addition to the relationship between the working carer and the care receiver, other eligibility criteria, such as minimum service periods, employer size and notice requirements also vary across jurisdictions. There is no minimum service period in British Columbia, Quebec or New Brunswick, but other jurisdictions have a minimum service period, ranging from as little as two weeks (Ontario) to as much as six consecutive months (Prince Edward Island). In Ontario, the only jurisdiction where employer size is an

Table 6.1: Carer leave schemes, Canada (November 2023)

Leave details				Eligibility					
Leave name and introduced	Leave duration	Compensation		Worker/employee status	Qualifying period	Person needing care	Evidence	Notice period and process
Family Responsibility Leave, 1995	Varies across provinces but typically 3–5 days per annum	Unpaid		Workers in specific industries	Varies across provinces	Child or other immediate family members[a]	–	Varies across provinces
Compassionate Care Leave, 2004	Varies across provinces but 8–28 weeks per annum	Eligible for partial income replacement through EI; 55% of usual earnings to maximum		All	600 insured hours of work in the 52 weeks before the start of their claim	Family member for whom the employee is caring be diagnosed with a serious medical condition with a significant risk of death within 26 weeks	Medical certificate	Varies across provinces
Critical Illness Leave for Children, 2017	37 weeks per annum	Eligible for partial income replacement through EI; 55% of usual earnings to maximum		All	600 insured hours of work in the 52 weeks before the start of their claim	Child under 18 who is a family member or 'like family'	Medical certificate	Varies across provinces
Critical Illness Leave for Adults, 2017	17 weeks per annum	Eligible for partial income replacement through EI; 55% of usual earnings to maximum		All	600 insured hours of work in the 52 weeks before the start of their claim	Family member or 'like family'	Medical certificate	Varies across provinces

Note: [a] Varies across provinces.

eligibility criterion, FRL is available only to family carers who work for an employer with 50 or more employees.

Eligible employees are generally expected to give their employer reasonable notice and sufficient information for the employer to ascertain that the employee is entitled to take the FRL, but the details vary. British Columbia has no notice requirements; Ontario requires only verbal notification; Saskatchewan, Manitoba, New Brunswick, Nova Scotia and Prince Edward Island require written notice as soon as possible; and Newfoundland requires written statements outlining the nature of any leave exceeding three days.

For working carers who are entitled to FRL and meet the eligibility criteria, the duration of the leave also varies across jurisdictions from 3 (Manitoba, New Brunswick, Nova Scotia, PEI) to 12 (Saskatchewan) days per year, with most jurisdictions providing 3 to 5 days per year. Most eligible employees can take time off work to attend to family responsibilities without jeopardising their job. Employers are not required to pay wages or benefits during the FRL, unless stated in an employment contract or collective agreement.

Longer-term leaves

In Canada, there are three other legislated longer-term leaves that are designed to support working carers: Compassionate Care Leave, Critical Illness Leave for Children and Critical Illness Leave for Adults. In this section we first describe the intent and duration of each of these extended leaves, then their eligibility criteria, which are the same for all three leaves, but with minor variations across jurisdictions.

Compassionate Care Leave

Compassionate Care Leave (CCL) is intended to support employees caring for a family member who has a serious medical condition with a significant risk of death within 26 weeks. It was first introduced in 2004 through amendment of the Canada Labour Code. Most provinces amended their own labour codes at about the same time, though Alberta was the last province to implement CCL, in February 2014. Corresponding changes also were made to the Employment Insurance Act to enable the Compassionate Care Benefit. The CCL and compassionate care benefit have been amended over the years, expanding the definition of eligible family member and increasing the length of the leave and the benefit. Every jurisdiction in Canada requires that the family member for whom the employee is caring be diagnosed with a serious medical condition with a significant risk of death within 26 weeks. Most jurisdictions provide 27–28 weeks of job-protected CCL within a 52-week period to working carers who meet the eligibility criteria, although this varies across jurisdictions: as few as 8 weeks in Nunavut; 16 weeks in Quebec; 27 weeks in Alberta, BC, Northwest Territories; and 28 weeks in Manitoba, New Brunswick, Newfoundland, Nova Scotia, Ontario, Prince Edward Island, Saskatchewan and Yukon as well as for workers in federally regulated industries. Self-employed workers have been eligible for CCL since 2010. The leave can be taken more than once in an employee's career but they must have accrued the required insurable hours each time. In 2018, one in seven employed carers reported that they had ever taken some CCL (Magnaye et al, 2023).

Critical Illness Leaves

Two Critical Illness Leaves (CILs) were introduced more recently as part of the 2017 Budget Implementation Act (Bill C-63) in which the Government of Canada made significant amendments to the Canada Labour Code. The CILs are intended to support employees caring for a critically ill or injured person whose 'baseline state of health has changed significantly'. If the care receiver is already living with a chronic medical condition, working carers are not eligible for CIL unless this person's health changes significantly because of a 'new and acute life-threatening event'. Working carers who meet the eligibility criteria are able to take up to 37 weeks of leave within a 52-week period to provide care or support to a critically ill child who is under age 18, or up to 17 weeks of leave to provide care or support to a critically ill family member who is age 18 or older. The leave can be taken more than once in an employee's career but they must have accrued the required insurable hours each time. Ontario also has a Family Caregiver Leave of up to eight weeks for each specified family member.

All employees covered by the Canada Labour Code (those working in federally regulated industries) or by provincial employment standards legislation are eligible for the CCL and CIL. Employment standards legislation protects employees against dismissal, lay-off, suspension, demotion or discipline because of taking leaves of absence for the purposes of compassionate or critical care. Members of certain professions/jobs (for example, healthcare professionals, embassy workers, commission sales persons, farm labourers and so on) are not covered by this legislation.

To be eligible for CCL and CIL, regardless of jurisdiction, employees must have accumulated 600 insured hours of work in the 52 weeks before the start of their claim, equivalent to 15 weeks of full-time work at 40 hours per week. While there is no minimum length of service for eligibility in some jurisdictions (Federal, British Columbia, Ontario, New Brunswick, Prince Edward Island, Yukon, Northwest Territories, Nunavut), other jurisdictions require a minimum employment period ranging from 30 days (Manitoba, Newfoundland) to 13 consecutive weeks (Saskatchewan). In addition, to be eligible for the CIL, working carers' regular weekly earnings from work must have decreased by more than 40 per cent for at least one week because the employee needs to take time away from work to provide care or support to a critically ill family member. Self-employed individuals are also eligible if they have registered for access to Employment Insurance (EI) Special Benefits for self-employed people and meet the following eligibility criteria: waited at least 12 months from the date of confirmed programme registration to apply; have experienced a 40 per cent reduction in the amount of time spent on their business for at least one week because they need to provide care or support; and have earned a minimum amount of self-employed earnings during the preceding calendar year (reduced temporarily from CA$7,555 in 2020 to CA$5,289 in 2021–22, due to the pandemic).

Most jurisdictions use the same broad and inclusive definition of 'immediate family' that includes close kin and 'like family' relationships for both the shorter FRL and longer CCL and CIL leaves. In all cases and jurisdictions, a family member's critical illness, critical injury or significant risk of death must be certified in writing by a medical doctor or nurse practitioner.

Employer notification for CCL and CIL is required 'as soon as possible' in nine jurisdictions (Federal, British Columbia, Saskatchewan, Quebec, Nova Scotia, Prince Edward Island, Yukon, Northwest Territories and Nunavut). Manitoba requires notice of one pay period unless circumstances necessitate a shorter period, whereas Alberta and Newfoundland require two weeks' notice unless there is a valid reason otherwise. Ontario requires employees to advise their employer in writing. New Brunswick requires employees to advise their employers of anticipated commencement date and duration.

Analysis and discussion of the adequacy of carer leave policies and programmes

In this section, we assess and discuss the adequacy of short- (FRL) and longer-term (CCL and CIL) carer leaves in Canada. Key characteristics that enhance the utility of family carer leave policies include their equity or inclusivity, flexibility, job protection and income security (Canadian Human Rights Commission, 2014; Keating et al, 2014; Blum et al, 2023).

Equity and inclusivity

There is great diversity among the 5.2 million employed family carers in Canada. Yet public policies tend to ignore such differences, seeking simple, fiscally conservative and comprehensive solutions to problems that are often complicated in order to meet the most needs possible. Equity refers to the breadth of people eligible for a given carer leave: who is supported and who is not? The structure of Canada's government system continues to result in substantial variability across federal, provincial and territorial jurisdictions. Gender equity is an explicit value of the current federal government, and carer support legislation and programmes are expressed in gender-neutral language, such that carer leaves make it more possible for all carers to maintain employment alongside care responsibilities. At the same time, other long-standing gender inequities are reinforced: the gendered nature of care, persistent gender wage gap and the low partial income replacement rate of the Employment Insurance programme result in the lower-income earner in a family (the majority of whom are women) taking all or most of the leave and economic hit. In the following paragraphs we elaborate on the inequities in Canadian carer leave policies that arise from geography, job conditions and the nature of care itself.

As noted earlier, Canada's federated government structure results in substantial variability in policy and programme provisions. While the carer leaves already described are legislated in all jurisdictions (with the exception of FRL in the Northern Territories), the specific provisions, including eligibility and duration, vary substantially across jurisdictions. The result is inequity for working carers living in different geographic regions of the country. For example, carers eligible for CCL who live in Nunavut receive as few as eight weeks' job-protected leave while those who live elsewhere (governed by labour legislation for Federal, Manitoba, New Brunswick, Newfoundland, Nova Scotia, Ontario, Prince Edward Island, Saskatchewan and Yukon governments) receive more than three times that amount at 28 weeks of job-protected leave.

While the location in which carers live in Canada will determine the length of benefit period, where carers live in proximity to those for whom they provide care does not affect access to the benefit. Whether the dyad lives in the same town, health region, province or even country is not an eligibility criterion. If working carers need to leave Canada to provide care or support to a person who is critically ill or injured or needing end-of-life care, they may still be eligible to receive EI benefits, submitting the same type of proof that is required for care receivers living in Canada. This feature is important to those transnational carers who live in Canada but are supporting critically ill or end-of-life family members in other countries.

Another source of inequity arises from the fact that workers in some occupations are not eligible for the leaves described earlier, at least under the Canada Labour Code. Similarly, minimum hours of service required to be eligible for the CCL and CIL (and FRL in some provinces) are often beyond the reach of those with non-standard employment, such as those who work in part-time, temporary, casual or seasonal jobs (Prince, 2015; Cox, 2019). In fact, those with part-time or non-standard employment are less likely to accumulate the required number of hours of insurable employment because of their work pattern, resulting in significantly lower eligibility rates

(Canada Employment Insurance Commission, 2021). Working carers in low-pay, low-benefit, low-autonomy jobs that lack inherent flexibility are similarly disadvantaged. When faced with high levels of care needs, these carers are more likely to have to leave the paid labour force to provide unpaid care work.

The dyadic relationship between the carer and care receiver determines eligibility for a given programme. One key shortcoming identified in an early evaluation of the CCL programme was a narrow definition of immediate family member (Osborne and Margo, 2005). Over time, the eligibility criteria for FRL, CCL and CIL have broadened beyond nuclear families of parents and children to be more inclusive and encompass a diverse network of extended family and 'family-like' relationships, better reflecting the diversity and complexity of families across the lifecourse.

The definition of immediate family used in the enabling legislation for these leaves is now very broad, and so inclusive on the surface. However, the gendered nature of care and a persistent wage gap continue to result in decisions about division of responsibility for paid and unpaid work within families that perpetuates gender inequity in earnings (Fortin et al, 2017; Goldin, 2021). Women also are more likely than men to work part time (Patterson, 2018), reflecting women's greater responsibilities for childcare and further reinforcing gender inequity. Women's labour force participation was particularly hard hit during the global pandemic, when women bore the brunt of family care responsibilities, including home schooling and eldercare (Desjardin et al, 2020; Goldin, 2022). When families must make choices as to who will take a carer leave, financial imperatives will most often dictate that the lower wage earner (most often women) will be the logical 'choice'. This is evidenced in part by the fact that most claimants in the 2019–20 fiscal year were women for the CCL (70.5 per cent), CIL for children (77.8 per cent) and CIL for adults (67.9 per cent) (Canada Employment Insurance Commission, 2021).

One evaluation of the Compassionate Care Benefit (CCB) also suggests that older carers are over-represented among CCL claimants. Employed carers aged 45–54 and 55 years old and over represent 20.6 per cent and 21.6 per cent of the labour force, respectively, but received 31.7 per cent and 35.6 per cent of the total amount paid for CCB. Conversely, carers aged 25–45 years comprise 43.5 per cent of the labour force, but they received only 31.2 per cent of all benefits paid (Canada Employment Insurance Commission, 2021). These figures are congruent with recent research showing that baby-boomer carers contribute the most to care in Canada, as compared to other generational cohorts (Fast et al, 2023).

Other inequities arise from the conditions underlying the need for carer leaves and the age of the care receiver. Over time, eligible health conditions have been expanded to include not only end-of-life care but also critical illness or injury. While the longer carer leaves described earlier cover only working carers who are providing care to family members with the most serious health conditions, carers of family members with ongoing chronic conditions, who comprise the majority of carers in Canada, are left out (Armstrong and O'Grady, 2004). They are not eligible for either CCL or CIL leaves unless the care receiver's chronic condition deteriorates substantially. As a result, the much shorter FRL is the only option available to those supporting someone with a chronic condition. Further changes to extend CCL for up to three weeks beyond the death of a family member through a Private Member's Bill, Bill C-220, an Act to amend the Canada Labour Code (Bereavement Leave), passed unanimously in the federal House of Commons and the Senate in the spring of 2021 and became law in September 2021 after receiving Royal Assent (Jeneroux, 2021). While the CIL is available to care for both children and adults, the length of leave is more than double if caring for children under the age of 18, than if caring for adults, reflecting a greater value placed on supporting young families than on families later in the lifecourse.

Flexibility

Flexibility refers to the capacity of policy instruments to permit some leeway in how legislation is applied to benefit and support target users. Among the legislated leaves described earlier, there are several features that provide flexibility to working carers: the ability to share leaves, the ability to take leaves of varying durations and the opportunity for leaves to be taken more than once.

The CCL, CIL and their associated benefits can be shared by two or more employees who are caring for the same family member. When first introduced as part of the CCL, this was applauded as the first official acknowledgement that care receivers are surrounded by care networks (Fast et al, 2004). When shared, the total number of weeks of leave taken by all carers, either at the same time or sequentially, cannot exceed the maximum allowable 28 weeks within a 52-week period. In fiscal year 2019–20, less than one out of ten CCL claims approved (7.2 per cent) were shared among qualifying carers, consistent with the previous three fiscal years (6.4 per cent, 6.9 per cent and 7.5 per cent, respectively) (Canada Employment Insurance Commission, 2021).

Leaves are also flexible in the sense that they can be taken in shorter 'chunks'. For example, FRL can be taken in one-day increments. However, in some jurisdictions, any part of a day taken as FRL counts as a full day of time off unless the employer and employee agree otherwise. This condition may limit the flexibility that working carers need to manage their paid work and care work responsibilities, penalising those who need only a few hours off, for example to take immediate family members to medical appointments. Furthermore, days of FRL cannot be carried over from year to year or otherwise banked. CCL and CIL also are flexible in that the leave can be taken in separate, non-consecutive, one-week increments by the same carer, up to the maximum allowable within a 52-week period.

Finally, while the CCL is intended to support care at the end of life, a few jurisdictions recognise that death is difficult to predict. While the need is uncommon, the CCL can be taken more than once in two jurisdictions (British Columbia and Ontario) if the family member does not die within 26 weeks. Federally, it is also possible for an employee to take CCL more than once. However, the employee must wait until the expiry of the initial 52 weeks before taking another 28 weeks of leave. If the leave is interrupted, or a second leave is applied for after the initial 52-week period, a new medical certificate is required.

Relatedly, the medical certificate requirement may affect carers' ability or willingness to apply for the CCL or CIL. Carers may be unable to gauge how much time they have left with a family member and be uncertain about how to time their application for CCL. They also may be reluctant to seek a document that declares their family member to be at imminent risk of death or to have a life-threatening condition. Further, healthcare providers have been shown to be reluctant to issue such prognoses and to be poor predictors of these outcomes (Christakis and Lamont, 2000; Lamont and Christakis, 2001). Approximately one-third of applicants for CCL did not receive benefits, with absence of a medical certificate among the primary reasons for disentitlement (Canada Employment Insurance Commission, 2021).

Job protection

Job protection affords employees job security while they are absent from work, either when they are ill or when caring for a family member. The Canada Labour Code and provincial Employment Standards legislation for all the leaves already described provide job security, requiring employers to guarantee that employees who take such leaves are able to return to an equivalent job on conclusion of the leave. The employee must be reinstated in their former position or be given a comparable position in the same location and with the same wages and benefits. An employer may not dismiss, suspend, lay off, demote or discipline an employee because the employee has taken or intends to take CCL or CIL. The employer also cannot take such leaves into account in any decision to promote or train an employee. This has been articulated by the Employment Standards Tribunal and is well established in case law. Furthermore, Canadian human rights law prohibits discrimination on the protected ground of family status. This means that people who need to provide care to family members also have a right to participate fully in the labour force, and employers have a legal obligation and duty to accommodate these employees, unless it causes 'undue hardship' to the organisation (Canadian Human Rights Commission, 2014). That said, the cross-jurisdictional variability already described results in job protection for most, but not all, working carers in Canada.

Yet uptake of available carer leave programmes remains low, even among those who are eligible. In fact, the utilisation rate of the CCL fell for two consecutive fiscal years between 2018–19 and 2019–20 (Canada Employment Insurance Commission, 2021). Perhaps the most fundamental hurdle to effective and comprehensive carer support policy is the low level of awareness about care as a social issue and as a legitimate workplace and policy issue, and about programmes and benefits that might be available to carers. As always, many people fail even to identify themselves as carers (Milligan and Morbey, 2013). Administrative hurdles also may make working carers ineligible, or discourage them from applying, for available programmes. The need for a doctor's declaration that the care receiver is at end of life, or has a life-threatening illness, has been a significant barrier (Employment and Social Development Canada, 2016).

Income security

Income security refers to a person's ability to pay for their basic needs without fear of losing their income source. For many working carers in Canada, loss of income accompanies most absences from work to attend to family care responsibilities. The negative impact of caregiving on employment is well documented and includes missing days of paid work, reducing hours of paid work and exiting the labour force altogether (Keating et al, 2014; Magnaye et al, 2023). While the question has not been asked in national surveys of Canadian carers, findings from Australia, Japan, UK and US report that care-related employment consequences result in financial hardship for many carers (Friss Feinberg and Skufca, 2020; National Alliance for Caregiving and AARP, 2020; Spann et al, 2020; Kikuzawa and Uemura, 2021; Furnival and Cullen, 2022). In the following paragraphs we analyse the impact of legislated leaves on carers' income security.

Half of carers in Canada (51 per cent in 2018) experienced absenteeism because of their caregiving, with women missing 9.7 consecutive days on average and men missing 6.8 consecutive days annually (Magnaye et al, 2023). This exceeds the FRL days provided by most jurisdictions. One Canadian study (Fast and Dosman, 2013) estimated the earnings losses associated with care-related absenteeism for individual caregivers (age 45+) caring for older adults for the periods 1997–2002 and 2003–08. They reported that workers who needed to take whole or part days away from paid work in order to provide care to an older person experienced wage losses that ranged from just over CA$100 to approximately CA$550 annually. These costs were generally higher in later life, during peak earning years and for men relative to women. Population-level aggregate annual care-related income losses associated with absences were found to have grown substantially between the two time periods studied: CA$37.6 million for women and CA$27.0 million for men during the period 1997–2002 and CA$83.7 million for women and CA$49.2 million for men during the later period 2003–08.

Many employed carers use their sick days, personal days, banked overtime and/or vacation time to manage their paid work and care work responsibilities and to avoid these income losses (Williams et al, 2011). While FRL affords job protection, most carers who take FRL do so without pay unless covered by their employer as part of an employment contract or collective agreement. For employees covered by the Canada Labour Code, the first three (of five) days are paid at the employee's regular rate if they have worked for the same employer for at least three consecutive months.

While the CCL and CIL themselves are unpaid, eligible employees may apply for CCB or Family Caregiving Benefits (FCB), respectively, which are delivered through the federal EI Special Benefits programme. The EI programme is essentially an insurance programme which replaces, in part, claimants' lost employment income while on leave. The CCB and FCB address carers' income security to some extent and reduce some of the financial stress associated with providing care (Williams et al, 2011). However, the relatively low benefit rate has been a long-standing criticism of the programme and is not reflective of the full costs associated with providing end-of-life or critical care (Osborne and Margo, 2005; Flagler and Dong, 2010; Williams et al, 2011). While the EI benefit amount is 55 per cent of pre-leave salary to a *maximum* of CA$650 per week in December 2022, the *average* weekly benefit paid is much lower (CA$482 for CCB, CA$449 for FCB for adults and CA$462 for FCB for children in the 2019–20 fiscal year) (Canada Employment Insurance Commission, 2021). Similarly, the *average* duration of benefits is much lower than the legislated *maximum* (11.0 weeks for CCB, 10.6 weeks for FCB for adults and 15.4 weeks for FCB for children in the 2019–20 fiscal year). For CCB specifically, 61 per cent of claimants received six weeks of benefits, while only 17.3 per cent received the maximum 26 weeks of benefits. The main reason for leaves shorter than the maximum allowed is the death of the care receiver. A Private Member's Bill that extends CCB benefits by ten days following the death of a care receiver became law in September 2021 (Jeneroux, 2021).

An evaluation of the former EI Parents of Critically Ill Children (PCIC) Benefit showed that this benefit eased financial stresses associated with caring for a critically ill or injured child, provided some flexibility in managing family and work responsibilities, reduced divorce or separation rates among recipients and helped keep recipients attached to the paid labour force

(Employment and Social Development Canada, 2017). This benefit has since been replaced by the Family Caregiver Benefit for Children, which was intended to address some of the original PCIC programme's shortcomings, but no evaluation of the new benefit has yet been published. The one-week waiting period (equivalent to the deductible for other types of employment insurance), which remains for the new FCB benefit, adds to the inadequacy of income replacement for these leaves, and is a substantial disincentive to apply for the benefit, especially among carers with higher incomes. While the legislation does allow employers to top up EI benefits, a 2012 study showed that few employers did so for family carers (10 per cent), in stark contrast to those that provided a top-up for EI or Quebec Parental Insurance Program maternity (41 per cent), parental (30 per cent) or paternity (24 per cent) leave benefits (Lero et al, 2012). It has been argued that making the CCB independent from Canada's Employment Insurance Program would make it more effective and foster a more compassionate programme that supports all carers (Flagler and Dong, 2010).

Another, probably more substantial, source of income insecurity for family carers in Canada is a failure to address future income losses that arise from care-related labour force exits and reduced working hours. In 2018, 15 per cent of employed Canadian carers reported that they reduced their hours of paid work and another 6 per cent reported that they had quit, retired or were fired from their jobs in the previous year because of their care responsibilities (Magnaye et al, 2023). The annual aggregate wage losses from leaving the labour force because of caring was estimated at CA$81.9 million for women and CA$53.8 million for men during the period 2003–08, while the annual aggregate wage losses arising from reducing working hours from full-time to part-time were estimated at CA$54.9 million for women and CA$13.3 million for men (Fast and Dosman, 2013). In both cases, eldercare-related wage losses were substantially higher during the 2003–08 period than in the previous six-year period from 1997 to 2002. However, it should be noted that these figures were based on care provided by carers aged 45 years and over to older people only, who comprise less than half of all carers. In addition, women are more likely to experience these income losses during childbearing/rearing years and in the years leading up to retirement (Ehrlich et al, 2020).

The Canada Pension Plan (CPP), one of three pillars of Canada's retirement income system, is a contributory plan such that retirement benefits received are affected by claimants' length of service and level of earnings. Employer pension plans also are increasingly defined contribution rather than defined benefit plans, which also are affected by length of service and earnings. In both cases, care-related labour force exits and reduced hours of work reduce pension plan contributions, and so also reduce retirement benefits (Evandrou and Glaser, 2003). Women are still more likely than men to take leaves, reduce labour force participation or exit the labour force altogether and experience more substantial cumulative financial consequences by doing so (Smith et al, 2020). Recommendations that would address Canadian carers' income insecurity in the longer term by providing a CPP caregiving drop-out provision akin to the long-standing CPP child-rearing drop-out have had no uptake. Pension amounts are adjusted for certain months in which employees have low or no income. The child-rearing and general drop-out provisions result in years of low or no earnings being dropped automatically from the calculation of average earnings on which the benefit calculation is based. The child-rearing drop-out applies to the period when a taxpayer is raising children under age seven. The general drop-out provision, intended to compensate for periods spent in education, unemployment or care-related labour force absences, now allows up to 17 per cent of the taxpayer's lowest earning years to be dropped from the calculation (up to eight years for those who work from age 18 to 65). However, for many taxpayers this does not cover all these periods of low or no earnings (Clemens and Emes, 2016).

COVID-19 pandemic response and implications for employed carers

In 2020, the COVID-19 global pandemic brought the plight of family carers (and professional carers) into sharp public focus. Barely a day went by without media stories about rampant outbreaks in long-term care facilities, carers overburdened with new or radically altered care responsibilities, work-from-home mandates and significant job losses. Home care shortages increased the workload for carers; family members in need of care moved in with their carers; other family carers were locked out of residential care facilities to reduce the risk of virus transmission (Parmar et al, 2021). The pandemic response restrictions intensified family carers' isolation and stress, reduced their ability to obtain much-needed outside support and increased their financial burden (Kent et al, 2020; Ontario Caregiver Organization, 2020). The federal government responded by making two temporary programmes available to support families with care responsibilities who needed financial assistance.

Temporary changes to the EI programme improved access to FCB (described earlier) for carers who needed to take time away from work to provide care or support to a critically ill or injured person or someone needing end-of-life care. To qualify for benefits, an employed or self-employed worker needed 120 insured hours in a 52-week period (down from 600) during the first year of the pandemic, but this was later increased to 420 insured hours. The 52-week period to accumulate insured hours was also extended for those who received the Canada Emergency Response Benefit (available to workers who lost income as a result of the COVID-19 pandemic from 15 March to 3 October 2020). Eligible applicants received a minimum benefit of CA$500 per week before taxes, but could receive financial assistance of up to 55 per cent of usual earnings, to a maximum of CA$595 per week. This programme ran for two years, from 27 September 2020 to 24 September 2022.

The Canada Recovery Caregiving Benefit (CRCB) provided income support to employed and self-employed workers who were unable to work for at least half of the week because they had to care for a child under age 12 or a family member who needed supervised care. This situation may have arisen because schools, day care or care facilities were closed due to COVID-19 or because the child or family member was sick, was required to quarantine or was at high risk of serious health consequences because of COVID-19. Administered by the Canada Revenue Agency, the CRCB provided *households* with CA$500 (CA$450 after taxes were withheld) weekly. Recipients had to apply every week for a maximum of 26 weeks. The 26 weeks did not need to be taken consecutively and could be applied retrospectively up to 60 days after a period ended. Implemented in September 2020, this programme was suspended in May 2022.

Provincial jurisdictions across Canada also introduced new or strengthened existing unpaid job-protected leaves for workers affected by COVID-19. British Columbia, Alberta, Saskatchewan, Manitoba, Ontario, Newfoundland and New Brunswick provided an unpaid, job-protected infectious disease or public health emergency leave for employees who were unable to perform their job duties for reasons related to COVID-19. Nova Scotia made emergency leave available when the provincial government declares an emergency under the Emergency Management Act or Health Protection Act or when the Medical Officer of Health issues a directive or order. The Yukon government introduced a new regulation that allows an employee to take leave without pay for a period of up to 14 days if they require it and complements the 10-day COVID-19-related rebate available to employers who pay employees to take time off for sick leave or self-isolation due to COVID-19. In all jurisdictions, the leave applies as long as the circumstances set out in the legislation apply.

Other support measures for carers

Recent Canadian case law has begun to establish carers' right to request flexible working arrangements, under human rights legislation. More recently, the federal government has enacted right to request flexible working legislation that conveys this right to all Canadians employed in federally regulated industries. Its intent is to allow employees to more flexibly balance work and home life (Government of Canada, 2022). None of Canada's ten provinces or three territories have yet followed suit, but workers in provincially regulated industries can still rely on human rights legislation to pursue this right.

In contrast, Canada does relatively poorly on other forms of carer support not tied to employment. In 2011, the province of Manitoba enacted its Caregiver Recognition Act, the only jurisdiction in Canada to do so. Its purpose is to acknowledge the vital role of carers and to set out general principles for governments and agencies to promote. While the Act requires that the government of Manitoba reports periodically on the situation of its constituent carers and establishes an annual carer recognition day and an inventory of carer supports and services, no tangible supports or services are enabled by it and the promised carer recognition and support framework has yet to materialise at the time of writing.

Continuing care policy clearly favours community-based care over institutional/residential care, though this also is consistent with care receivers' and carers' preferences for ageing in the community. Home care and continuing care programmes deliver services to those in need of care in all Canadian jurisdictions, though there are substantial variations across jurisdictions in the 'basket' of goods and services that are covered, in eligibility criteria for cost subsidies and in the amount of subsidy provided (Canadian Home Care Association, 2011). Yet resource allocation decisions are incongruent with this policy priority, with only 4 per cent of total public spending on healthcare services going to the home and community care sector (Canadian Institute for Health Information, 2021). While home care services were originally developed to support older people and others with chronic conditions to continue living in the community, increasing demand for and cost of delivering health and continuing care services have resulted in policy changes that prioritise what has become known as post-acute care (medical services that support a patient's continued recovery after acute care hospital discharge). As a result, home care services for persons with chronic conditions are severely rationed, based on an expectation that family carers will continue to provide the bulk of the care. Of course, this fails to recognise that the escalating burden on carers means they will have greater difficulty maintaining paid work alongside their care work despite the availability of a range of carer leaves accompanied by partial income replacement.

Some provincial jurisdictions have implemented self-managed care programmes which provide cash benefits to care recipients with which they can purchase the services they need. In some jurisdictions, care recipients may use these funds to compensate family members or friends for the care they provide. While these schemes are popular and appealing, implying as they do greater choice and the opportunity to support family carers, they come with two substantial barriers. First, there are severe shortages of trained care workers in Canada, such that many care receivers who would prefer to hire a personal care aide have difficulty finding one. And second, the care receiver (or their carer) must take on all the administrative responsibilities of an employer (hiring, firing, payroll, tax withholding and so on). A few jurisdictions have addressed the latter challenge by delegating these administrative responsibilities to a third party.

Nova Scotia is the only Canadian jurisdiction that provides a Caregiver Benefit to carers who provide more than 20 hours per week of care to a low-income care receiver with significant care needs. The maximum benefit in 2023 is CA$400 per month. Given that carers must be providing a minimum of 20 hours per week of care, the maximum implicit wage amounts to CA$4.65/hour, or one-third of Nova Scotia's minimum wage. The federal government also has introduced a set of non-refundable tax credits that can be used to reduce the carer's income tax liability. The amount depends on the carer's relationship with the care receiver, the care receiver's living situation and net income, and whether other credits are being claimed for that person. In 2018, only 8 per cent of carers reported receiving federal tax credits (Hango, 2020).

Legislation is not the only way carer leave can be provided, and governments are not the only providers of carer support measures. Employers, trade unions and collective agreements may also include/provide carer leaves, or other carer supports. Some Canadian employers are aware of the challenges that their working carers face in balancing paid work and care work responsibilities, but relatively few are taking targeted action to support them. The few existing Canadian investigations of workplace practices for assisting working carers have found that some employers are aware that family care is becoming a workplace issue, but are less aware of its magnitude – for example, that some 35 per cent of the Canadian workforce experience this work–family challenge. Few employers report addressing the issue directly or with formal workplace policies, instead dealing with it on a case-by-case basis and assuming that flexible working arrangements provided to all employees will meet the need (Lero et al, 2012; Employer Panel for Caregivers, 2015). A new voluntary Carer-Inclusive and Accommodating Organizations Workplace Standard has been developed (Canadian Standards Association, 2017) to guide employers and offer them a set of tools (practical solutions, information and case studies) to help them implement policies and programmes aimed at creating more accommodating workplaces.

Conclusion

Workers in Canada do relatively well when it comes to carer leaves. Legislation establishes a range of leaves that apply to a variety of caring circumstances – shorter and longer durations and for critical junctures in the care trajectory. An inclusive definition of family means that they also apply to most working carers. Importantly, other employment legislation provides partial income replacement for eligible employed carers, though the income replacement rate of 55 per cent to a maximum has been widely criticised for being inadequate.

The emphasis on policy instruments that support carers' employment is consistent with Canadian governments' political ideologies and values that prioritise the health of the economy as a strategy for achieving social as well as economic goals. This is increasingly evident as governments are building post-pandemic recovery with a strong commitment to 'deliver jobs and growth across the economy' (Department of Finance Canada, 2021). Carer leaves protect working carers' employment and earning capacity while simultaneously supporting the labour market.

Several federal policy measures were implemented during the pandemic to support carers, extending existing leaves and income support instruments. These were introduced as temporary responses but were extended as new waves of the pandemic hit. Despite advocates encouraging policy makers to make these measures permanent, all of them were discontinued as of September 2022, suggesting that Canada's poor history with respect to seizing opportunities to support carers prevails and the ongoing challenges faced by employed carers in Canada remain open for another 'window of opportunity.'

References

Armstrong, P. and O'Grady, K. (2004) 'Compassionate Care Benefits not compassionate enough', *The Canadian Women's Health Network–Network Magazine*, 64.

BCLI (2007) 'Report on the Parental Support Obligation in Section 90 of the Family Relations Act'. Available from: https://www.bcli.org/sites/default/files/Parental_Support_FRA_section_90_Report.pdf [Accessed 2 July 2021].

Bélanger, A., Martel, L. and Caron-Malenfant, E. (2005) 'Population projections for Canada, provinces and territories, 2005–2031'. Available from: https://www150.statcan.gc.ca/n1/en/pub/91-520-x/91-520-x2005 001-eng.pdf?st=5ZpvwGrh [Accessed 14 April 2021].

Blum, S., Dobrotić, I., Kaufman, G., Koslowski, A. and Moss, P. (2023) *International review of leave policies and research 2023*. Available from: http://www.leavenetwork.org/lp_and_r_reports/ [Accessed 14 April 2021].

Canada Employment Insurance Commission (2021) 'Employment insurance monitoring and assessment report for the fiscal year beginning April 1, 2019 and ending March 31, 2020.' Available from: https://www.canada.ca/en/employment-social-development/programs/ei/ei-list/reports/mon itoring2020.html [Accessed 3 May 2021].

Canadian Centre for Caregiving Excellence (2022) 'Giving care: an approach to a better caregiving landscape in Canada'. Available from: https://canadia ncaregiving.org/giving-care/ [Accessed 14 November 2022].

Canadian Home Care Association (2011) 'Access to quality health care: the home care contribution'. Available from: https://cdnhomecare.ca/wp-cont ent/uploads/2020/03/Access-to-Quality-Health-Care-CHCA-June-2011-English.pdf [Accessed 24 January 2024].

Canadian Human Rights Commission (2014) 'A guide to balancing work and caregiving obligations: Collaborative approaches for a supportive and well-performing workplace'. Available from: https://www.chrc-ccdp.gc.ca/sites/default/files/2020-07/a_guide_to_balancing_work.pdf [Accessed 24 January 2024].

Canadian Institute for Health Information (2021) 'National health expenditure trends, 2021 – snapshot'. Available from: https://www.cihi.ca/en/national-health-expenditure-trends-2021-snapshot [Accessed 8 June 2022].

Canadian Standards Association (2017) 'B701–17 Carer-inclusive and accommodating organizations'. Available from: https://www.csagroup.org/store/product/2425673/ [Accessed 24 January 2024].

Christakis, N. and Lamont, E. (2000) 'Extent and determinants of error in doctors' prognoses in terminally ill patients: prospective cohort study', *British Medical Journal*, 320(7233): 469–72.

Clemens, J. and Emes, J. (2016) 'Rates of return for the Canada Pension Plan'. Available from: https://www.fraserinstitute.org/sites/default/files/rates-of-return-for-the-canada-pension-plan.pdf [Accessed 24 January 2024].

Cox, M. (2019) 'Where's the compassion in Canada's compassionate care benefit program?' Moncton, sn.

Department of Finance Canada (2021) 'Supporting Canadians through the recovery'. Available from: https://www.canada.ca/en/department-fina nce/news/2021/12/supporting-canadians-through-the-recovery.html [Accessed 8 June 2022].

Desjardin, D., Freestone, C. and Powell, N. (2020) 'Pandemic threatens decades of women's labour force gains'. Available from: https://thoughtlea dership.rbc.com/pandemic-threatens-decades-of-womens-labour-force-gains/ [Accessed 14 April 2021].

Dymond, B. and Hart, M. (2004) 'Canada and the new American empire: asking the right questions'. Available from: https://policyoptions.irpp.org/magazines/north-american-integration/canada-and-the-new-american-empire-asking-the-right-questions/ [Accessed 14 April 2021].

Ehrlich, U., Möhring, K. and Drobnič, S. (2020) 'What comes after caring? The impact of family care on women's employment', *Journal of Family Issues*, 41(9): 1387–419.

Employer Panel for Caregivers (2015) 'When work and caregiving collide: how employers can support their employees who are caregivers'. Available from: https://www.canada.ca/en/news/archive/2015/01/minis ter-wong-releases-report-employer-panel-caregivers.html [Accessed 24 January 2024].

Employment and Social Development Canada (2016) 'Stakeholder roundtable summary: Employment Insurance Special Benefits consultations.' Available from: https://publications.gc.ca/site/eng/9.840467/publication.html [Accessed 29 June 2022].

Employment and Social Development Canada (2017) 'Evaluation of the Employment Insurance Parents of Critically Ill Children Benefit'. Available from: https://www.canada.ca/en/employment-social-development/corporate/reports/evaluations/parents-critically-ill-children-benefit.html [Accessed 24 January 2024].

Evandrou, M. and Glaser, K. (2003) 'Combining work and family life: the pension penalty of caring', *Ageing & Society*, 23(5): 583–601.

Fast, J. and Dosman, D. (2013) 'Monetizing the costs of eldercare-related employment consequences', Final report provided to Human Resources and Skills Development Canada.

Fast, J., Duncan, K.A., Keating, N. and Kim, C. (2023) 'Valuing the contributions of family caregivers to the care economy', *Journal of Family and Economic Issues*, https://doi.org/10.1007/s10834-023-09899-8

Fast, J., Keating, N., Otfinowski, P. and Derksen, L (2004) 'Characteristics of family/friend care networks of frail seniors', *Canadian Journal on Aging*, 23(1): 5–19.

Flagler, J. and Dong, W. (2010) 'The uncompassionate elements of the Compassionate Care Benefits Program: a critical analysis', *Global Health Promotion*, 17(1): 50–9.

Fortin, N., Bell, B. and Bohm, M. (2017) 'Top earnings inequality and the gender pay gap: Canada, Sweden and the United Kingdom', *Labour Economics*, 47: 107–23.

Friss Feinberg, L. and Skufca, L. (2020) 'Managing a paid job and family caregiving is a growing reality', Washington DC: AARP Public Policy Institute.

Furnival, A. and Cullen, D. (2022) 'Caring costs us: the economic impact on lifetime income and retirement savings of informal carers', Sydney: Carers Australia and the National Carer Network.

Gardiner, H. (2011) 'My parents' keeper'. Available from: https://www.canadianlawyermag.com/news/general/my-parents-keeper/268141 [Accessed 14 April 2021].

Goldin, C. (2021) *Career and family: Women's century-long journey toward equity.* Princeton, NJ: Princeton University Press.

Goldin, C. (2022) 'Understanding the economic impact of COVID-19 on women', *Brookings Papers on Economic Activity (Spring)*: 65–110. Available from: https://scholar.harvard.edu/goldin/publications/understanding-economic-impact-covid-19-women [Accessed 11 October 2023].

Government of Canada (2022) 'Flexible work arrangements for federally regulated employees'. Available from: https://www.canada.ca/en/emp loyment-social-development/corporate/portfolio/labour/programs/lab our-standards/flexible-work-arrangements.html [Accessed 8 June 2022].

Hango, D. (2020) 'Insights on Canadian Society: Support received by caregivers in Canada'. Available from: https://www150.statcan.gc.ca/n1/pub/75-006-x/2020001/article/00001-eng.htm [Accessed 24 January 2024].

Jeneroux, M. (2021) 'Bill C-220 – Analysis of changes to my Private Members' Bill'. Available from: https://mattjeneroux.ca/bill-c220/ [Accessed 24 January 2024].

Keating, N., Fast, J., Lero, D., Lucas, S. and Eales, J. (2014) 'A taxonomy of the economic costs of family care to adults', *Journal of the Economics of Ageing*, 3: 11–20.

Kent, E., Ornstein, K. and Dionne-Odom, J. (2020) 'The family caregiving crisis meets an actual pandemic', *Journal of Pain Symptom Management*, 60(1): e66–e69.

Kikuzawa, S. and Uemura, R. (2021) 'Parental caregiving and employment among midlife women in Japan', *Research on Aging*, 43(2): 107–18.

Lamont, E. and Christakis, N. (2001) 'Prognostic disclosure to patients with cancer near the end of life', *Annals of Internal Medicine*, 134(12): 1096–105.

Lero, D., Spinks, N., Fast, J., Hilbrecht, M. and Tremblay, D.-G. (2012) 'The availability, accessibility and effectiveness of workplace supports for Canadian caregivers', s.l.: Final report provided to Human Resources and Skills Development Canada.

Lohmann, H., Peter, F.H., Rostgaard, T. and Spiess, C.K. (2009) 'Towards a Framework for Assessing Family Policies in the EU', OECD Social, Employment and Migration Working Papers No. 88, Paris: Organization for Economic Cooperation and Development.

Magnaye, A., Kim, C., Eales, J. and Fast, J. (2022) 'Snapshots of aging: who are employed caregivers in Canada?' Available from: https://rapp.ualberta. ca/snapshot-of-aging/ [Accessed 16 December 2022].

Magnaye, A., Kim, C., Eales, J. and Fast, J. (2023) 'Snapshots of aging: how does caregiving impact paid work for employed women and men?' Available from: https://rapp.ualberta.ca/snapshot-of-aging/ [Accessed 23 January 2023].

Milligan, C. and Morbey, H. (2013) *Older men who care: Understanding their support and support needs*, Lancaster: Lancaster University Centre for Ageing Research.

Moore, M. (2016) 'Identical origins, divergent paths: Filial responsibility laws in Canada and the United States', Master of Laws thesis, Queens University, Kingston.

Moyser, M. (2017) *Women and paid work*, Ottawa: Statistics Canada (catalogue no 89-503-X2015001).

National Alliance for Caregiving and AARP (2020) 'Caregiving in the U.S. 2020', Washington, DC: National Alliance for Caregiving and AARP. [Online]

Natural Resources Canada (2020) 'Ten key facts on Canada's natural resources'. Available from: https://natural-resources.canada.ca/science-and-data/data-and-analysis/key-facts-and-figures-on-the-natural-resources-sector/16013 [Accessed 14 April 2021].

OECD (2023) 'Life expectancy at birth (indicator), Canada'. Available from: https://data.oecd.org/healthstat/life-expectancy-at-birth.htm#indicator-chart [Accessed 24 January 2024].

Olsen, G.M. (2007) 'Toward global welfare state convergence: family policy and health care in Sweden, Canada and the United States', *Journal of Sociology and Social Welfare*, 34(2): 143–64.

Ontario Caregiver Organization (2020) '2020 spotlight on Ontario caregivers – COVID-19 edition'. Available from: https://ontariocaregiver.ca/spotlight-report/ [Accessed 24 January 2024].

Osborne, K. and Margo, N. (2005) 'Compassionate Care Benefit analysis and evaluation'. Available from: https://publications.gc.ca/collections/collection_2007/hcc-ccs/H174-10-2005E.pdf [Accessed 24 January 2024].

Parmar, J. and Anderson, S. (2021) 'A tale of two solitudes experienced by Alberta family caregivers during the COVID-19 pandemic'. Available from: https://acfp.ca/wp-content/uploads/2021/02/751-Anderson_A-TALE-OF-TWO-SOLITUDES-EXPERIENCED-BY-ALBERTA-FAMILY-CAREGIVERS-DURING-THE-COVID-19-PANDEMIC.pdf [Accessed 8 June 2022].

Patterson, M. (2018) 'Who works part time and why?' Available from: https://www150.statcan.gc.ca/n1/en/pub/71-222-x/71-222-x2018002-eng.pdf?st=-M14-qJf [Accessed 2 July 2021].

Prince, M. (2015) 'Canada's Compassionate Care Benefit needs a rethink'. Available from: https://www.theglobeandmail.com/opinion/canadas-compassionate-care-benefit-needs-a-rethink/article24164935/ [Accessed 24 January 2024].

Sheets, D. and Gallagher, E. (2013) 'Aging in Canada: state of the art and science', *The Gerontologist*, 53(1): 1–8.

Smith, P., Cawley, C., Williams, A. and Mustard, C. (2020) 'Male/female differences in the impact of caring for elderly relatives on labor market attachment and hours of work: 1997–2015', *Journals of Gerontology Series B: Psychological Sciences and Social Sciences*, 75(3): 694–704.

Spann, A., Vicente, J., Allard, C., Hawley, M., Spreeuwenberg, M. and de Witte, L. (2020) 'Challenges of combining work and unpaid care, and solutions: a scoping review', *Health and Social Care in the Community*, 28(3): 699–715.

Statistics Canada (2015) 'The surge of women in the workforce'. Available from: https://www150.statcan.gc.ca/n1/en/pub/11-630-x/11-630-x2015 009-eng.pdf?st=CzuSH4H- [Accessed 24 January 2024].

Statistics Canada (2017) 'Age and sex, and type of dwelling data: key results from the 2016 Census'. Available from: https://www150.statcan.gc.ca/n1/daily-quotidien/170503/dq170503a-eng.htm [Accessed 24 January 2024].

Statistics Canada (2022a) 'Labour force characteristics by age group, monthly, seasonally adjusted'. Available from: https://www150.statcan.gc.ca/t1/tbl1/en/tv.action?pid=1410028702&pickMembers per cent5B0 per cent5D=1.1&pickMembers per cent5B1 per cent5D=3.3&cubeTimeFrame.startMonth=04&cubeTimeFrame.startYear=2022&referencePeriods=20220401 per cent2C20220401 [Accessed 6 May 2022].

Statistics Canada (2022b) 'Population projections for Canada, Provinces and Territories, 2021 to 2068'. Available from: https://www150.statcan.gc.ca/n1/pub/91-520-x/91-520-x2022001-eng.htm [Accessed 22 November 2023].

Statistics Canada (2023a) 'Canada's population estimates: record-high population growth in 2022', *The Daily*, 22 March. Available from: https://www150.statcan.gc.ca/n1/en/daily-quotidien/230322/dq230322f-eng.pdf?st=kNZg7OiA [Accessed 23 June 2023].

Statistics Canada (2023b) 'Labour force survey, December 2022'. Available from: https://www150.statcan.gc.ca/n1/daily-quotidien/230106/dq2301 06a-eng.htm [Accessed 23 January 2023].

The Petro-Canada CareMakers Foundation (2021/2022) 'Family caregiving in Canada: addressing systemic challenges and identifying opportunities for action', Toronto: Author. Available from: https://www.caremakers.ca/resources [Accessed 23 January 2023].

Williams, A.M., Eby, J.A., Crooks, V.A., Stajduhar, K., Giesbrecht, M. Vuksan, M. et al (2011) 'Canada's Compassionate Care Benefit: is it an adequate public health response to addressing the issue of caregiver burden in end-of-life care?' *BMC Public Health*, 11: 335.

7

Germany

Katja Knauthe and Andreas Hoff

Introduction

In Germany, five million people need long-term care as defined by the Long-Term Care Insurance Act. Most (83.5 per cent) of those in need of care and support are aged 65 years or older, with 33.3 per cent aged 85 years or older. Most (62 per cent) are women (Stat. Bundesamt, 2022a). The German care regime rests on the subsidiarity principle[1] that explicitly encourages care at home, primarily by family members (for example, Anttonen and Sipilä, 1996). Accordingly, German Long-Term Care Insurance (LTCI) legislation states: 'LTCI is meant to support with their benefits primarily home care and the willingness of family members and neighbours to give care in order to allow those in need of care to stay in their homes for as long as possible' (Deutscher Bundestag, 1994, authors' translation). Indeed, most people in Germany prefer to be cared for at home (Kuhlmey et al, 2010; Hayek et al, 2018). The law supports this wish with benefits from LTCI. The proportion of people cared for at home has increased by 10 per cent since 2000 (from 70 per cent to 80 per cent) (BMG, 2021b, 2021c). There are an estimated four to five million carers in Germany.[2] Three out of four carers under the age of 65 are still working. The majority are women (75 per cent) who combine care and work (Geyer et al, 2014; Knauthe and Deindl, 2019; Eggert et al, 2021).

Research has highlighted the challenges related to reconciling the conflicting demands of care and employment. Difficulties for working carers include time conflicts that lead to an increased propensity to work part time, often in less well-paid jobs, and an inability to participate in training or to attend social events important for promotion. There are a number of adverse effects of caring on work performance, including absenteeism, lateness, increased use of sick leave, lack of energy, higher propensity to make mistakes and so on, as is well documented (for example, Hoff et al, 2014; Eggert et al, 2021).

The question of who should be responsible for implementing measures aimed at enabling a successful reconciliation of family care and employment has been controversial for many years (FMFSWY, 2011, 2019; Geyer et al, 2014; ZQP, 2018). If long-term care (LTC) is a societal challenge, there are those who argue that the government ought to pass appropriate legislation (INTERVAL, 2018; FMFSWY, 2019). However, it has also been suggested that because employers can benefit from a successful reconciliation, particularly in the light of severe skilled labour shortages in many German industries, they should facilitate the combination of work and care.

This chapter provides an overview of the most important legal measures intended to contribute to a better reconciliation of caring and paid work. The focus is explicitly on care for older people – and not on childcare. The next section sets the scene by providing background information on the political context, state of the economy/labour market situation and demographic structure. This is followed by a section examining various laws influencing the circumstances of working carers. The effect of the COVID-19 pandemic on working carers is then discussed. This is followed by a critical review of existing policies and the chapter ends with some concluding remarks.

National context

This section provides key information about the political background and the German welfare state, the current state of the economy/labour market and demographic change.

Political background

Germany is often referred to as a 'social market economy' that is, a market economy that 'combines the principle of the market with that of social compensation' (Müller–Armack, 1976: 243, author's translation). Esping-Andersen (1990) categorised Germany as a conservative-corporatist welfare state regime, indicating the strong role of corporatism in labour market affairs as well as the dominance of conservative family norms and values in family policy and caregiving. With the emergence of care regime classifications, Germany was specified as 'a care regime reliant on unpaid care (though partly compensated for by the government)' (Anttonen and Sipilä, 1996).

German government revenues amounted to around €1.6 trillion in 2020 (Statista, 2022b). Most of this comes from taxation and social insurance contributions. In 2020, the volume of social welfare state expenditure was around €1.1 trillion. This corresponds to around 33.6 per cent of gross domestic product (GDP), which represents an increase of 3.3 percentage points as compared to 2019, which is primarily due to higher expenditure as a result of the COVID-19 pandemic (BMAS, 2021b).

Germany is a federal republic consisting of 16 federal states (*Bundesländer*). This is important, since the federal states are responsible for implementation of legislation at regional level and have additional legislative power. Thus, LTC planning and delivery vary widely across federal states.

Economic and labour market context

Germany is the largest economy in the European Union (EU) and the fourth-largest in the world after the United States, China and Japan. Whereas Germany experienced high levels of unemployment during the 1990s and 2000s – with 6–9 per cent in West Germany and 14–19 per cent in East Germany – unemployment dropped to 4 per cent in West Germany and 6 per cent in East Germany by the end of 2019 (bpb, 2020). However, the COVID-19 pandemic halted the decline in unemployment: in 2022 the unemployment rate averaged around 5.2 per cent, recovering slightly from 5.7 per cent a year earlier (2021) (Statista, 2022a).

With regard to the development of unemployment (as a result of the COVID-related lockdowns), there were hardly any gender-specific differences. Men and women were equally affected by a (short-term) increase in unemployment during the pandemic. In the first year of the pandemic in Germany, in 2020, the unemployment rate for women rose from 5.4 to 6.1 per cent. Afterwards, there were signs of this further easing, so that in April 2022 only 4.8 per cent were registered as unemployed. The development was similar for men. While before 2020 the unemployment rate was 6.2 per cent, it rose to 6.8 per cent during the pandemic but fell to 5.3 per cent in 2022 (Bundesagentur für Arbeit, 2022).

The situation is different when it comes to work–life balance. As a result of kindergarten and school closures and contact bans, established informal care networks were significantly weakened, leaving childcare and school learning entirely the responsibility of parents. The main burden of childcare during the lockdown was borne by mothers. For them, the duration of childcare on weekdays increased from 2.9 hours before the pandemic to 9.6 hours. In contrast, childcare time for fathers also increased – but only by 2.5 hours per weekday compared to before the pandemic (Fuchs-Schündeln and Stephan, 2020; Zinn et al, 2020; Haupt et al, 2022). There are no comparable studies for family carers providing care for adults.

Demographic structure

Germany is the most populous country in the EU, with 83.2 million inhabitants (Eurostat, 2020; Stat. Bundesamt, 2022c). The number of deaths has exceeded the number of births since 1972. Average life expectancy at birth has increased to 78.6 years for boys and 83.4 years for girls (Stat. Bundesamt, 2022e). Birth rates have fallen since the mid-1960s. Although there has been a slight increase in birth rates in recent years, a total fertility rate of 1.53 children per woman (2019) is still well below the population maintenance level of 2.1 children per woman (Huinink and Schröder, 2019; Stat. Bundesamt, 2022d, 2022e). So far, net immigration has been the main factor preventing a population decline (BMG, 2021c: 13). The falling birth rate has contributed to a rapidly ageing society. The median age in Germany is 45.9 years (2021), making it the 'second oldest' country in Europe after Italy (47.6 years) (Statista, 2022c).

The current age structure predicts a decline in the working-age population and an increase in the number of people in retirement over the next 20 years. The number of people aged 67 and over will increase from 16 million (19 per cent) in 2018 to over 21 million in 2060. The working-age population is expected to shrink from 52 million currently to about 40–46 million in 2060. The number of people aged 80 and over is predicted to rise from 5.4 million (6 per cent) at present to 7.8–9.9 million (9–13 per cent) in 2060 (Stat. Bundesamt, 2019, 2022d). The risk of needing LTC rises with age from 1.6 per cent for those under 60 to 8 per cent for people aged 60 to 80, reaching 39.9 per cent for those older than 80 years (BMG, 2021b, 2021c).

There is a correlation between the need for care and the degree of disability. The rate of severe disability is highest among people aged 65 and over. According to the Federal Statistical Office, the rate of severely disabled people over the age of 65 was 24.7 per cent. Looking at women over the age of 65, the rate is 60 per cent. It is similarly high for men at 56 per cent. Almost half of all severely disabled people in Germany are aged between 55 and 74 years (Stat. Bundesamt, 2022b, 2022f).

Care leave policies

Before the introduction of the Caregiver Leave Act in 2008, there were only a few options for employees to look after relatives in need of care. As a rule, employees had to apply for vacation days or unpaid leave to care for their relatives. However, there were also some collective agreements that gave employees the opportunity to take time off work for a limited period to look after relatives in need of care. These regulations were not universal, though, and applied only to certain sectors and occupational groups. In addition to these mostly unpaid leave options, Germany has had the Part-Time and Fixed-Term Employment Act (TzBfG) since 2001. It enables employees to reduce their working hours, for example to meet family obligations, including caring for relatives. Employees are generally entitled to part-time work if the company has more than 15 employees. But the employer can reject the part-time application for operational reasons. This and the next section focus on support options for family carers. They explain the German laws and present official funding options as well as indirect ways, such as paid sick leave, to reconcile care and work. The focus is on care leave policies.

However, other LTC policies are considered too. First and foremost, the LTCI is the central piece of legislation in this field. Since it influences the financial situation of people in need of care considerably, it affects working carers too and will be looked at first.

Long-term Care Insurance

The German LTCI was introduced more than 25 years ago in 1995 and was the first such social insurance scheme worldwide. It aimed to mitigate the financial and social impact of LTC risk, to sustainably improve the situation of people in need of LTC and their families and to create incentives to expand LTC provision in Germany (BMG, 2021c: 11 ff). LTCI did not change the family's obligation to provide care – if anything, it reinforced it by adding a *legal* obligation to the moral obligation for families to provide care.

LTCI follows a similar rationale to that of Health Insurance (HI) (*Krankenversicherung*). Everybody living in Germany is obliged to take out both types of insurance – either in the statutory (89 per cent of the population) or private system (11 per cent) (BMG, 2021c). Statutory LTCI is funded by employee and employer insurance contributions. The contribution to LTCI is levied together with the contribution to HI and currently amounts to 3.4 per cent (as of 1 June 2023). Contributions are paid on a parity basis, that is, employers and employees each pay half. The surcharge for those without children is 0.6 per cent. There is an exemption for children under the age of 18. If the child is not yet in education, this is extended to the age of 23. They are generally insured free of charge with their parents. The same applies to family members. In addition to children, this may include spouses who have no income of their own (Althammer et al, 2021; EC, 2021; BMG, 2023).

LTCI is administered by 'long-term care funds' (*Pflegekassen*) established under the existing umbrella of the 'health insurance funds' (*Krankenkassen*). LTCI benefit amounts are calculated according to care need and care arrangement (home care versus residential care), corresponding to an LTC grade. Access to LTC benefits expanded significantly following a major LTCI reform in 2017, with two main changes: (1) the equalisation of care need caused by dementia to a physical disability and (2) the replacement of the previous three LTC degrees (*Pflegestufen*) with five distinct LTC grades (*Pflegegrade*). Instead of the previous approach of calculating the amount of time in minutes needed for caregiving, the 'need of care' (*Pflegebedürftigkeit*) is now determined by the degree of an individual's autonomy, independence, impairments or incapacitation in six fields (modules), which are weighted as follows: mobility (10 per cent), cognitive and communicative abilities, behaviour patterns and psychological problems (15 per cent), level of self-sufficiency (40 per cent), health restrictions, demands and stress due to

Table 7.1: LTCI benefit payments per month by grade and type of care

LTCI grade	LTCI benefit for informal care per month	LTCI for formal home care per month	LTCI for residential care per month
Grade 1	€125	€125	€125
Grade 2	€316	€724	€770
Grade 3	€545	€1,363	€1,262
Grade 4	€728	€1,693	€1,775
Grade 5	€901	€2,095	€2,005

Source: BMG (2022), using the German country profile in the European Commission's long-term care report 2021 (EC, 2021) as a template for translating the German LTCI terminology into English

therapies (20 per cent) and structure of everyday life and social contacts (15 per cent). The grade of care is determined by the Medical Services of the Statutory Health Insurance Funds (*Medizinischer Dienst der Gesetzlichen Krankenkassen*) or by its private counterpart (EC, 2021; Jacobs et al, 2021). Cash payments to 'informal' carers are always considerably lower than payments for professional carers (Table 7.1). It is possible to combine them.

Cash payments for respite care (*Verhinderungspflege*) (up to six weeks per year) or short-term care (*Kurzzeitpflege*) (up to eight weeks per year) are not included in Table 7.1. Furthermore, residents in sheltered accommodation are entitled to a monthly supplement of €214 (BMG, 2022).

First steps towards carer leave schemes

Conflicts related to the reconciliation of caring and paid work existed well before the introduction of LTCI and reflected the German care regime that assumes primary family responsibility for care. Although that has not changed as the underlying principle, today female employment is the norm: 76 per cent of women aged 20–64 are employed, as compared to 83 per cent of men (Statista, 2022a). Legislation aimed at promoting a better reconciliation of employment and care for dependent children was thoroughly reformed in 2007 through the introduction of a paid carer leave scheme (*Elternzeit/ Elterngeld*) and 2015 (*Elternzeit Plus/Elterngeld Plus*). In contrast, family caregivers in LTC are still waiting for equivalent legislation.

The first step in this direction was undertaken with the Care Time Act (*Pflegezeitgesetz*) in 2008, which created two unpaid carer leave schemes for working carers: (1) Care Leave (*Pflegezeit*), which allowed full or partial leave of absence to care for a family member for up to six months and (2) Short-term Prevented Work Absence (*Kurzzeitige Arbeitsverhinderung*) for up to ten working days, which was intended to provide working carers with time to organise LTC or to find a place in a residential care home.

In this context, regulations on social security (payments towards pension entitlements) for carers were also included in LTCI. In 2011 Care Leave was complemented by a third leave scheme. The 2011 Family Care Leave Act introduced (3) Family Care Leave (*Familienpflegezeit*), which allows partial leave of absence for up to two years. All three leave schemes were reformed in 2015. They are introduced in detail in the following sections.

Short-Term Prevented Work Absence and Care Support Allowance

Short-Term Prevented Work Absence (*Kurzzeitige Arbeitsverhinderung*) for up to ten working days was introduced with the intention of giving family members a legal entitlement to leave of absence for organising LTC when the need arises. If a close relative[3] of an employee urgently needs care, s/he has the right to be absent from work for up to ten working days to organise care or to provide care during this time. This helps relatives to organise care at short notice, for example, after a stroke. Employees are obliged to inform their employer immediately of their inability to work and the expected duration of their absence. Under the 2015 reforms the Care Support Allowance (*Pflegeunterstützungsgeld*) was established, which for the first time provides a *paid* carer leave scheme, albeit for a very short time period. The benefit is paid by the long-term care fund (*Pflegekasse*) with whom the person in need of care is insured. The gross care support allowance is 90 per cent of the lost net pay, in most cases. The entitlement period is a maximum of ten working days per person in need of care; in the event of several cases at the same time, the entitlement is divided up between them (FMFSWY, 2011; BMG, 2021a, 2021b).

Longer-term carer leave schemes

There are two longer-term leave schemes to enable family carers to provide LTC which are regulated by two different sets of legislation: Care Leave (*Pflegezeit*) and Family Care Leave (*Familienpflegezeit*). The two schemes differ essentially in that the former consists of a full or partial release from work for a maximum of six months, while the latter provides for a temporary reduction in working time to an average of at least 15 hours per week for a maximum of 24 months. In other words, whereas Care Leave focuses on care provision and enables family carers to reduce their working hours to zero if necessary to provide care, Family Care Leave specifically aims at a better reconciliation of caregiving and employment. Unless someone maintains employment for at least 15 hours per week s/he will not be entitled to Family Care Leave. In both cases, employees enjoy protection against dismissal from the time of announcement (but no more than 12 weeks before the announced start) until the end of the Care Leave.

In contrast to Short-term Prevented Work Absence, which is universally available, there is no legal entitlement to Care Leave and Family Care Leave when someone is employed in a small or medium-sized company (SME) with fewer than 16 employees (Care Leave) or 26 employees (Family Care Leave), respectively. This exception was achieved after intensive lobbying by the employers' associations, arguing that this was necessary to protect SMEs. This decision has significant implications, given that 56 per cent of employees in the private sector are employed in SMEs – 18 per cent in small companies with fewer than 10 employees and 21.5 per cent in small companies with fewer than 50 employees (Statista, 2022d).

Care Leave (Pflegezeit)

Entitlement to Care Leave is granted to employees who provide home care. Eligibility extends to carers of close relatives in need of LTC or in the final phase of their lives (the last three months). It is a socially insured leave of absence from work, not paid by the employer, in whole or in part, for a period of up to six months (BMJ, 2008). The entitlement applies only to employers with more than 15 employees. An employee must prove the need for care by submitting a certificate from the LTCI fund or the medical service of the health insurance fund (or the private insurance equivalent). In case of close relatives who are minors in need of care, there is also an entitlement to leave of absence if care is provided outside the home. If leave has been requested for a shorter period, it may later be extended up to a maximum of six months with the employer's consent. In addition, employees may claim full or partial leave from work for up to three months to care for a close relative in the final phase of life (BMG, 2021a, 2021b). In this case, too, employees must prove the necessity of care by the close relative to their employer by means of a medical certificate.

In 2015, the German Government introduced an interest-free loan for carers taking advantage of either Care Leave or Family Care Leave. Recipients may apply for a loan at the Federal Office for Family and Civil Society Tasks, which is a subordinate agency of the Federal Ministry for Families, Senior Citizens, Women and Youth (FMFSWY, 2011).

Family Care Leave (Familienpflegezeit)

Family Care Leave was introduced in 2015. Since then, employees have had a legal entitlement to partial leave for home care of up to 24 months with a minimum weekly working time of 15 hours (BMJ, 2011). The legal entitlement to partial leave under the Family Care Leave Act does not apply to employers with 25 or fewer employees.[4] In order to be able to care for close relatives who are minors in need of care, whether at home or in a residential care facility, employees also have the option of taking leave under the Family Care Leave Act. The notice period for the leave of absence is eight weeks. At this time, it must be stated for what period and to what extent leave from work will be taken. The desired number of working hours must also be stated. A written agreement must be signed between employer and employee. An employer is obliged to comply with the employee's wishes unless there are urgent operational reasons to the contrary.

Combining care leaves and social insurance

Family carers can also take combined leave under the Care Leave Act and the Family Care Leave Act. The total duration of all leave options combined is a maximum of 24 months. Leaves can also be shared in parallel or taken consecutively (BMJ, 2011; BMG, 2021b). This is the case, for example, when siblings share the care for a parent at the same time or take over the care responsibilities from each other.

A crucial question in relation to carer leave schemes was whether carers would continue to be covered by social insurance during that period. Since 1 January 2017, the following applies: anyone who cares for one or more people in need of care in a care degree 2 to 5 in their home environment for at least ten hours a week is a caregiver for the purposes of LTCI. The LTCI pays social insurance contributions for these caregivers (BMJV, 2021).

Table 7.2 summarises the carer leave options available to working carers in Germany.

Further support measures for carers

In addition to the official leave schemes there are other legal entitlements that indirectly work towards a better reconciliation of care and work. Moreover, individual agreements with employers or collective agreements as part of collective bargaining between trade unions and employers' associations provide alternative options.

Working part time

Employees who have been employed for more than six months can apply to reduce their working hours in companies with more than 15 employees in accordance with the Part-Time and Fixed-Term Employment Act (*Teilzeit-und Befristungsgesetz*). This must be at least 20 per cent. The reduction in working hours must be for a period of at least one year and the employer must be notified at least three months in advance. The employer is obliged to agree to the reduction in working hours unless there are operational reasons to the contrary. Entitled employees can reduce their working hours

Table 7.2: Carer leave schemes, Germany (November 2023)

| Leave details | | | | Eligibility | | | |
Leave name and introduced	Time period	Compensation	Worker/employee status	Qualifying period[a]	Person needing care	Evidence	Notice period and process
Short-Term Prevented Work Absence, 2012	10 days per annum	90% of pay through Carer Support Allowance	All employees	–	Close relative	Need for care/no care degree	Notify employer ASAP
Care Leave, 2008	Full or partial leave up to six months	Interest-free loan (BAFzA)	All employees of companies with 15+ employees	–	Close relatives	Proof of a care degree	10 days, written agreement with employer
Family Care Leave, 2015	Reduce working time for up to 24 months	Interest-free loan (BAFzA)	All employees of companies with 25+ employees	–	Close relatives who are minors	Proof of a care degree	Eight weeks, written agreement with employer

Note: [a] Entitlement to Short-Term Prevented Work Absence Care Leave and Family Care Leave is not dependent on duration of employment, but Care Leave and Family Care Leave are not available to those working for SMEs.

for a limited period of time and return to their original working hours once the part-time phase has ended. The minimum duration of the reduction in working hours is one year, the maximum five years (BMAS, 2000, 2019).

Another opportunity applies to older workers only. Employed persons aged 55 and older may take advantage of 'part-time work for older workers' (*Altersteilzeit*) if they were employed for at least 1,080 calendar days within the last five years before the start of partial retirement and have a full social insurance contribution record allowing for early retirement. The agreement is made on a voluntary basis between the employee and their employer. Two models are often preferred: either the equal distribution model, in which working time is reduced by half, or the block model, in which employees continue to work the same hours as before and retire fully after half of the agreed time span (BMAS, 2021a).

Flexible solutions for working hours and workplace

Several programmes and initiatives are designed to motivate employers to offer variable working hours and home office or remote work. Companies that offer family- and care-sensitive working hours can be awarded the quality seal 'Work and Family Audit'. The audit, which can be used in all sectors regardless of company size, documents the status quo of the family-sensitive measures already on offer, systematically reviews and develops a company's potential and ensures that family awareness is anchored in the corporate culture with binding target agreements. There are various certificate programmes for companies that are committed to improving the compatibility of family, care and work. A nationally recognised example of employer branding is the work and family audit. It applies to all sizes of companies, although it can be seen from the list of companies already certified that approximately one third are SMEs, with the rest being large companies. There is also a company network called *Erfolgsfaktor Familie* (Success Factor Family), of which companies that implement compatibility measures can become members. In both programmes, however, there are no uniform minimum standards that must be met in order to be considered family friendly.

Additional support for everyday life

Services such as household help, shopping services, laundry services or meals-on-wheels usually must be financed privately. A subsidy by the employer can effectively relieve some of this burden on carer employees. German employers can claim subsidies for household-related services as tax-deductible business expenses (BMJ, 2022). Cooperation with social service providers, such as outpatient and inpatient care facilities, can also give carers easy and quick access to reliable providers. This is the case if a company cooperates with a care service from the region or provides a hotline or contact person on site who can answer employees' questions. As a large company, the Mercedes Benz Group, for example, offers a telephone hotline with care experts as well as free consultation hours and care courses for caring relatives.

However, it is not sufficient to offer measures such as those outlined – working carers need to be encouraged to use them. The measures need to be offered with the intention that they will actually be used, without fear of negative consequences. Survey data show that 58 per cent of companies do not have any specific offers for better reconciling caregiving and employment (ZQP, 2018). This is because companies doubt the bureaucracy, costs and sustainability of the measures, as only be a small group of employees will take advantage of them. For many companies and the German employers' association, the legal measures are sufficient. They see no need for any extension such as paid leave for carers (FMFSWY, 2019).

Sick leave/sick pay as informal means of reconciliation

Employees are entitled to sick leave (*Krankschreibung*)/sick pay (*Lohnfortzahlung im Krankheitsfall*). Employers have to continue payment of wages in the event of illness for a period of up to six weeks (BMJ, 1994). This also applies to measures of preventive medical care or rehabilitation. In light of the high physical and psychological strain on working carers, they are more likely to fall ill than other people (Eurocarers, 2017). Thus, sick leave can become an informal form of care leave that does not require much administrative effort – just a doctor's sick certificate. Likewise, sick pay can become an informal payment for the duration of sick leave. This covers the entirety of the salary of the working carer for six weeks. If these six weeks are followed by an extension of the medically certified incapacity for work, the person concerned receives sickness benefit (*Krankengeld*) from the HI fund (*Krankenkasse*). The amount of sickness benefit equates to 70 per cent of the previous gross monthly income – but no more than 90 per cent of the net income – and is payable for a total of up to 78 weeks (§ 47 SGB V). If family carers use this, it means that they will lose part of their wages – but not as much as if taking Care Leave or Family Care Leave without any payments.

COVID-19 pandemic response and implications for employed carers

The COVID-19 pandemic alerted the wider public to common deficiencies in the LTC sector. However, public attention focused mainly on the formal care sector – mainly on hospitals and residential care homes. In contrast, carers became even less visible than before, while their difficult circumstances were aggravated by temporary unavailability of auxiliary services such as day-care centres or service providers (for example, home help, cleaning services, meals on wheels) (Eggert et al, 2021; Ehrlich et al, 2022). Studies conducted during the pandemic identified various stress indicators that had a negative impact on everyday caring and thus increased the burden of care for carers. An important concern was the risk of contracting COVID-19 or that the care recipient would contract the virus. Furthermore, the loss of paid care services and lack of time for oneself were named as extremely stressful (Eggert et al, 2021; Theurer et al, 2022). In contrast, a very recent publication based on German Ageing Survey data concluded that the perceived care burden did not increase on average during the pandemic for working carers specifically – the greatest burden during the pandemic was reported by high-intensity carers who had abandoned employment due to their high care pressures, followed by working carers with high-intensity care duties (Ehrlich et al, 2022).

Other research shows that social support and well-being have changed because of the pandemic. Personal well-being declined as the pandemic continued. The greatest changes were among women and the very old, who were already at increased risk of loneliness before the pandemic, and this risk increased further (Brandt et al, 2021; Budnick et al, 2021). A considerable number of respondents in such surveys stated that they no longer received sufficient support or were no longer able to provide sufficient support to others. In particular, older people withdrew from supporting others, mainly because of (mutual) fear of infection (BMG, 2021c; Eggert et al, 2021; Jacobs et al, 2021).

The data indicate a change in the reconciliation of care and work. Two-thirds of the working carer respondents in such surveys reported more problems with work/care reconciliation since the beginning of the pandemic, as they had to increase their support to people in need of care (BMFSFJ, 2021; BMG, 2021c; Budnick et al, 2021; Eggert et al, 2021). In addition, there were occupational changes. Above all, many employees worked from home or in a home office – some of them exclusively. What may appear as a relief initially quickly turned into a disadvantage for some, with the realisation that focused work is much more difficult when care is urgently needed at the same time in the same household.

Ehrlich et al (2022) found that more people – predominantly women – contributed to care tasks during the first wave of the pandemic. However, this changed during the second wave. Somewhat unexpectedly, they found that the pandemic did not result in a significant reduction of employment of working carers. Policy makers recognised the particular burden placed on family caregivers during the pandemic and introduced acute assistance in May 2020 (extended until the end of April 2023) to simplify the reconciliation of caring and employment. Details of this are outlined in the following section (BMFSFJ, 2021).

Better support to reconcile caregiving and employment in an acute care situation

The Care Support Allowance (*Pflegeunterstützungsgeld*) could be claimed for up to 20 working days instead of 10 days previously if an additional care need arose that only the family carer could provide. Likewise, carers were entitled to 20 days' short-term absence from work instead of 10 days previously. The prerequisite was that there was a pandemic-related acute care situation that had to be dealt with, for example, if day care facilities had closed due to the pandemic or outpatient care services had been curtailed.

Flexibility of Family Care Leave and Care Leave

Working carers were given more flexibility in using both leave schemes with the employer's consent. Those who had not yet exhausted the legal entitlement period of 24 and 6 months, respectively, were able to use the remainder at short notice, provided they did not exceed the total duration of 24 months. Furthermore, they had to give notice to their employer only ten days in advance (instead of eight weeks) for Family Care Leave. Moreover, the minimum working time of 15 hours per week could be temporarily reduced. Notification to the employer in text form was sufficient.

Additional entitlement for interest-free loan

The interest-free loan under the Family Care Leave Act was adjusted. Months with income losses due to the pandemic could be disregarded when determining the loan amount upon application. The repayment of loans was made easier. This acute aid was extended until the end of April 2023. There is little indication that employers extended their respective leave schemes during the pandemic. In a survey conducted by the Centre for Quality in Care (ZQP), of a total of 520 respondents, no one had used extended short-term absence from work (Eggert et al, 2020).

Adequacy of care leave policies

In this section we critically review the adequacy of current care leave policies, focusing on two influential reports exploring this subject.

Increased risk of poverty due to caregiving

Family carers commonly experience wage losses – and thus accumulate lower pension income – in the long run. This has significant gender implications, since family carers are predominantly women. Family caregiving for young children as well as for ageing parents thus becomes a major (financial) lifecourse risk for women. Moreover, the insistence on the subsidiarity principle results in privatisation of care-related costs – financially and otherwise.

Low uptake of interest-free loan and Care Leave/Family Care Leave

Data are patchy on the take-up of the care support allowance in relation to the Short-term Prevented Work Absence for up to ten days as well as the uptake of the interest-free loan for the duration of Care Leave/Family Care Leave. For the first time in 2017, the micro-census asked who was using Care Leave and Family Care Leave. In 2017, their numbers were 82,000 persons. The number of people who applied for the interest-free loan to compensate for lost wages was extremely low. In 2018, just 867 applications were approved (INTERVAL, 2018; FMFSWY, 2019). The take-up rate thus fell far short of the government's expectations.

Family carers pay for 70.7 per cent of care-related expenses from their earned income, 55.3 per cent from the care recipient's Care Allowance (*Pflegegeld*), 46.3 per cent from their own savings, 28.5 per cent from the pension of the care recipient and 16.3 per cent from the earned income of other family members (FMFSWY, 2019: 45). The Care Support Allowance is used by 9,000–13,000 people per year (INTERVAL, 2018; Deutscher Bundestag, 2019; FMFSWY, 2019). However, only about half of those who applied for these leave schemes were granted Care Support Allowance.

The recommendations of the Independent Advisory Board for the Reconciliation of Caregiving and Employment

In 2015, the Independent Advisory Board for the Reconciliation of Caregiving and Employment (*Unabhängiger Beirat für die Vereinbarkeit von Pflege und Beruf*) started its work as mandated in the Family Care Act (*Familienpflegezeitgesetz*) (BMJ, 2011). It was charged to address issues related to the reconciliation of caring and employment and to monitor the implementation of relevant legislation and its effects. The Board has 21 members from relevant interest groups, including two academics with research expertise. Other members include representatives of the umbrella organisations of trade unions, employers' associations, independent welfare associations, statutory and private health insurance/LTCI and interest groups for family carers. The Board is required to write a report on the current state of affairs every four years.

In 2019, the Advisory Board submitted its first report to the German Government with recommendations for action which effectively represents a critical review of the Care Leave/Family Care Leave legislation. Its key recommendations focused on the continuous development of relevant legislation, financial support for working carers and greater control for carers over their working time. Furthermore, it also discussed improvements of the support infrastructure, including accessibility to transparent advice, as well as the use of assistive technologies to help better reconcile caring and employment. At the beginning of the report, the Board set out the seven overarching principles that guide its work:

1. LTC is considered a societal task. Care is not an individual issue; rather it is a social responsibility. The need for care and care tasks are neither individual fates nor exclusively family tasks. In order to strengthen the overall social responsibility for care work, it is necessary to place the refinancing of care costs on broader shoulders in order to ensure the financial stability of LTCI and its benefits.
2. Every individual decision in favour or against caring should be respected. In Germany, the principle of 'outpatient before inpatient' applies. This means that LTCI services are primarily intended to support home care and the willingness of relatives and neighbours to provide care so that those in need of care can remain in their home environment for as long as possible. If a relative decides against this principle and instead makes use of professional or inpatient care, this should not be judged negatively.
3. Carers should be supported to prevent them from giving up their jobs. If that is not possible, then to prevent them from giving up their jobs permanently. The job provides a meaningful element and offers both distance and variety from the care work. It also provides important social contacts.
4. There should be more measures encouraging a gender-equal division of labour in caring. A gender-equitable balance between care and work can help to ensure that women and men are equally able to care for their relatives and work at the same time.
5. Operational feasibility in companies should be considered. Small companies with few employees find it more difficult to compensate for absences due to family care. Care must be taken here to adapt the law in future so that small companies are not excessively burdened but their employees can also benefit from the regulations on care leave. Future reports will therefore focus primarily on SMEs.
6. The specific circumstances of the self-employed will be considered. The Caregiver Leave Act applies only to employees who are in an employment contract. This means that the self-employed have not yet been able to take advantage of it. In future, adjustments are to be made to improve the compatibility of care and work for the self-employed.
7. Recommendations for action must not fall behind existing legislation.

This acknowledgement is important since some principles address persisting challenges (5 and 6); others are in contrast to the traditional care regime that may no longer be in line with most people's views but is nevertheless still enshrined in law (1–4). Among the recommendations made were:

1. The introduction of a paid carer leave scheme equivalent to the scheme available for parents of dependent children (*Elterngeld/Elterngeld Plus*) for 36 months. This would replace the interest-free loan mentioned earlier, which was heavily criticised because of its very low uptake.
2. For Family Care Leave the minimum working hours of 15 per week should be extended to 36 months. Working carers should be able to reduce their working hours to zero for up to six months.
3. The Short-term Prevented Work Absence and Care Support Allowance should be extended to ten days per year.
4. Care Leave and Family Care Leave should be combined in one piece of legislation.
5. There should be improvement and extension of the professional care infrastructure.
6. Support measures for working carers should be easily and swiftly accessible, flexible and reliable.

However, not all members of the Advisory Board agreed on these recommendations. The Confederation of German Employers' Associations (*Bundesvereinigung der Deutschen Arbeitgeberverbände*) submitted a substantial minority opinion with the report, emphasising its opposition to the proposed *paid* leave scheme. This opinion was endorsed by the Federal Confederation of Municipal Umbrella Organisations (*Bundesvereinigung der kommunalen Spitzenverbände*) and the Confederation of Municipal Employers' Associations (*Vereinigung der kommunalen Arbeitgeberverbände*). Furthermore, the private healthcare insurance/LTCI body opposed the proposition of introducing it regardless of company size (FMFSWY, 2019).

The Alliance for Good Care (Bündnis für gute Pflege)

Several lobby organisations are trying to improve the public representation of carers. The largest organisation is the Alliance for Good Care, which has 13.6 million members and represents 23 welfare associations, trade unions, professional carer workers' associations and self-help organisations that are active nationwide (Bündnis für gute Pflege, 2021). It has been campaigning for ten years for better pay and working conditions for care professionals, as well as better services and support for care recipients and family carers. In addition, the Alliance states that current state support services should be evaluated regularly to measure their effectiveness. Overall, its key recommendations are similar to those of the Independent Advisory Board, namely (1) general improvement of the situation of family carers, (2) sustainable financial support, (3) comprehensive information and advice, (4) an improved care infrastructure and (5) investment in digital and technical solutions to support family carers. These recommendations and demands have not yet been implemented by politicians. The COVID pandemic took precedence. However, the recommendations will no doubt be pursued further.

Conclusion

In Germany, the ageing of the population will continue. By the mid-2030s, the number of people of retirement age (67 years and older) will increase by about 4 million to at least 20.0 million. The number of people aged 80 and over will remain stable until the mid-2030s and then increase sharply. Their share of the population will rise from 7 per cent in 2022 to 12 per cent, which corresponds to about 10 million people (Stat. Bundesamt, 2022a, 2022d). This is also expected to increase the need for care. Nevertheless, German care regimes still rest on the subsidiarity principle assuming primary responsibility of the family for care. However, the majority of working-age women and men are employed and these individuals often need to combine caring with their employment. Given the increasing shortages of skilled labour in many German industries, the successful reconciliation of employment and caregiving is vital for the German economy.

But many family carers are unable to reconcile care and employment. This leads to restrictions on gainful employment and, conversely, to an increased risk of poverty in old age as well as to (income) dependence on a possible full-time working partner. A change in this traditional division of labour is not sufficiently promoted in Germany. Mechanisms such as marital break-up, free family co-insurance and inadequate public services promote the preservation of traditional family patterns. Thus, primarily female lifecourses are characterised by interruptions due to caring. Viewed over the entire working life, the interruption effect (due to caring for relatives) has a stronger impact on income and thus on later pensions than the gender effect due to stereotypes and gender bias (BMFSFJ, 2017; Knauthe and Deindl, 2019). It remains questionable to what extent politicians are willing to change 'familialism' in favour of public care provision. This would entail considerable additional financial expenditure.

For family carers in Germany, a mixed care arrangement consisting of professional care services and informal care responsibilities would be the most effective. The current focus on a family-based care system could be replaced in favour of a service-based care system. The consistent design of mixed care arrangements is a central condition for ensuring that family carers have a realistic chance of developing their gainful employment biography in addition to informal care work. Mixed care arrangements of outpatient and (partly) inpatient support services that are available at short notice and accessible in the neighbourhood would be crucial. In order for considerations on mixed care arrangements to be put into practice, it would be necessary to turn away from the primacy of informal care, which is currently hidden behind the positive-law requirement of 'homecare before residential care'.

Notes

[1] The principle of subsidiarity states that a task (for example, care for a relative) should be undertaken by the smallest 'responsible' unit if possible (for example, family). Higher-level units should intervene only if the lower units cannot.

[2] These are family members who care for their relatives. People who do not receive benefits from LTCI are not covered by the system. Thus, the numbers of people in need of care as well as informal caregivers are only estimates.

[3] Close relatives are, in particular: grandparents, parents, parents-in-law, step-parents, spouses, civil partners, partners in a marriage-like or civil partnership-like community, siblings, spouses of siblings and siblings of spouses, civil partners of siblings and siblings of civil partners, children, adopted or foster children, the children, adopted or foster children of the spouse or civil partner, children-in-law and grandchildren (FMFSWY, 2011).

[4] The fact that the entitlement to care leave is linked to different preconditions depending on the size of the company is not sufficiently justified by the legislative instance and is therefore often criticised (FMFSWY, 2019).

References

Althammer, J., Lampert, H. and Sommer, M. (2021) *Lehrbuch der Sozialpolitik* (10th rev edn), Berlin: Springer Gabler. https://doi.org/10.1007/978-3-662-56258-1

Anttonen, A. and Sipilä, J. (1996) 'European social care services: is it possible to identify models?' *Journal of European Social Policy*, 6(2): 87–100. https://doi.org/10.1177/095892879600600201

BMAS (2000) *TzBfG: Gesetz über Teilzeitarbeit und befristete Arbeitsverträge (Teilzeit- Befristungsgesetz)*, Bundesministerium für Arbeit und Soziales. https://www.gesetze-im-internet.de/tzbfg/BJNR196610000.html [Accessed 24 January 2024].

BMAS (2019) *Rund um das Gesetz zur Teilzeit*, Berlin: BMAS. [Available from: https://www.bmas.de/DE/Arbeit/Arbeitsrecht/Teilzeit-flexible-Arbeitszeit/Teilzeit/teilzeit-rund-um-das-gesetz.html [Accessed 24 January 2024].

BMAS (2021a) *Altersteilzeit: Schrittweise in den Ruhestand*, Berlin: BMAS. Available from: https://www.bmas.de/DE/Arbeit/Arbeitsrecht/Teilzeit-flexible-Arbeitszeit/Teilzeit/altersteilzeit-artikel.html [Accessed 24 January 2024].

BMAS (2021b) *Sozialbericht*, Bonn: BMAS. Available from: https://www.bundesregierung.de/breg-de/service/gesetzesvorhaben/sozialbericht-2021-1948452 [Accessed 24 January 2024].

BMFSFJ (2017) *Zweiter Gleichstellungsbericht der Bundesregierung*, Berlin. Available from: https://www.gleichstellungsbericht.de/de/topic/2.zwei ter-gleichstellungsbericht-der-bundesregierung.html [Accessed 24 January 2024].

BMFSFJ (2021) *Akuthilfen für pflegende Angehörige sind verlängert*. Available from: https://www.bmfsfj.de/bmfsfj/aktuelles/alle-meldungen/akuthil fen-fuer-pflegende-angehoerige-sind-verlaengert-160232 [Accessed 24 January 2024].

BMG (2021a) *PflegeZG: Freistellung nach Pflegezeitgesetz*. Berlin: Bundesministerium für Gesundheit. Available from: https://www.bunde sgesundheitsministerium.de/leistungen-der-pflege/vereinbarkeit-von-pfl ege-und-beruf.html [Accessed 24 January 2024].

BMG (2021b) *Ratgeber Pflege: Alles was Sie zum Thema Pflege wissen sollten*. Berlin: Bundesministerium für Gesundheit. Available from: https://www. bundesgesundheitsministerium.de/service/publikationen/details/ratgeber-pflege.html [Accessed 24 January 2024].

BMG (2021c) *Siebter Pflegebericht: Entwicklung der Pflegeversicherung und den Stand der pflegerischen Versorgung in der Bundesrepublik Deutschland*. Berlin: Bundesministerium für Gesundheit. Available from: https://www. bundesgesundheitsministerium.de/fileadmin/Dateien/3_Downloads/ P/Pflegebericht/Siebter_Pflegebericht_barrierefrei.pdf_ [Accessed 24 January 2024].

BMG (2022) *Pflegeleistungen zum Nachschlagen*. Berlin: Bundesministerium für Gesundheit. Available from: https://www.bundesgesundheitsminister ium.de/service/publikationen/details/pflegeleistungen-zum-nachschlagen. html [Accessed 24 January 2024].

BMG (2023) *Finanzierung der sozialen Pflegeversicherung*. Finanzierung der Pflegeversicherung (bundesgesundheitsministerium.de)

BMJ (1994) *§. 3. EntgFG: Entgeltfortzahlungsgesetz*. Berlin: Bundesministerium für Justiz. Available from: https://www.gesetze-im-internet.de/entgfg/ __3.html [Accessed 24 January 2024].

BMJ (2008) *PflegeZG: Gesetz über die Pflegezeit (Pflegezeitgesetz)*. Berlin: Bundesministerium für Justiz. https://www.gesetze-im-internet. de/pflegezg/ [Accessed 24 January 2024].

BMJ (2011) *FPfZG: Gesetz über die Familienpflegezeit (Familienpflegezeitgesetz)*. Berlin: Bundesministerium für Justiz. Available from: https://www.gesetze-im-internet.de/fpfzg/BJNR256410011.html [Accessed 24 January 2024].

BMJ (2022) *EStG § 4 Abs. 4: Einkommensteuergesetz*. Berlin: Bundesministerium für Justiz. https://www.gesetze-im-internet.de/ estg/__4.html

BMJV (2021) *Pflegezeitgesetz (PflegeZG)*. Available from: www.gesetze-im-internet.de/pflegezg/ [Accessed 24 January 2024].

bpb (2020) *Statistik der Bundesagentur für Arbeit. Arbeitslosigkeit im Zeitverlauf: Datenstand November 2019.* Bonn.

Brandt, M., Garten, C., Grates, M., Kaschowitz, J., Quashie, N. and Schmitz, A. (2021) 'Veränderungen von Wohlbefinden und privater Unterstützung für Ältere: ein Blick auf die Auswirkungen der COVID-19-Pandemie im Frühsommer 2020' [Changes in well-being and private support for older people: a closer look at the impact of the COVID-19 pandemic in early summer 2020], *Zeitschrift fur Gerontologie und Geriatrie*, 54(3): 240–46. https://doi.org/10.1007/s00391-021-01870-2

Budnick, A., Hering, C., Eggert, S., Teubner, C., Suhr, R., Kuhlmey, A. and Gellert, P. (2021) 'Informal caregivers during the COVID-19 pandemic perceive additional burden: findings from an ad-hoc survey in Germany', *BMC Health Services Research*, 21(1): 353. https://doi.org/10.1186/s12913-021-06359-7

Bundesagentur für Arbeit (2022) *Tabellen: Arbeitslosigkeit im Zeitverlauf: Entwicklung der Arbeitslosenquote: Strukturmerkmale*, Nürnberg.

Bündnis für gute Pflege (2021) *10 Forderung zur Bundestagswahl 2021*. Available from: http://www.buendnis-fuer-gute-pflege.de/ [Accessed 24 January 2024].

Deutscher Bundestag (1994) *Gesetz zur sozialen Absicherung des Risikos der Pflegebedürftigkeit (Pflegeversicherungsgesetz)*, Berlin.

Deutscher Bundestag (2019) *Wirksamkeit des Gesetzes zur besseren Vereinbarkeit von Familie, Pflege und Beruf*, Berlin.

EC (2021) *Long-term care report. Trends, challenges and opportunities in an ageing society*, Publications Office of the European Union. Available from: https://op.europa.eu/de/publication-detail/-/publication/b39728e3-cd83-11eb-ac72-01aa75ed71a1 [Accessed 24 January 2024].

Eggert, S., Budnick, A., Gellert, P. and Kuhlmey, A. (2020) *Pflegende Angehörige in der COVID-19-Krise: Ergebnisse einer Bundesweiten Befragung*, Berlin. Available from: https://www.zqp.de/produkt/analyse-corona-angehoerige/?hilite=Corona [Accessed 24 January 2024].

Eggert, S., Teubner, C., Budnick, A. and Gellert, P. (2021) 'Vereinbarkeit von Pflege und Beruf: generelle und aktuelle Herausforderungen Betroffener', in K. Jacobs, A. Kuhlmey, S. Greß, J. Klauber and A. Schwinger (eds), *Pflege-Report: Vol. 2021. Sicherstellung der Pflege: Bedarfslagen und Angebotsstrukturen*, Springer, pp 59–70.

Ehrlich, U., Kelle, N. and Bünning, M. (2022) *Pflege und Erwerbsarbeit: Was ändert sich für Frauen und Männer in der Corona-Pandemie?* (02/22), Berlin.

Esping-Andersen, G. (1990) *The three worlds of welfare capitalism*, Cambridge: Polity Press.

Euro Carers (2017) *The impact of caregiving on informal carers' mental and physical health*. Available from: https://eurocarers.org/publications/the-impact-of-caregiving-on-informal-carers-mental-and-physical-health/ [Accessed 24 January 2024].

Eurostat (2020) *Population and population change statistics*. Available from: https://ec.europa.eu/eurostat/statistics-explained/index.php?title=Population_and_population_change_statistics [Accessed 24 January 2024].

FMFSWY (2011) *Better reconciliation of family, care and work*, Berlin. Available from: https://www.bmfsfj.de/bmfsfj/meta/en/publications-en/bessere-vereinbarkeit-von-familie-pflege-und-beruf-englisch-96102 [Accessed 24 January 2024].

FMFSWY (2019) *First Report of the German Independent Advisory Board on Work–Care Reconciliation*, Berlin.

Fuchs-Schündeln, N. and Stephan, G. (2020) *Bei drei Vierteln der erwerbstätigen Eltern ist die Belastung durch Kinderbetreuung in der Covid-19-Pandemie gestiegen*, IAB-Forum.

Geyer, J. and Schulz, E. (2014) *Who cares? Die Bedeutung der informellen Pflege durch Erwerbstätige in Deutschland PDF Logo*, Berlin. Available from: https://www.econstor.eu/handle/10419/96168 [Accessed 24 January 2024].

Haupt, M., Zimmermann, S. and Müller, L. (2022) *Auswirkungen der COVID-19-Pandemie auf die Geschlechterverhältnisse*, Bonn.

Hayek, A., Lehnert, T., Wegener, A., Riedel-Heller, S. and König, H.-H. (2018) 'Langzeitpräferenzen der Älteren in Deutschland: Ergebnisse einer bevölkerungsrepräsentativen Umfrage', *Gesundheitswesen*, 80(8–9): 685–92.

Hoff, A., Reichert, M., Hamblin, K.A., Perek-Bialas, J. and Principi, A. (2014) 'Informal and formal reconciliation strategies of older peoples' working carers: the European carers@work project', *Vulnerable Groups & Inclusion*, 5(1): 24264. https://doi.org/10.3402/vgi.v5.24264

Huinink, J. and Schröder, T. (2019) *Sozialstruktur Deutschlands*, UVK Verlag.

INTERVAL (2018) *Abschlussbericht zur Untersuchung der Regelungen des Pflegezeitgesetzes und des Familienpflegezeitgesetzes in der seit 1. Januar 2015 geltenden Fassung unter Einbeziehung der kurzzeitigen Arbeitsverhinderung und des Pflegeunterstützungsgeldes (unveröffentlicht)*.

Jacobs, K., Kuhlmey, A., Greß, S., Klauber, J. and Schwinger, A. (eds) (2021) *Pflege-Report: Vol. 2021. Sicherstellung der Pflege: Bedarfslagen und Angebotsstrukturen*, Springer.

Knauthe, K. and Deindl, C. (2019) *Altersarmut von Frauen durch häusliche Pflege: Gutachten im Auftrag des Sozialverband Deutschland e. V*, Berlin.

Kuhlmey, A., Dräger, D. and Winter, M. (2010) *COMPASS: Versichertenbefragung zu Erwartungen und Wünschen an eine qualitativ gute Pflege. Informationsdienst Altersfragen*. Available from: https://search.gesis.org/publication/dzi-solit-000187229 [Accessed 24 January 2024].

Müller-Armack, A. (1976) *Wirtschaftsordnung und Wirtschaftspolitik. Studien und Konzepte zur Sozialen Marktwirtschaft und zur Europäischen Integration* [Translation: Economic order and economic policy. Studies and concepts on the social market economy and European integration], Bern: Haupt Verlag AG.

Stat. Bundesamt (2019) *Bevölkerung im Wandel: Annahmen und Ergebnisse der 14. koordinierten Bevölkerungsvorausberechnung.* Available from: https://www.destatis.de/DE/Presse/Pressekonferenzen/2019/Bevoelkerung/pressebroschuere-bevoelkerung.pdf?__blob=publicationFile [Accessed 24 January 2024].

Stat. Bundesamt (2022a) *15. koordinierte Bevölkerungsvorausberechnung: Annahmen und Ergebnisse*, Stat. Bundesamt. Available from: https://www.destatis.de/DE/Themen/Gesellschaft-Umwelt/Bevoelkerung/Bevoelkerungsvorausberechnung/begleitheft.html [Accessed 24 January 2024].

Stat. Bundesamt (2022b) *7,8 Millionen schwerbehinderte Menschen leben in Deutschland.* Available from: https://www.destatis.de/DE/Presse/Pressemitteilungen/2022/06/PD22_259_227.html [Accessed 24 January 2024].

Stat. Bundesamt (2022c) *Bevölkerungsstand: Amtliche Einwohnerzahl Deutschlands 2021.* Available from: https://www.destatis.de/DE/Themen/Gesellschaft-Umwelt/Bevoelkerung/Bevoelkerungsstand/_inhalt.html [Accessed 24 January 2024].

Stat. Bundesamt (2022d) *Bevölkerungsvorausberechnung.* Available from: https://www.destatis.de/DE/Themen/Gesellschaft-Umwelt/Bevoelkerung/Bevoelkerungsvorausberechnung/_inhalt.html [Accessed 24 January 2024].

Stat. Bundesamt (2022e) *Geburten.* Available from: https://www.destatis.de/DE/Themen/Gesellschaft-Umwelt/Bevoelkerung/Geburten/_inhalt.html [Accessed 24 January 2024].

Stat. Bundesamt (2022f) *Verteilung von Schwerbehinderungen in Deutschland,* Schwerbehinderungen – Verteilung in Deutschland nach Altersgruppen und Geschlecht 2021. Available from: https://de.statista.com/statistik/daten/studie/246334/umfrage/verteilung-von-schwerbehinderungen-in-deutschland-nach-altersgruppen/ [Accessed 24 January 2024].

Stat. Bundesamt (2022g) *Pflegestatistik.* Available from: https://www.destatis.de/DE/Themen/Gesellschaft-Umwelt/Gesundheit/Pflege/Publikationen/_publikationen-innen-pflegestatistik-deutschland-ergebnisse.html [Accessed 24 January 2024].

Statista (2022a) *Arbeitsmarkt in Deutschland.* Available from: https://de.statista.com/statistik/studie/id/53842/dokument/arbeitsmarkt-in-deutschland/ [Accessed 24 January 2024].

Statista (2022b) *Bruttoinlandsprodukt und Wirtschaftswachstum: Industrien und Märkte.* Available from: https://de.statista.com/statistik/studie/id/6973/dokument/bruttoinlandsprodukt-und-wirtschaftswachstum-statista-dossier/ [Accessed 24 January 2024].

Statista (2022c) *Europäische Union: Durchschnittsalter der Bevölkerung in den Mitgliedstaaten im Jahr 2021.* Available from: https://de.statista.com/statistik/daten/studie/248994/umfrage/durchschnittsalter-der-bevoelkerung-in-den-eu-laendern/ [Accessed 24 January 2024].

Statista (2022d) *Kleine und mittlere Unternehmen (KMU) in Deutschland.* Available from: https://de.statista.com/statistik/studie/id/46952/dokument/kleine-und-mittlere-unternehmen-kmu-in-deutschland/ [Accessed 24 January 2024].

Theurer, C., Rother, D., Pfeiffer, K. and Wilz, G. (2022) 'Belastungserleben pflegender Angehöriger während der Coronapandemie' [Burden experienced by caregiving relatives during the corona pandemic]. *Zeitschrift fur Gerontologie und Geriatrie*, 55(2): 136–142. https://doi.org/10.1007/s00391-022-02026-6

Zinn, S., Kreyenfeld, M. and Bayer, M. (2020) *Kinderbetreuung in Corona-Zeiten: Mütter tragen die Hauptlast, aber Väter holen auf: SOEP-CoV-Studie Nr. 51*, Berlin: DIW aktuell.

ZQP (2018) *Vereinbarkeit von Beruf und Pflege: Analyse.* Available from: https://www.zqp.de/beruf-pflege-unternehmen/ [Accessed 24 January 2024].

8

Japan

Shingou Ikeda

Introduction

For decades, Japanese governments have attempted to create support to prevent people exiting the labour market ('job leaving') due to caring responsibilities. Yet, as is still often said, Japan is a familialist welfare society in which families are expected to take a key role in providing care (Kröger and Yeandle, 2013; Shinkawa, 2014). The main pillars of the support provided for working carers in Japan are its legislation the Child and Family Care Leave Act established in 1995 and the Long-term Care Insurance (LTCI) system which came into force in 2000.

The Child and Family Care Leave Act, which was amended in 2016, requires employers to provide long-term care leave, annual short-term care leave (time off for family care) and exemption from overtime work for their employees. It also introduced flexible working arrangements, including reducing scheduled working hours, flexitime and staggered working time to address varied situations at different stages of providing care. The Act indicated the government's strong will to support family carers to combine work and care (Sodei, 1995; JILPT, 2006; Ikeda, 2013, 2021a, 2023). The Ministry of Health, Welfare and Labour (MHLW, 2023) has proposed that in the next amendment of the Child and Family Care Leave Act employers should inform their employees about the support system for combining work and family care such as care leave so as to make the system easy to use in the workplace.

Following the introduction of the LTCI in 2000, it appeared that Japan was intending to defamilialise care by expanding care services for older people (Ikeda, 2000, 2002). The Japanese Government has developed care services as an important measure in supporting people to combine work and care (Prime Minister's Office of Japan, 2015; Cabinet Office, 2016; JILPT, 2020; Ikeda, 2021a, 2023). Indeed, since the government's declaration that they would endeavour to eliminate labour market exit due to family care in 2015, it seems to have been an unwavering government policy to support the reconciliation of work and care through the defamilialisation of care for older people.

The LTCI system nevertheless faces serious financial difficulties due to the increased number of people using services. Provision and use of home care services has increased under the LTCI system, although (compared with home care services) there have been few cutbacks in the provision of care in specialised facilities (Shimoebisu, 2015). It has also been found that timetables for delivering home care are often inconvenient for working carers (MHLW, 2015). Consequently, 'refamilialisation' of care for older people (Fujisaki, 2009), the opposite of defamilialisation, has in fact increased in a context of financial pressure on the LTCI system arising from the rapid increase in the number of people requiring care (JILPT, 2020; Ikeda, 2021a, 2023). One result of restricted access to LTCI services has been the introduction of workplace measures to support employees to combine work and care in the form of the major amendment of Child and Family Care Leave Act in 2016, which can be seen as a means of facilitating the refamilialisation of the care of older people.

In sum, the Japanese Government's policy on combining work and care is caught between defamilialisation in principle and refamilialisation in practice. Care leave policy has been viewed as an opportunity to address these issues and to provide working carers with workplace measures to support their continued employment. This chapter outlines care leave policy in Japan in the early 2020s and its background and considers future issues in the context of the defamilialisation and refamilialisation of care for older people in Japan.

National context

Social context

Japan is one of the most aged countries globally, primarily as a result of rapid population ageing after World War II. The Annual Report on the Ageing Society (Cabinet Office, 2022) showed that approximately 30 per cent of the population was aged over 65. People in this age group are insured under the LTCI through compulsory contributions from the age of 40. By 2036, it is expected that one third of the population will be aged 65 or older and that there will be many centenarians (Cabinet Office, 2022). The number of people using LTCI-supported services exceeded 6.5 million in 2019, and has increased consistently since implementation of the LTCI in 2000 (Cabinet Office, 2022). Japanese society also faces acute population change from 2025, when the 'baby boomers' born in the late 1940s reach the age of 75 or older (the age at which the Japanese medical insurance system defines them as the 'old-old').

The Japanese government views this trend as a problem; an increasing number of people are giving up work to care for elderly parents, reducing the size of the available workforce and threatening the nation's economic growth (Cabinet Office, 2016; Ikeda, 2019, 2021a). Japan is often characterised as a familialist welfare society, in which adult children and older parents support and care for each other (Kröger and Yeandle, 2013; Shinkawa, 2014). Nevertheless, it established a social security system for older people after World War II, which was later expanded during the subsequent period of high economic growth. After the 1973 oil crisis, however, the government began to emphasise mutual support between older parents and adult children. High levels of adult children living with their older parents and reciprocity between the generations were promoted, with housework and childcare support from grandparents while they are relatively young subsequently 'repaid' by care from adult children to their ageing parents (Sodei, 1989; Yokoyama, 2002).

Women's full-time employment after becoming mothers has often been supported in Japan by co-resident parents providing childcare. Studies have shown, however, that women often withdraw from the labour market when their co-resident parents or parents-in-law need long-term care (Maeda, 1998); some argue that Japan's familialist welfare society places the main burden of care on women (Kasuga, 2001; Yamato, 2008). However, it has also been argued that families in Japan cannot undertake long-term care entirely without external support. Government policy turned to the 'defamilialisation' (Esping-Andersen, 1999) of care for older people through the LTCI scheme set up in 1997, which expanded provision of care services by private businesses. It has been shown that after the LTCI came into force in 2000, it became more common for older people to use formal care services (Ikeda, 2002).

After the LTCI was introduced, the supply of care services for older people, financed by insurance contributions, expanded rapidly. Yet although use of LTCI-financed care services has become widespread, many families still provide unpaid care. Residential care services, such as nursing home provision, have not expanded and admission criteria have become more stringent. Home care (or domiciliary care) is similarly rationed. Based on analysis of restrictions on home-visit nursing care services following an amendment of the LTCI Act in 2005, Fujisaki (2009) called this tightly controlled provision the 'refamilialisation of elderly care'.

Even though the LTCI expanded social care services with the aim of defamilialising care for older people, demand for support continues to exceed supply. To compensate for insufficient care services, families' care roles have expanded again. Population ageing will further increase the gap between demand for and supply of care services, while access to support funded by the LTCI has become more tightly restricted. In this sense, despite the aspiration for defamilialisation, refamilialisation of care for older people may still be increasing (Ikeda, 2021a, 2021b, 2023).

Economic inequalities also influence the degree to which family members undertake care for older people. Some working carers have the means to purchase costly private care services, supplementing the insufficiency of LTCI care services, while others – to save money in the context of a system where co-payment of LTCI services may be up to 30 per cent of their total costs – undertake the care themselves.

Care for persons with disabilities has not received the same degree of political attention in Japan as support for the old, even though the Child and Family Care Leave Act does not explicitly exclude persons with disabilities. Japanese governments have focused attention on demographic trends and population ageing with economic and fiscal management policies, rather than adopting a more inclusive welfare approach.

However, the latest working group on statutory care leave and other measures brought up the issues on working parents of children with disabilities (MHLW, 2023). It might be the first step in expanding the support system for working carers of families with disability in the future.

Economic context

Japan's labour market is characterised by long-term employment, a wage system based on seniority and labour unions organised at the company level (Abegglen, 1958; Dore, 1973; Inagami, 2005). Companies hire new graduate students and continue to employ them, typically, until mandatory retirement age. A seniority wage system means long-term job continuation in the same organisation is economically advantageous. Seniority wage system and long-term employment within a single organisation are also linked, with managers and executives generally selected from long-term employees. These employment and income security systems are protected by labour unions organised on a company basis. This means most employees aim to remain with the same company for as long as possible to develop their careers and increase their income. Employees who leave the labour market to provide care or look after their families find re-entering the workforce difficult. Many women who leave their jobs when they have a child, or to support child rearing, re-enter the labour market as non-regular workers with low incomes and in unstable employment with poor security, even if, prior to exit, they were expected to become managers or executives.

Japan's employment model is male dominated and work centred (Osawa, 1993; Hazama, 1996; Inagami, 2005). Employment and income security through long-term employment and the seniority wage system was traditionally applied to male employees as 'breadwinners', while women were considered secondary earners, with less employment and income security. Prior to the expansion of women's employment in the 20th century, it was common for women to leave their jobs on marriage or first childbirth to devote themselves to housework and childcare. Until recently, a result of women's labour market exit on marriage or when children were born was the 'M-shaped curve' of women's labour force participation rate by age, in which women re-entered the labour market after childbirth (Imada, 1996; Imada and Ikeda, 2007). Although the Act on Equal Opportunity and Treatment between Men and Women in Employment (EEO Act) established in 1985 prohibited gender discrimination, and the Child Care Leave Act (the predecessor of Child and Family Care Leave Act) established in 1991 supported labour market participation after childbirth, it remains difficult for workers with family responsibilities to stay in the Japanese workplace, as a work-centred culture, based on the assumption that male workers have a full-time housewife to undertake all housework, childcare and family care, remains (Imada and Ikeda, 2007).

It is common for male Japanese workers to work overtime and to take few periods of annual paid leave. Female workers seeking to develop their careers find they also need to adopt this work-focused approach. Even if they can take childcare leave, the work-centred culture ultimately prevents women with family responsibilities from continuing in their jobs. It is thus argued that reforming workplace culture is crucial to support combining work and family care (Takeishi, 2006; Takeishi and Takasaki, 2020).

With regard specifically to care for older people, there are increasing numbers of male workers who provide care to their frail old parents or wives (Tsudome and Saito, 2007). The expanding prevalence of caring responsibilities among male employees may become a catalyst for change in the traditional work-centred culture, although even today most working carers are still non-regular female employees (that is, part-time workers and fixed-term contract workers with lower income and weak employment security). The second-largest number of employed family carers are regular male employees including managers, executive, and high skilled workers, while female regular employees are the third largest (Employment Status Survey, Statistics Bureau, 2017; Ikeda, 2021a, 2023). Growing diversity among carers thus makes combining work and care an increasingly common concern for employees. This represents a risk to the core Japanese labour force, if carers are an increasingly diverse group that includes men, and leave the labour market due to family care. Further, more female regular employees are remaining in their jobs and developing their careers by moving into management positions. In this context, Japanese employers are gradually recognising that care for older people is a business challenge and beginning to arrange support for combining work and care (Ikeda, 2021a).

Political context

Japan is almost a one-party state in which, since 1955, the Liberal Democratic Party (LDP) has been in government for decades (sometimes in coalition with the Komeito or other parties since the late 1990s). The LDP is often described as a catch-all party, covering liberal and conservative policies. In fact, LDP-led governments have stressed both expanding social security for older people and the importance of traditional family ties in the context of restricted care services.

The LDP government established the National Health Insurance in 1958, the National Old Age Pension System in 1959 and the Act on Social Welfare for the Elderly (which regulates care services for older people) in 1963. These policies were introduced against a backdrop of high economic growth in the mid-20th century, although in the late 20th century (in response to low economic growth following the 1973 'oil crisis') the government turned again to stress family care. Policy makers emphasised mutual support between adult children and their older parents in the context of both childcare and eldercare. It was expected that older people would receive care from their adult children in return for care of their infant grandchildren, and, despite an increase in nuclear families and single person households, a high level of co-residence of adult children and their parents.

With changes to older people's households, governments began to recognise the importance of expanding social care services. The LTCI system established in 1997 was designed to reduce the amount of care families provide to older people by providing insurance-financed care services (Ikeda, 2000, 2002). Care for older people nevertheless still relies heavily on family support, due to insufficient provision of both services and funding (Shimoebisu, 2015).

In sum, LDP governments have supported both defamilialisation and refamilialisation of care for older people. Compared with some Anglo-Saxon countries, the Japanese government has established a comparatively generous system of long-term care and carer support (for example, the US and the UK have, respectively, no nationally legislated public care services and no long-term care leave with income security). Yet, compared with Scandinavian countries such as Sweden and Denmark (which have sufficient nursing facilities), the Japanese government has not expanded nursing or residential care facilities but has instead increased home care services under the LTCI. In this sense, the Japanese Government still depends on family care to supplement home care services. This is why, in the context of most international comparisons of welfare states, Japan is positioned as a familialist society.

Carer leave policies

Japanese care leave policy was legislated as a means of promoting gender equality, itself a core focus of the EEO Act 1985, which ratified the 1979 United Nations Convention on the Elimination of all forms of

Discrimination Against Women. Japan's care leave policy is also deeply influenced by the country's changing demography, notably its decreasing birth rate and increasing numbers of older adults. As a countermeasure against demographic labour force shortages, successive Japanese prime ministers (perhaps most notably Shinzo Abe, prime minister 2012–20) have emphasised the importance of labour participation for all adults, including women and older people, and, since 2015, prime ministers have focused political efforts on preventing exit from the labour market to provide care for family members (Cabinet Office, 2016).

Japan's first care leave legislation, the Child Care Leave Act established in 1991, responding to the falling fertility rate, obliged employers to accept employees' care leave applications. At the time it was common in Japan for women to leave their jobs after childbirth and the government was concerned that young working women would avoid having children so as not to give up their occupations and careers. The government's 'Angel Plan' in 1995 expanded nurseries for infants and spread childcare leave to support mothers' labour force participation. In practice, the childcare leave and nurseries had a demonstrably positive impact on mothers' continued labour market participation (Imada and Ikeda, 2007). The Child Care Leave Act in 1991 was expanded in scope to include male employees. However, the number of fathers taking leave has been much lower than that of mothers. The government promoted fathers' use of childcare leave based on the understanding that some men's lack of engagement in child rearing was influencing the falling birth rate (MHLW, 2002).

Japan also faced issues regarding care of older people, influenced by rapid population ageing after World War II. To support women's job continuation, it was thus also important to have policies to address long-term care. In 1995, the Child Care Leave Act was reformed as the Child and Family Care Leave Act. This established care leave for long-term care, in addition to leave to care for children (Sodei, 1995), and was also how the Japanese government ratified the International Labour Organization's 1981 Workers with Family Responsibilities Convention (ILO, 1985).

In sum, the care leave policy embodied in the Child and Family Care Leave Act was originally aimed at promoting the welfare of female workers and gender equality. Since the mid-2000s, however, care leave policies have been regarded as economic measures, with the ultimate aim of improving labour force retention (Expert Research Committee on Work–Life Balance, 2008). Former Prime Minister Shinzo Abe stressed the labour force participation and career development of women (Cabinet Office, 2013), as also embodied in the Women's Advancement Promotion Law established in 2015. He also focused on long-term care and declared prevention of job leaving for long-term care as an economic measure as well as a social security policy priority (Cabinet Office, 2016).

Japan has enacted statutes for both short-term and long-term leave, and for flexible working arrangements (MHLW, 2017; Ikeda, 2019, 2021a). Some details of these follow.

Short-term leave

Statutory short-term care leave allows workers to take time off work to care for eligible family members with an injury, physical or mental disability and associated issues (in provisions of the Child and Family Care Leave Act). Workers who take care of eligible family members in need of care can take up to five days off a year (ten days if there are two or more such family members). The worker can take this leave in one-hour increments or for one whole day. Workers whose work makes it difficult for them to take time off in one-hour increments can enter a labour-management agreement to take their leave in one-day increments. The worker is not paid or otherwise compensated for loss of earnings during this type of leave.

All employees (except day labourers) caring for a spouse, parents, children, parents-in-law, grandparents, siblings or grandchildren are eligible for this time off. The care provided must be because of an injury, illness or physical or mental disability that requires at least two weeks of constant care. Workers covered in labour-management agreements are not eligible for the leave if:

- the worker has been employed at the current workplace for less than six months;
- the worker works two scheduled days or less a week;
- the worker is engaged in jobs unsuitable for time off in an hourly increments.

Notice must be given in writing, or by phone on the day, if the working carer is unable to apply in advance.

Long-term leave

Long-term care leave was designed to enable workers to address a situation involving the person they care for and to make longer-term arrangements for combining work and care, rather than to provide care directly. Based on this premise, the Child and Family Care Leave Act allows workers to take long-term leave for a maximum of 93 days (per relevant family member) to care for a family member needing care due to injury, illness or physical or mental disability that requires more than two weeks of constant care. 'Family member' includes a partner (including a common-law partner), parents, children (in a legal parent–child relationship, including adopted children), parents of the partner, grandparents, siblings and grandchildren. The 93 days' leave can be split into one, two or three instalments. This long-term care leave applies to all employees, again excluding day labourers. Workers with fixed-term contracts, to be eligible, must:

- have worked at their current workplace for a year or more;
- have at least 93 days and six months left on their contract from the start date of the care leave.

Workers covered in labour-management agreements are not eligible for the leave if:

- the worker has been employed at the current workplace for less than a year;
- the worker works two scheduled days or less a week;
- the worker's contract ends within 93 days after application for the Family Caregiver Leave.

The worker must apply in writing to their employer at least two weeks before the planned start date of the leave. The worker can defer the leave once, within the scope of the 93 days, by applying at least two weeks before the planned end date of the leave.

Table 8.1 shows the maximum length of long-term care leave that workplaces such as offices, factories or shops provide according to their work rules. Many workplaces (82.9 per cent) limit the care leave up to 93 days based on the statutory provision, although over 10 per cent accept the leave for one year or more.

Table 8.2 shows how working carers use long-term care leave in practice. It shows that about half of employed working carers who take long-term care leave return to work within under one month (49.2 per cent); 55.5 per cent of male long-term care leave takers return to work within one week, although about one third of female long-term care leave takers need over three months. While some workplaces will accept workers taking care leave over the statutory 93 days if needed, the majority of employed working carers are adequately supported with using the 93 days divided into three portions.

Table 8.3 summarises the carer leave options available in Japan.

Other support measures

Flexible working arrangements

Workers may also request exemption from overtime work, or limitation of overtime and working late at night, until the end of long-term care for family members who need support due to injury, illness or physical or mental disability that requires more than two weeks of constant care. 'Family member' includes a partner (including common-law partner), parents,

Table 8.1: Maximum length of long-term care leave in work rules of workplace

	Up to 93 days in total	Over 93 days and under 6 months	6 months	Over 6 months and under 1 year	1 year	Over 1 year	Total
Work place with regulation on the maximum length of long-term care leave	82.9%	3.2%	2.9%	0.9%	8.2%	2.0%	100.0%

Source: MHLW (2022)

Table 8.2: Percentage of employed workers who returned from long-term care leave

	Under 1 week	1 week or more and under 2 weeks	2 weeks or more and under 1 month	1 month or more and under 3 months	3 months or more and under 6 months	6 months or more and under 1 year	1 year or more	Total
Total	26.1%	5.8%	17.3%	25.3%	7.4%	11.0%	7.1%	100.0%
Female	12.1%	4.0%	17.7%	32.5%	8.1%	15.3%	10.3%	100.0%
Male	55.5%	9.8%	16.4%	10.2%	5.9%	1.9%	0.4%	100.0%

Note: Every number rounds off to the second decimal place.

Source: MHLW (2022)

Table 8.3: Carer leave schemes, Japan (November 2023)

Leave details			Eligibility					
Leave name and introduced	Time period	Compensation	Worker/employee status	Qualifying period	Person needing care	Evidence	Notice period and process
Short-term care leave, 2009	5 days (10 days if there are 2 or more such family members) per annum	Unpaid	All employees (but not day labourers)	Not eligible: working individuals in a labour-management agreement; people employed at the current workplace for less than 6 months and working 2 days or less per week	Spouse, parents, children, parents-in-law, grandparents, siblings or grandchildren	–	Notice given in advance in writing or over the telephone on the day in emergencies
Long-term care leave, 1995	A total of 93 days per family member (the 93 days can be split into up to three separate blocks)	Unpaid but can receive up to 67% of salary through employment insurance system	All employees (but not day labourers); limited-term contract workers need a certain period left on their contract before the leave starts	Not eligible: working individuals in a labour-management agreement; people employed at their current workplace for less than 1 year; if the contract will end within 93 days after the application is made; people working 2 days or less per week	'Family member' includes a partner (including a common-law partner), parents, children (in a legal parent–child relationship, including adopted children), parents of the partner, grandparents, siblings and grandchildren	–	Application in writing to their employer at least two weeks before the planned start date of the leave

children (in a legal parent–child relationship, including adopted children), parents of the partner, grandparents, siblings and grandchildren.

Additionally, employers are required to introduce flexible working arrangements, within specified options. These include arrangements to reduce scheduled working hours; flexitime; staggered time; and a financial subsidy to support use of care services that enable workers to care for a family member for at least three years. Workers can use the system twice or more within the three-year period.

Analysis of survey data on working carers conducted by the Japanese Institute for Labour Policy and Training (JILPT) in 2019 showed that long-term care leave, exemption from overtime and staggered time may have positive implications for carers' ability to remain in employment until their caring role ends, as Table 8.4 shows. In multivariate analysis, reducing scheduled working hours and flexitime time did not seem to have such an effect. Findings nevertheless indicate that exemption from overtime might be replaced by staggered time. As for systems of reducing scheduled hours, this may require redesign, in terms of hourly care leave, as hourly short-term care leave is available from 2021 (Ikeda, 2023). In sum, research has highlighted the importance of paying attention to the variety of ways in which short-term care leave, long-term care leave and flexible working arrangements can be combined to enable workers to address the various challenges they face when providing care.

COVID-19 pandemic response and implications for employed carers

In April 2020, during the global COVID-19 pandemic, the labour force participation rate in Japan reached a low of 61.5 per cent (rising to 62.2 per cent in August 2021). The (pre-pandemic) 2.4 per cent unemployment rate (February 2020) rose to a peak of 3.1 per cent in October 2020, and was 2.8 per cent as of August 2021, based on the Statistics Bureau of Japan's Labour Force Survey (e-stat, 2023).

COVID-19 created additional demands on services, including childcare and care for older and disabled people. Nursery and school closures were mandated by an emergency declaration of the government in 2020, creating challenges for those combining work and childcare. Home care services for older people were also reduced to curb infection rates, but the implications for combining work and care for older people seem not to have been as severe (NHK, 2020).

The government established special support for COVID-19 in the form of a subsidy to prevent labour market exit from small and medium-sized enterprises (SMEs). The subsidy covered the cost of paid leave for care for up to 20 days. SMEs received ¥200,000 if employees took the paid leave

Table 8.4: Determinant factors of quitting jobs at the start of providing care by the end of providing care

Explained variable (yes=1, no=0)	Job quitting by the end of providing care							
	Estimation1				Estimation2			
	β	SE	EXP(β)		β	SE	EXP(β)	
Sex (male=1, female=0)	-.589	.176	.555	**	-.609	.178	.544	**
Age at the start of providing care	.021	.007	1.021	**	.021	.007	1.021	**
Education (BM: high school)								
Junior college	-.256	.172	.774		-.283	.173	.753	
College or graduate school	-.211	.172	.810		-.222	.173	.801	
Terms of providing care	.213	.017	1.238	**	.215	.017	1.239	**
Jobs at the start of providing care								
Employment types (regular=1, non-regular=0)	-.293	.179	.746		-.316	.180	.729	
Job categories (BM: clerical work)								
Professionals or managers	.272	.195	1.312		.259	.196	1.296	
Sales or services	.235	.185	1.265		.232	.186	1.261	
Blue-collar	-.187	.212	.830		-.191	.214	.826	
Number of employees at company (100 and more=1,under 100=0)	.084	.141	1.087		.064	.143	1.066	
Daily working hours (including overtime work)	.064	.037	1.066		.066	.037	1.069	
Support system for balancing work and family care								
Long-term care leave	-.505	.215	.603	*	-.466	.227	.628	*

(continued)

Table 8.4: Determinant factors of quitting jobs at the start of providing care by the end of providing care (continued)

Explained variable (yes=1, no=0)	Job quitting by the end of providing care					
	Estimation1			Estimation2		
	β	SE	EXP(β)	β	SE	EXP(β)
Exemption from overtime work	-.660	.324	.517 *	-.523	.362	.593
Reducing scheduled working hours		–		.021	.280	1.021
Flexitime		–		.387	.252	1.473
Staggered working hours		–		-.682	.283	.506 *
Constant	-3.067	.489	.047	-3.036	.491	.048 **
Chi-square		230.78	**		237.54	**
Df		13			16	
N		1410			1410	

method: logistic regression   Yes=1, no=0   ** p<.01, * p<.05

Note: BM = Bench Mark.

Source: Ikeda (2023: 89), using Survey on Work and Long-term Family Care (JILPT, 2019)

for more than five and less than ten days. If employees took the paid leave for ten days or more, the SME received ¥350,000.

A similar subsidy was available for parental leave to deal with the temporary closure of elementary schools in emergency situations. During the pandemic, parents faced challenges, caring for their children by themselves at home when elementary schools closed to prevent the spread of infection (Takami, 2021). The rationale for the subsidy for family care leave was based on the premise that carers of older people faced similar challenges to those experienced by parents needing to arrange childcare. In general, the system for supporting care for older people introduced in the Child and Family Care Leave Act and related measures follows similar support previously introduced for childcare. The subsidies for childcare and family care are based on the same idea, with the emergent situation related to childcare instigating the development of support for family care.

Adequacy of care leave policies

Equity/inclusivity

The Child and Family Care Leave Act was specifically designed to protect employees with permanent contracts with their employer, and thus excludes self-employed workers and people on temporary or fixed-term contracts. This has implications in terms of inequalities of coverage, as most full-time employees with long service records are male, while part-time and temporary workers are predominantly female. As a result, the Child and Family Care Leave Act may have the effect of widening the gender gap in employment security among working carers. Furthermore, current care leave policy does not support young carers who have not yet entered the labour market, although they experience challenges related to accessing education and in finding employment. Japanese care leave policy currently focuses on a rather narrow cohort of carers, lending support to the argument that the Japanese government should reform the policy to provide more comprehensive support for carers, including bringing more diverse groups of working carers, and young carers, within its remit.

Flexibility

In Japan, workers typically opt to use statutory paid annual leave (20 days per year, which can be carried over for up to one year) to provide periods of unpaid care (Sodei, 1995; JILPT, 2006). It was claimed that this reflects the greater flexibility, compared with the care leave policies, of the annual leave system (Sodei, 1995; JILPT, 2006; Nishimoto 2012). Responding to this, in 2009 the Child and Family Care Leave Act established annual short-term care leave (time off for family care) of up to five days, in addition to the original long-term care leave. In 2016 the Child and Family Care Leave Act was further amended to make long-term care leave more flexible by allowing recipients to divide it into three periods of time, addressing issues related to providing care for a prolonged period of time. Under regulations governing the Act, its provisions must be reviewed five years after enforcement of any previous amendment. In 2019, short-term care leave was also reformed to allow people to take time off in one-hour increments. Both short- and long-term care leave are nevertheless still compensated at less than full salary, unlike annual leave (see next section).

Job protection and income security

Workers who apply for, or who take, either short-term or long-term care leave are protected from disadvantageous treatment, such as dismissal, under the Child and Family Care Leave Act. Workers are not compensated at their full salary for either short-term leave or long-term leave. Instead, when taking long-term family care leave, they receive compensation (up to 67 per cent of normal salary) through the employment insurance system.

Other support measures applicable to carers

The Japanese government released 'Model measures in workplace to prevent job leaving due to family care' (MHLW, 2014), which includes pamphlets for employers and employees focused on preventing labour market exit due to long-term care. The pamphlets emphasised the importance of communication between employers and employees, encouraging the former to provide information about the support for working carers available to their employees. Identifying working carers is challenging for employers, as many workers try to combine work and care without telling their companies (Nishikubo, 2015; Ikeda, 2016); employers are therefore encouraged to create an open working environment (Nishikubo, 2015; Ikeda, 2016). Government has recommended that employers design their workplace policies in ways that reflect the lived experience of working carers, suggesting introducing surveys of their employees before designing measures to support them (Sato and Yajima, 2014). The Promotion and Research Project on Work–Life Balance and Diversity Management (2013, 2014, 2022), in the business school of Chuo University, undertakes employee surveys in response to employers' requests in order to highlight the challenges related to providing support to facilitate the combination of work and family care.

Employees also need to communicate with others who are part of their caring networks, including care recipients, other family members and care workers before leaving the labour market, and we recommend that the government should provide further guidance to support these discussions.

Conclusion

At a glance, care leave and other support systems for combining work and care look comprehensive in Japan and seem to be focused on the defamilialisation of care. There is statutory long-term care leave of up to 93 days; annual short-term care leaves of up to five days a year; and flexible working arrangements for up to three years, as well as exemption from overtime work until the end of long-term care. The long-term family care leave provides income replacement at 67 per cent of recipients' wages.

However, it is not clear that these care leave policies are sufficient for working carers. The numbers who take either short or long-term care leave are very small, arguably because the framework for the care leave does not fit with the realities of working carers' needs (JILPT, 2006; Ikeda, 2010, 2017a; MHLW, 2015). It is also possible that the LTCI reduced the need for long-term family care leave, which is supposed to be taken before care recipients begin to use care services (Ikeda, 2010). On the other hand, family carers need to be able to change their working hours flexibly after the expansion of home care services, which are more widely available since the introduction of the LTCI and intended to release family carers from the daily provision of care (Shimizutani and Noguchi, 2005; JILPT, 2006; Ikeda, 2010). It is often said the provision of care services through the LTCI is insufficient, especially for full-time working carers, as there is a mismatch between the usage time frames of home care services and the working hours of family carers. In response, the government expanded the usage time frame of home care services and improved flexible working arrangements (MHLW, 2015; JILPT, 2020; Ikeda, 2021a, 2021b; 2023).

In an attempt to fill the gap between the care leave policy and the realities of working carers' needs, the 2016 amendment of the Child and Family Care Leave Act allowed workers to divide the leave period over the course of the year, enabling them to return to their workplace as soon as possible. The amendment did not oblige employers to reduce the scheduled working hours, as is required in cases of childcare, however; instead, an exemption from overtime work was introduced. Reducing scheduled working hours, along with optional flexible working arrangements such as flexitime and staggered working time, is still based on the assumption that changes in scheduled working hours must be adapted to the varied situations of people providing care (MHLW, 2015; Ikeda, 2019, 2021a). It is true that some working carers are eager to reduce their scheduled working hours, even if their income or opportunities at work are similarly reduced; however, others prefer staggered time or flexitime, keeping the overall length of their working hours, if they need to change their start or end time of work to provide care (JILPT, 2015; MHLW, 2015; Ikeda, 2021a, 2021b).

Looking to the future, the LTCI system may face further challenges with continued ageing of the population. The challenges faced by the childcare sector, where insufficient nursery places have led to an increased need for extended periods of leave to care for children, may also become applicable to care for older people as demand for care outstrips supply. The leave policy for the care of older people is modelled on care for children in Japan; as such, it presumes the highest level of care will be required in the initial phases. This, however, overlooks differences between care for children and care for older adults. Care for children is broadly predictable and diminishes over time, whereas the support needed by older adults can be unpredictable, often with increased demands on carers over time. A reduction of working hours for three years, for example, is less likely to facilitate care for an older person than for a child. Some have argued that a longer period of support, instead of flexible working, is more appropriate for carers of older people (Ikeda, 2017b). The need for shorter working hours reflects differences between childcare and care for older people. Typically, older people with care needs can live by themselves or be left for periods, whereas young children require constant supervision (Winicott, 1965). It has also been argued that carers should not help older people in receipt of care too much, to avoid compromising their independence and autonomy (Hirayama, 2014, 2017). This autonomy-oriented care approach could reduce the need for care leave or for reduced scheduled working hours (Ikeda, 2021a, 2021b). It is therefore important that care leave policies for carers of older adults factor in different considerations than for policies that support the care of children.

Furthermore, it is important to highlight that it remains unclear whether current statutory care leave policies in Japan adequately address working carers' difficulties in combining work and care. The Child and Family Care Leave Act focuses on the conflict between work and providing care in terms of attendance during working hours. Although many working carers have caring demands that conflict with working schedules, there are also care tasks that fall during non-working hours and through the night, leading to fatigue. This issue, which affects carers' health, is particularly acute in care for older people (Ikeda, 2014, 2015, 2017b), and pent-up fatigue, due to providing care at night, sometimes causes presenteeism in the workplace (Ikeda, 2015), where working carers are not absent but do not work at their full capacity or potential. The Child and Family Care Leave Act, in its focus on time management between work and providing care, does not address this problem.

To gain further insight into the challenges carers of older adults face, in contrast to those with childcare responsibilities, the government has recommended that employers survey their workforce to find out about workers' care responsibilities and what support would be most appropriate. Carers' experiences and perspectives are diverse, with some appreciating the ability to take leave to provide care, while others would like respite care. For others, to ensure the care they provide is sustainable, work provides a form of opportunity to distance from the people they care for and taking care long-term leave in order to be devoted to providing care would have adverse effects for job continuation. Thus, the appropriateness of care leave is influenced not only by the amount of time made available, but also by the flexibility workers have to reconcile work and care as they prefer. In this sense, the Japanese government is still working towards creating the optimal support system for combining work and care. The current support system is insufficient for certain groups of working carers, for example, carers of disabled adults and part-time or temporary workers who also provide care. To address this, the government would need to take steps to provide support to diverse groups of working carers currently unable to benefit from the available policies.

References

Abeggglen, J.C. (1958) *The Japanese factory: Aspects of its social organization*, Glencoe, IL: Free Press.

Cabinet Office (2013) 'Basic policies for economic and fiscal management and reform: ending deflation and revitalizing the economy'. Available from: https://www5.cao.go.jp/keizai1/2013/20130614_2013_basicpol icies_e.pdf [Accessed 24 January 2024].

Cabinet Office (2016) 'Basic policy on economic and fiscal management and reform 2016'. Available from: https://www5.cao.go.jp/keizai1/basicp olicies-e/archives.html [Accessed 24 January 2024].

Cabinet Office (2022) 'Annual report on the ageing society' [Published in Japanese]. Available from: https://www8.cao.go.jp/kourei/whitepaper/ w-2022/zenbun/04pdf_index.html [Accessed 24 January 2024].

Dore, R. (1973) *British factory – Japanese factory: The origins of national diversity in industrial relations*, Berkeley and Los Angeles: University of California Press.

Esping-Andersen, G. (1999) *Social foundations of post-industrial economies*, Oxford: Oxford University Press.

e-stat (2023) *Labour force survey*. Available from: https://www.e-stat.go.jp/ en/stat-search/files?page=1&layout=datalist&toukei=00200531&tstat= 000000110001&cycle=1&year=20200&month=12040604&tclass1=00000 1040276&tclass2=000001040277&result_back=1&tclass3val=0 [Accessed 23 November 2023].

Expert Research Committee on Work–Life Balance (2008) 'Merit for enterprise to tackle work life balance, Council for Gender Equality, Cabinet Office'. [Published in Japanese]. Available from: https://www.gender.go.jp/ kaigi/senmon/wlb/pdf/wlb-0.pdf [Accessed 24 January 2024].

Fujisaki, H. (2009) 'The long-term care insurance and defamilization and refamilization of elderly care', *Japanese Journal of Welfare Studies*, 6: 41–57. [Published in Japanese]

Hazama, H. (1996) *The thought which made the Japanese economic miracle: Labor ethos in high economic growth*, Tokyo: Bunshin-do. [Published in Japanese]

Hirayama, R. (2014) *In the face of the age of sons giving care: An insight from the lives of 28 caregivers*, Tokyo: Kobunsha. [Published in Japanese]

Hirayama, R. (2017) *Sons who care: A blind side of masculinities and analyzing care from the perspective of gender*, Tokyo: Keiso Shobo. [Published in Japanese]

Ikeda, S. (2000) 'The principle of subsidiarity and long-term care insurance', *Journal of Social Security Research*, 36(2): 200–9. [Published in Japanese]

Ikeda S. (2002) 'The thought and system of long-term care insurance', in W. Ohmori (ed), *Elderly care and support for independence: The aims of long-term care insurance*, Kyoto: Minerva Shobo, pp 115–43. [Published in Japanese]

Ikeda, S. (2010) 'Leaving jobs for long-term care and the need for family care leave: the need for consecutive time off and factors determining leaving employment', *Japanese Journal of Labour Studies*, 599: 88–103. [Published in Japanese]

Ikeda, S. (2013) 'A new issue of supporting combining work with care: addressing working caregivers' fatigue'. JILPT Discussion Paper 13-01. [Published in Japanese]

Ikeda, S. (2014) 'Working carers' fatigue and taking time off', *Japanese Journal of Labour Studies*, 643: 41–8. [Published in Japanese]

Ikeda, S. (2015) 'The impacts of working caregivers' health on their work. In combining work and care', *JILPT Research Report*, 170: 70–88. Tokyo: JILPT. [Published in Japanese]

Ikeda, S. (2016) 'Addressing the issue of fatigue among working carers: the next challenge after reforming the family care leave system', *Japan Labor Review*, 13(2): 111–26.

Ikeda, S. (2017a) 'Family care leave and job quitting due to caregiving: focus on the need for long-term leave', *Japan Labor Review*, 14(1): 25–44.

Ikeda, S. (2017b) 'Supporting working carers' job continuation in Japan: prolonged care at home in the most aged society', *International Journal of Care and Caring*, 1(1): 63–82.

Ikeda, S. (2019) 'Combining work and family care in Japan: Part II: What is the challenge after reforming the long-term care leave system?' *Japan Labor Issues*, 3(5): 18–23.

Ikeda, S. (2021a) *Combining work and family care*, Diversity Management Series, Tokyo: Chuo-Keizai-Sha.

Ikeda, S. (2021b) 'The necessity of reduced working hours under the re-familization of elderly care', *Japan Labor Issues*, 5(30): 16–33.

Ikeda, S. (2023) 'Structure of job quitting for caregiving: workers' needs for support to balance work and long-term care under the Child and Family Care Leave Act', JILPT 4th term Project Research Series No.4.

Imada, S. (1996) 'Women's employment and job continuity', *The Japanese Journal of Labour Studies*, 433: 37–48. [Published in Japanese]

Imada, S. and Ikeda, S. (2007) 'The problem of women's job continuity and the childcare leave system', *Japan Labor Review*, 4(2): 139–60.

Inagami, T. (2005) *Post-industrial society and Japanese corporate society*, Kyoto: MINERVA Shobo. [Published in Japanese]

International Labour Organization (1985) *ILO's Convention on Workers with Family Responsibilities Convention, 1981 (C156)*. Available from: https://www.ilo.org/century/history/iloandyou/WCMS_213324/lang--en/index.htm [Accessed 29 November 2023].

Japan Institute for Labour Policy and Training (JILPT) (2006) 'For expanded use of family care leave system: report on the Study of Utilization of Family Care Leave System and Related Matters', JILPT Research Report (73). [Published in Japanese] Summary in English available from: https://www.jil.go.jp/english/reports/documents/jilpt-research/no73.pdf [Accessed 24 January 2024].

JILPT (2015) 'Combining work and care', JILPT Research Report (170). Tokyo: JILPT. [Published in Japanese] Summary in English available from: https://www.jil.go.jp/english/reports/jilpt_research/2015/no.170.html [Accessed 24 January 2024].

JILPT (2019) 'Survey on Work and Long-term Family Care', JILPT Research Report (204). Tokyo: JILPT. Available from: https://www.jil.go.jp/english/reports/jilpt_research/2020/no.204.html [Accessed 2 January 2024].

JILPT (2020) 'Combining work and care under the re-familization of elderly care in Japan', JILPT Research Report (204). Tokyo: JILPT. [Published in Japanese] Summary in English available from: https://www.jil.go.jp/english/reports/jilpt_research/2020/no.204.html [Accessed 24 January 2024].

Kasuga, K. (2001) *Sociology of long-term care issues*, Tokyo: Iwanami Shoten. [Published in Japanese]

Kröger, T. and Yeandle, S. (eds) (2013) *Combining paid work and family care: Policies and experiences in international perspective*, Bristol: The Policy Press.

Maeda, N. (1998) 'The effects in the extended household on women in work force', *The Japanese Journal of Labour Studies*, 459: 25–38 [Published in Japanese]

MHLW (Ministry of Health, Welfare and Labour) (2002) *The further countermeasures against falling birthrate*. [Published in Japanese] Available from: https://www.mhlw.go.jp/houdou/2002/09/h0920-1.html?msclkid= e4fd51fdceb011ec918ba9a4c14995bf [Accessed 24 January 2024].

MHLW (2014) 'Model measures in workplace to prevent job leaving due to family care', Tokyo: MHLW.

MHLW (2015) 'Report of working group on support for work family balance in the future', Tokyo: MHLW. [Published in Japanese.]

MHLW (2017) 'Annual health, labour and welfare report 2017'. [Published in Japanese.] Summary in English available from: https://www.mhlw.go.jp/english/wp/wp-hw11/dl/summary.pdf [Accessed 24 January 2024].

MHLW (2022) *Basic survey of gender equality in employment management.* Available from: https://www.mhlw.go.jp/toukei/list/71-23.html [Accessed 24 November 2023].

MHLW (2023) 'Report of working group on balance support between work and child care and family care in the future'. [Published in Japanese] Available from: https://www.mhlw.go.jp/content/11909500/001108929.pdf [Accessed 24 January 2024].

NHK (2020) *Close up gendai*, 23 April.

Nishikubo, K. (2015) *Crisis of elderly care: How Japanese companies can prepare for the risk of loss of human resources*, Tokyo, Jumpo-sha. [Published in Japanese]

Nishimoto, M. (2012) 'Taking family leave from employment: does a system compatible with family care and employment exist?' *Japanese Journal of Labour Studies*, 623: 71–84. [Published in Japanese]

Osawa, M. (1993) *Beyond enterprise-centered society: Reading contemporary Japan from gender perspective*, Tokyo: Jiji-Tsushin-Sha. [Published in Japanese]

Prime Minister's Office of Japan (2015) *Revising Japan revitalization strategy 2015.* Available from: https://www.kantei.go.jp/jp/singi/keizaisaisei/pdf/dai1en.pdf [Accessed 26 November 2023].

Promotion and Research Project on Work–Life Balance and Diversity Management (2013) 'Problems on companies' support system on combining work and family care which enable employees' job continuation: research report on employees' needs of support for family care 2011–2012', Business School of Chuo University. [Published in Japanese]

Promotion and Research Project on Work–Life Balance and Diversity Management (2014) 'Problems in supporting employees who have possibilities of facing family care or who actually face the family care: survey on combining work and family care 2014', Business School of Chuo University. [Published in Japanese]

Promotion and Research Project on Work–Life Balance and Diversity Management (2022) 'Problems of employees combining work and Family Care in 3 participant companies', Business School of Chuo University. [Published in Japanese]

Sato, H. and Yajima, Y. (2014) *Protecting employees from job leaving due to family care: A new problem of work–life balance*, Rodo Chosa Kai.

Shimizutani, S. and Noguchi, H. (2005) 'What accounts for the onerous care burden at home in Japan? Evidence from household data', *Keizai Bunseki*, 175: 1-32. [Published in Japanese]

Shimoebisu, M. (2015) 'Position of the family in care policies', *Japanese Journal of Family Sociology*, 27(1): 49–60. [Published in Japanese]

Shinkawa, T. (2014) *Turning point of welfare state reform: Labor, welfare, liberty*, Kyoto: Minerva-Shobo. [Published in Japanese]

Sodei, T. (1989) 'Women and elderly care', in M. Ozawa, N. Kumura and H. Ibu (eds), *Women's lifecycle: Comparing income security between Japan and US*, Tokyo: University of Tokyo Press, pp 127–49. [Published in Japanese]

Sodei, T. (1995) 'The issues and meanings of the family care leave system', *Japanese Journal of Labor Studies*, 427: 12–20.

Statistics Bureau (2017) *Employment status survey*. Available from: https://www.stat.go.jp/english/data/shugyou/index.html [Accessed 23 November 2023].

Takami, T. (2021) 'Working hours under the COVID-19 pandemic in Japan', *Japan Labor Issues*, 5(30): 2–10.

Takeishi, E. (2006) *Employment system and women's careers*, Tokyo: Keiso Shobo. [Published in Japanese]

Takeishi, E. and Takasaki, M. (2020) *Supporting womens' career development*, Diversity Management Series, Tokyo: Chuo-Keizai-Sha.

Tsudome, M. and Saito, M. (2007) *White paper on male carers*, Kyoto: Kamogawa-Press. [Published in Japanese]

Winicott, D.W. (1965) *The maturational processes and facilitating environment*, London: Hogarth.

Yamato, R. (2008) *The making of life-long carers in Japan: Reconstructed generational relationship and strong rooted gender relationships*, Tokyo: Gakubun-Sha. [Published in Japanese]

Yokoyama, F. (2002) *Postwar Japan's policies on women*, Tokyo: Keiso Shobo. [Published in Japanese]

9

Slovenia

Tatjana Rakar, Maša Filipovič Hrast and Valentina Hlebec

Introduction

This chapter provides an overview of existing carer leave and related policies in Slovenia. In the first part the national economic, social, political and welfare policy contexts are briefly explained to facilitate understanding of the corresponding carer-related policies already implemented. Existing carer leave policies in Slovenia are then described, as well as the changes introduced during the lengthy and politically contentious process of adopting and implementing different versions of the Long Term Care Act, which was initially adopted in 2021, with several subsequent amendments.[1] This section is followed by an analysis of the impact of COVID-19 on the care and well-being of older people in Slovenia. The final section provides an evaluation of the adequacy of carer leave policies in Slovenia. This draws on research on carers and highlights the unmet needs of many older people in need of care. The chapter concludes with suggestions for potential avenues for further research and policy recommendations.

National context

Economic and social context

Slovenia is a relatively small country, population of 2,110,547 (SURS, 2022), that was once part of Yugoslavia and gained its independence in 1991. It was one of the more economically developed countries within Yugoslavia and among the first Central and Eastern European countries to enter the European Union (EU) in 2004, and then the eurozone in 2007. Following independence, Slovenia experienced strong economic growth and rising gross domestic product (GDP) until the global economic downturn in 2008, when it experienced a prolonged recession. Growth resumed in 2014 but was adversely affected by the COVID-19 pandemic in 2020 (Figure 9.1). During the period of economic recovery, 2014–19, employment increased, public finances improved and the difference between the growth in Slovenia's GDP and the European average reduced (UMAR, 2021). The pandemic strongly affected the economy and although the government has tried to decrease its impact on households through several

Figure 9.1: Slovenia's real GDP growth rate (percentage change on previous years)

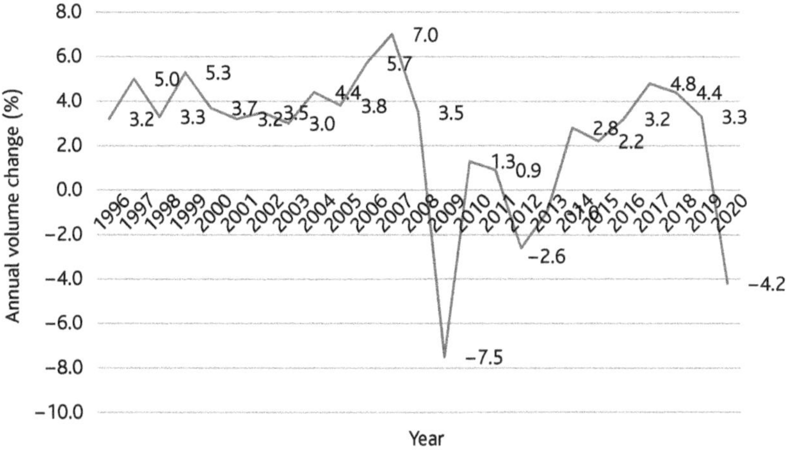

Source: SURS (2022)

targeted measures, the social situation has deteriorated. Real GDP fell by 5.5 per cent in 2020, although this reduction was less than the EU average (-6.2 per cent) (UMAR, 2021: 110).

At the beginning of the 1990s, Slovenia's economic restructuring led to high unemployment rates. Employment subsequently increased as the economy grew, but unemployment rose again after 2008. It began to fall again in 2014 and remains below the EU average (Table 9.1). In comparison to other Central and Eastern European countries, Slovenia's transition to a market economy was relatively smooth and inequalities did not become significantly pronounced. The size of the Gini coefficient increased only marginally, as compared to the pre-transition period (see Flere and Lavrič, 2003; Malnar, 2011; Filipovič Hrast and Ignjatović, 2012). Income inequality, as measured by the Gini index, has remained lower than the EU 27 average (Table 9.1).

However, despite positive growth and relatively low inequality levels, several indicators point to economic weaknesses. Purchasing power in Slovenia decreased from 2009 and recovered only gradually to reach the level of 2008 (Trbanc, 2020; UMAR, 2021). Furthermore, the Slovenian labour market has become increasingly segmented between those who have secure, permanent employment and those with less secure (temporary or part-time) jobs (Ignjatović, 2011; Kajzer, 2011; Trbanc, 2020). Young people, in particular, are increasingly likely to be employed in temporary jobs (Trbanc, 2020; UMAR, 2021). Furthermore, although the overall risk of poverty in Slovenia is below the EU 27 average (and has been decreasing since 2014), the poverty rate among the older population is higher than

Table 9.1: Employment and poverty data related to Slovenia

	2011	2012	2013	2014	2015	2016	2017	2018	2019	2020
Slovenia – total employment (per cent of total population)	73.9	74.4	74.3	74.6	75.4	75.6	78.0	78.9	79.3	78.7
EU 27 – total employment (per cent of total population)	74.4	74.9	75.3	75.7	76.1	76.5	77.0	77.5	77.8	77.1
Slovenia – female employment (per cent of total population)	70.2	70.9	70.3	70.8	71.5	72.5	74.9	75.6	76.2	75.9
EU 27 – female employment (per cent of total population)	67.7	68.5	69.0	69.6	70.0	70.6	71.2	71.6	72.1	71.4
Slovenia – employment 55–65 (per cent of total population)	33.0	34.8	35.7	38.1	39.3	40.9	45.3	49.1	50.5	51.9
EU 27 – employment 55–65 (per cent of total population)	48.6	50.5	52.3	54.1	55.7	57.6	59.3	60.7	61.8	62.3
Slovenia – female employment 55–65 years	23.5	26.3	26.8	30.9	32.7	35.0	39.3	43.6	45.7	48.0
Slovenia – part-time employment (per cent of total employed)	9.3	9.3	9.3	10.0	10.1	9.6	10.4	9.9	8.6	8.7
Slovenia – part-time employment (per cent of total employed) – female	12.3	12.7	12.9	14.0	13.9	13.7	14.8	14.7	12.9	12.7
EU 27 – part-time employment (per cent of total employed) – female	31.3	31.8	32.5	32.3	32.2	32.0	31.8	31.4	31.4	29.2
Slovenia – unemployment (per cent of labour force)	8.2	8.9	10.2	9.8	9.0	8.1	6.6	5.2	4.4	5.0
EU27 – unemployment (per cent of labour force)	9.8	10.8	11.3	10.8	10.0	9.0	8.0	7.2	6.6	7.0
Slovenia – unemployment (per cent of labour force) – female	8.2	9.5	11.0	10.7	10.2	8.6	7.4	5.8	4.9	5.6
Slovenia at risk of poverty rate	13.6	13.5	14.5	14.5	14.3	13.9	13.3	13.3	12.0	12.4
EU 27 at risk of poverty rate	16.9	16.9	16.8	17.3	17.4	17.5	16.9	16.8	17.2	17.1
Slovenia at risk of poverty rate 65+	20.9	19.6	20.5	17.1	17.2	17.6	16.4	18.3	18.6	19.4
EU 27 at risk of poverty rate 65+	15.1	14.2	13.3	13.2	13.7	14.3	14.7	15.5	16.9	17.3
GINI-EU 27	30.5	30.4	30.6	30.9	30.8	30.6	30.3	30.4	30.2	30.0
GINI-Slovenia	23.8	23.7	24.4	25.0	24.5	24.4	23.7	23.4	23.9	23.5

Note: Data on unemployment and part-time employment refer to age group 20–65 years.

Source: Eurostat (2022)

the EU 27 average (Table 9.1). This has implications for the ability of older people to pay for care.

High labour market participation among women has been traditional in Slovenia for more than half a century and is supported by a very well-developed network of childcare services, as well as relatively generous maternity and parental leaves. The female employment rate is high compared to the EU average (almost 76 per cent in 2020, compared to 71.4 per cent in the EU 27). Part-time employment, however, is relatively uncommon: only 8.7 per cent of the labour force were employed part time in 2020, and although the figure for women was slightly higher at 12.7 per cent, this percentage is substantially lower than the EU average (29.2 per cent of EU women were in part-time employment in 2020) (Eurostat, 2022).

Pension reforms, involving increasing the standard retirement age and abolishing early retirement schemes, have led to longer working lives. As Table 9.1 indicates, there has been a sharp rise in the employment rate of women aged 55–65 in Slovenia, from 23.5 per cent in 2011 to 48 per cent in 2020. On the other hand, compared to other European countries, levels of employment among the older age groups remain below the EU average, although the difference has decreased in the past 10 years (from 33 per cent in Slovenia and 48.6 per cent in EU 27 in 2011, to 51.9 per cent in Slovenia and 62.3 per cent in EU 27 in 2020) (Eurostat, 2022).

The full-time employment of women as well as increasingly prolonged working lives creates challenges for family carers in combining work and family care in the long term, especially given population ageing. Population projections indicate that in Slovenia the proportion of people aged 65 years or older will reach almost one third of the total population in 2060 (that is, 29.5 per cent) (UMAR, 2017: 10). This rising share will increase the burden on the state due to rising expenditure for pensions and health and long-term care, as well as increase the need for informal and formal care. Furthermore, it has been predicted that the share of GDP allocated to pensions will increase from 6 per cent to 16 per cent by the year 2070 (UMAR, 2021: 68).

Political and welfare policy context

Slovenia is a parliamentary democratic republic with a proportional electoral system and national legislative powers in all areas. The country is composed of 212 municipalities, 11 of which have urban status. The competencies of a municipality comprise local affairs, which may be autonomously regulated by the municipality.

Slovenia is a former socialist society with a tradition of a state socialist welfare system in which the state played a dominant role (Kolarič, Kopač and Rakar, 2009, 2011). In the post-independence transition period, reforms were implemented gradually rather than as 'shock therapy' as in some other post-socialist countries (Ferge, 2001; Kolarič, Kopač and Rakar, 2009), and followed a neo-corporatist development rather than the neoliberal paths found elsewhere (Bohle and Greskovits, 2007). The emerging Slovenian welfare system was thus a dual or hybrid model, combining the elements of the conservative-corporatist model and the social democratic model drawn from Esping-Andersen's (1990) typology. Characteristic of the conservative regime is that compulsory social insurance schemes are the main instrument for the provision of social protection. Similar to a social democratic regime, a strong public and state sector retained the status of the main service provider for all types of services to which all citizens are equally entitled (Kolarič, Kopač and Rakar, 2009, 2011).

After independence, welfare provision in Slovenia continued to develop gradually, with the state remaining heavily involved in service provision. However, in the period since the 2008 economic crisis, this well-developed welfare system came under increasing pressure. Slovenia was one of the countries that experienced the 'explosive cocktail' of high government deficit and demographic change (see Filipovič Hrast and Rakar, 2020; Greve, 2011). The 2008 economic crisis exposed critical weaknesses in Slovenia's pre-crisis economic performance, structural inconsistencies in its welfare system and the country's limited capacity for innovation (OECD, 2011: 17). This was exacerbated by political instability caused by the constant changes of left and right coalitions. Several Slovenian governments adopted gradual social policy reforms, while 2012 was marked by a complete reform of social legislation and changes in the regulation of non-contributory benefits, which came into force together with two austerity laws (Filipovič Hrast and Rakar, 2017, 2020). These pressures, coupled with the emphasis on austerity, have led to structural reforms of the welfare system, resulting in a step change in the reform process as well as social tensions reflected in public unrest and resistance to the reforms. Following the trends in welfare policy changes (Cantillon, 2011; Vandenbroucke and Vleminickx, 2011; Hemerijck, 2013; Van Kersbergen, Vis and Hemerijck, 2014), we can characterise the welfare state changes in Slovenia as predominantly moving towards austerity and cost containment (Filipovič Hrast and Rakar, 2017, 2020).

However, from 2014 onwards, there was a partial reversal of this trend, with earlier more universal or generous policies being partially expanded or reintroduced due to the economic recovery. Compared to social protection policies, which refer to social transfer policies, social investment policies relate to service delivery such as childcare measures, as well as policies for older people, and these have overall been less affected by government austerity measures (see Filipovič Hrast and Rakar, 2017). Reforms in line with a social investment strategy are being pursued (for example, active labour market policies), but remain relatively weak compared to those established in the past (for example, childcare and education) (Filipovič Hrast and Rakar, 2020).

In terms of Slovenia's care policies, there are substantial differences in arrangements for child and older people care (Filipovič Hrast and Rakar, 2021). Placing Slovenia on a continuum of care regimes ranging from defamilialised to familialised is difficult, with care for children being highly defamilialised (Chung, Filipovič Hrast and Rakar, 2018; Filipovič Hrast and Rakar, 2021) and older people's care highly familialised (Hlebec, Srakar and Majcen, 2016a; Filipovič Hrast, Hlebec and Rakar, 2020). Slovenia's childcare policies have been built upon a historically extensive system of public childcare provision and generous leave policies, together with a well-developed social protection system that targets families. These measures were retained and, in some cases, expanded up until the 2008 economic crisis, when in the following years certain austerity measures in terms of targeted selectivity and means testing were introduced (Filipovič Hrast and Rakar, 2017; Blum, Correia, Nygard, Rakar and Wall, 2020).

On the other hand, care policies for older people started to develop only later and, after initial growth, were relatively stagnant (especially the home care system). The austerity measures put in place during the Great Recession after 2008 and subsequent years seem to have produced a slowing effect on the sector's institutional design, with a stronger role played by private investors in both home care services as well as institutional care and increasing personal funds for care. Therefore, these changes toward greater defamilialisation via the market were seen in both the provision of institutional care and home care for older people. This is a considerable difference from the trends in family policy for children, an area which is almost the exclusive domain of the public sector (Hlebec and Rakar, 2017; Filipovič Hrast and Rakar, 2021). A comprehensive long-term care system is yet to be implemented and the recently adopted Long-Term Care Act (2021)[2] is part of ongoing public and political debates.

Carer leave policies

In Slovenia only one legislated measure directly supports carers' ability to balance work and care responsibilities, in the form of legislated short-term or emergency absence to respond to the urgent care needs of a family member. This paid sickness benefit or leave to care for sick family members was provided for in the Health Care and Health Insurance Act from 1992, with several later amendments.[3] However, this entitlement to benefit or leave was already in force during the socialist period of the Republic of Yugoslavia, before Slovenia gained independence in 1991.

Paid sickness benefit or leave to care for sick family members is intended for all insured persons. Insured persons are entitled to take leave to care for an immediate co-resident family member who is ill (spouse and children, biological or adopted). The leave does not apply to elderly parents and other relatives, as they are not defined as 'close family members'. In terms of benefits, leave is paid by the employer at 80 per cent of the individual's average gross earnings for all employment in the preceding calendar year. However, compensation cannot be lower than the guaranteed wage.[4] The duration of sickness benefit depends on the illness and is estimated individually, based on a medical certificate. In general, ten days of leave may be taken for each episode of illness per family member in need of care (or 20 days for children under seven and those with special needs). In exceptional cases the period may be extended up to 40 days (in the case of children under seven years and those with special needs) or up to 20 days for other close family members and up to six months in extreme cases. There are no regulations that limit the duration of the annual entitlement, only for each episode of leave taken. In the case of severe illness of a child, based on a request from the paediatric council, the leave can be extended until the child is 18 years old.

In terms of eligibility criteria, the leave is conditional: it applies only to insured persons in regular employment and excludes employees who are not insured. Self-employed persons need to insure themselves for such leave. Employees must provide their employer with a medical certificate. Care receivers are restricted to close family members living in the same household as the carer. There is no definition of a sick family member in the legislation; only the term 'close family member in need of care' is used. Job security is assured in that the law requires that leave can be taken without risk of job loss; this applies to all workers in regular employment.

In Slovenia there are no longer statutory leave options for people to provide care for older adults. Legislation relating to care leave applies only to those caring for children, in particular caring for a child with a serious mental or physical disability. However, measures concerning care for older relatives can be arranged via collective agreements. A good example at the company level is a collective agreement at ETI Elektroelement, d.o.o. (ETI), where 70 per cent of the workers are women. The company found that workers were taking sick leave to care for family members. The union proposed soft measures to address workers' work–life balance problems. Finally, three joint committees were established, including a representative of the trade union, the company's head of department and the company's head of human resources, which deal with cases such as young mothers (an extra day off), older people's care (annual leave should be a priority for those who care) and teleworking. As a result, the company was able to reduce sick leave, improve efficiency and contribute to greater employee well-being (Confederation Syndicate European Trade Union, 2019). Still, as concluded by a study of 20 sectoral collective agreements in Slovenia (in both the private and public sectors), the benefits available to working carers in collective agreements significantly lag behind those of working parents. Within the index of the importance of work–life reconciliation measures examined in this study, adjustments in case of workers caring for their older frail family members were found to receive no or very little attention in the collective agreements analysed (Kresal Šoltes et al, 2016).

However, in Slovenia there are other support measures to facilitate care for older people. In terms of direct financial support (for example, through a carer benefit, carer allowance or payments that a carer can use to hire or pay for a care service), there is a measure for 'family assistant' (carer).[5] It replaces full-time residential care with home care for those who are eligible for residential care and have opted for a family assistant instead of residential care. The carer must have competences for care work and must have the same permanent residence as the care recipient or be a close relative. A carer must leave their full-time employment with the intention of becoming a family assistant; however, they can continue to be employed part time. In addition to social security and healthcare insurance rights, the carer is entitled to a monthly payment for loss of income (or, in the case of part-time work, the proportionate part-time monthly payment). The carer fulfils the following tasks: personal care, medical care, social care and organisation of leisure activities and domestic help. It is intended for care of persons over 18 years old. However, family members who decide to remain in part-time employment cannot retain the full level of social security benefits; nor do they receive additional compensation for the loss of income (MDDSZ, 2022).

There are also measures in the form of self-managed or self-directed care schemes, where care recipients are provided with funds to hire help, with the option to pay or directly compensate family members. The 'care allowance for external care and assistance' is a cash benefit intended to pay for the expenses of a care recipient who needs constant help and care due to his or her permanent state of health. There are two different amounts, depending on the degree of need for assistance. In addition, there is also a 'care and assistance allowance' for the payment of expenses for people in need of permanent assistance and care due to a permanent state of health. There are three different amounts for this, depending on the need for assistance and the different types and categories of disability.

There are no statutory services for carers or services available to carers in their own right. Services and benefits are provided only to the care receiver. If the carer has their own healthcare needs in general, regardless of their care-giving role, they can access physicians and hospital services according to the rules of the national healthcare system.

After several years in preparation, in December 2021 a Long-Term Care Act[6] was finally adopted, which introduced drastic changes, especially in terms of long-term care financing. Additional changes relevant for this chapter are acknowledgement of the contribution of informal care and carers by introducing a policy measure of a family carer with social security rights, and also the right of a family carer to take leave and have care substituted, for up to 21 days of absence on a yearly basis (individual absence lasts a minimum of 7 days). However, the law has major flaws that virtually all organisations representing long-term care users and providers have highlighted. These critics emphasise that the law does not address the problem of long-term care in a comprehensive way and is not feasible in practice (STA, 2022). Moreover, the operation of the long-term system will depend largely on additional measures that have not yet been drafted.

The newly adopted long-term care measures cover institutional care, social home care, family carer and cash benefits. All forms of care, except institutional care, include the right to services to strengthen and maintain independence and e-care. The provisions of the Act will be phased in, planned to start in January 2023 with the rights to institutional care, while most of the rights relating to 'ageing in place' provisions were initially planned to come into force on 1 July 2024. These include the right to home care, the right to a caregiver for a family member and the right to cash benefits. The Act introduces the possibility to exercise the right to long-term care in the form of cash benefits. This means that the health insurance fund transfers a certain amount to the account of the person in need of long-term care. These rights are mutually exclusive. The person in need of care can therefore exercise only one of the two rights – as a benefit in kind or as a cash benefit.

However, in July 2022, the newly elected centre-left government extended the implementation of the Act for another year and will introduce important amendments, as it believes that more than a third of the Act needs to be changed because it is not feasible in practice. Therefore, a new Act will be drafted. In addition, oversight of the law has been transferred from the Ministry of Health to the Ministry of Labour, Family, Social Affairs and Equal Opportunities. Later it will be placed under the planned new Ministry for the Solidarity Future (MZ, 2022). The former ruling party and currently the largest opposition party, SDS (Slovenska demokratska stranka), believes that the decision of the ruling coalition to amend the Act, which also delays its implementation by one year, will harm older and vulnerable people, and therefore submitted a request for a referendum on the Act to Parliament (Hočevar, 2022). However, in November 2022, the majority of voters voted in favour of the amendments to the Long-Term Care Act, whereupon the implementation of the Act was delayed by one year. Thus, the future shape of long-term care in Slovenia remains one of the most politically contentious and ambiguous issues, leaving the urgently needed changes legally unresolved. Table 9.2 summarises the carer leave options available in Slovenia.

Table 9.2: Carer leave schemes, Slovenia (November 2023)

Leave details			Eligibility				
Leave name and introduced	Time period	Compensation	Worker/employee status	Qualifying period	Person needing care	Evidence	Notice period and process
Leave to care for sick family member, 1992	Depends on illness but typically 10 days' leave per episode (or 20 for children under 7/those with additional care needs). There are no limitations for annual entitlement.	80% of wages	All insured persons	–	Immediate co-resident family member (spouse and children, biological or adopted)	Medical certificate required	–

The impact of COVID-19

Older people were one of the most vulnerable groups at risk of infection during the pandemic in Slovenia, with those living in care homes among the worst affected. Measures to protect this vulnerable group in Slovenia, like elsewhere in Europe, included closing these facilities or limiting or preventing visits[7]; protocols for protection and reducing the risk of transmitting the virus; and reorganising homes into specific zones in the event of infection.[8] In the early stages of the pandemic, some appeals were made to families to take on the responsibility of providing care to their older family members and reduce the pressure on institutional care. According to media reports, this appeal was heeded by relatively few families.[9] The Community of Social Institutions (Skupnost socialnih zavodov) noted that the pandemic had accentuated years of neglect and insufficient development of long-term care in Slovenia[10] with its lack of skilled personnel and severe space constraints in care homes[11] (see Oven, 2020). This brought to the surface many existing problems in care homes, which at the time also led to public and political debates on staffing and lack of rooms in care homes (see Advocate of the Principle of Equality, 2021). Furthermore, the pandemic also reduced the accessibility of care homes as restrictions were placed on the ability of homes to accept new residents, leading to many beds being left unoccupied.

According to Eurofound (2022), many care arrangements during the pandemic shifted from formal to informal long-term care and saw the tightening of 'informal' care networks within a smaller family network, with many carers taking on more care work. In Slovenia there is no data on whether this has been the case. However, the conditions family carers faced during the pandemic increased their burden, and there were limited policies to address the needs of this group. From the carers' perspective, it was vital that all home care services (covering health and social care needs) continued during the pandemic, with additional safety measures and protocols.[12] However, staffing problems affected services, ranging from infections among staff, to quarantines and absences due to the need to care for children (with staff taking up their legal option of taking a leave of absence due to closing of childcare and school facilities in order to take care of the child during the pandemic). Provision of care was also difficult when older people and their carers were not living together, particularly in one period during the pandemic when free movement between municipalities was curtailed. Carers were, however, exempt from the restrictions; that is, an exception was the 'care and help to persons in need of help or support and care of family members' (Official Gazette, 2020).

The government also recognised the financial strain of the pandemic on vulnerable groups and provided a one-off solidarity supplement for pensioners in 2020,[13] as well as a one-off solidarity supplement for those registered as family assistants (carers).[14] The position of family carers has also recently improved due to the new Long Term Care Act, and in 2022 they received a higher salary replacement calculated at 1.2 times the minimum wage.[15] However, registered family carers continue to comprise a very small number of family carers in Slovenia, and therefore most family carers were not specifically targeted and supported during the pandemic. The care leave policies that were enacted were targeted only at parents caring for children, enabling access to a salary supplement in cases of leave to care for the child (due to closure of childcare facilities and schools), while not adding specific conditions and addressing other family carers, such as those caring for older people (see Rakar, Hlebec and Filipovič Hrast, 2022).

The sudden and unexpected circumstances presented by the COVID-19 pandemic saw the introduction of policy measures in the direction of refamilialisation (limited to the period of the pandemic) in care throughout Europe as well as globally, irrespective of care regime characteristics (see Eurofound, 2020a, 2020b; Blum and Dobrotić, 2021). The measures adopted to prevent COVID-19 infection (closure of childcare facilities and schools, limits on home care services, appeals to return nursing home occupants to their families, social distancing) shifted a large care burden for children and older people onto families or informal networks (see Eurofound, 2020a, 2020b, 2022). Meanwhile, the widespread adoption of flexible work arrangements may have facilitated the reconciliation of work and family life. However, on the other hand, together with the measures that closed childcare facilities, schools and limited home care services, it may have exposed families to a particularly difficult work–life balance, especially those from the 'sandwich generation'.

Adequacy of carer leave policies

Informal care in Slovenia is perceived as a cultural norm and an ordinary part of family life (Hlebec and Šircelj, 2011), rather than a policy-supported choice, as by law the family is legally obliged to provide financial support for the care for an older person and therefore when the costs become too high for the older people themselves, families are obliged to pay the costs. It is only when even families are unable to do so that the state subsidises the costs of care (Hlebec and Rakar, 2017). Additionally, there is a lack of focused research into family caring, the life situations of carers and systematic evaluations of care leave policies. There is, therefore, a lack of data by which to evaluate the uptake of measures to support carers. However, in recent years there have been both qualitative and quantitative explorations of pathways into informal care as well as insights into the coping strategies of carers, the potential negative consequence of caring and the unmet needs of older people, indicating gaps in the provision of formal and informal care for people 'ageing in place'.

In a cross-country comparative study of Slovenia and Austria, Rodrigues, Filipovic Hrast, Kadi, Hurtado Monarres and Hlebec (2022) found that transitions into informal care in these familialistic countries are a result of continuous cumulative processes, such as reciprocal intergenerational support, or a result of structurally determined cumulative processes triggered by turning points in life trajectories, such as divorce (followed by financial constraints and re-cohabitation of adult children with parents), serial caring roles or retirement of family carers.

One exploration of carers of older people who were ageing in place in Slovenia (Filipovič Hrast, Hlebec and Rakar, 2020) revealed a series of strategies employed by carers to meet the care needs of older people. External strategies were mostly linked to obtaining more care from formal sources or harvesting support from filial networks or friends and neighbours, whereas internal strategies included changing and adjusting work-related arrangements, withdrawal from leisure activities or giving up holidays. These strategies are largely a direct result of a lack of policy support measures for carers. The study also highlighted increased psychological distress and overburdening that carers may experience.

Another recent comparative study (van Aerschot, Kadi, Rodrigues, Filipovič Hrast, Hlebec and Aaltonen, 2022) focused on formal care for older people, addressing mostly measurable, task-oriented and instrumental care, which may not meet the emotional, psychological and relational needs of older people. Frequent changes in care workers who hurriedly carry out necessary (and accountable) care tasks sometimes leave older people upset and lonely. Unmet needs may lead to carers taking on more care responsibilities at the expense of their own social life and leisure activities. This study called for formal services to be structured in such a way as to not only optimise service provision but also enable older people to develop a personal relationship with care workers, develop and maintain social contacts and networks and pursue their own activities and interests.

The familialistic orientation of the Slovenian care regime is evident in the extensive nature of intergenerational care for older people as shown by Santini et al (2020). Of the six countries covered in this study, in Italy and Slovenia a substantial percentage of adolescent young carers provide care and support to their grandparents. Adolescent carers caring for grandparents are less likely to experience negative outcomes of caring, such as frustration or mental health problems. Rather, positive caring outcomes are possible, such as developing relational skills, higher resilience and maturity. An in-depth study (Santini et al, 2022) also revealed that adolescent young carers of grandparents may face both emotional and physical consequences from care activities, ranging from emotional distress to back pain due to heavy lifting.

Utilising SHARE (Survey of Health, Ageing and Retirement in Europe) data, another study has shown that the likelihood of having unmet care needs increases with age and is higher in rural areas than in urban areas, owing to fragmentation and lack of formal services for older people living in rural areas (Hlebec, Srakar and Majcen, 2016b).

Despite the lack of focused research on carers, compared to that on older people as care recipients, the studies mentioned indicate a need for in-depth studies of how informal care is integrated into carers' everyday lives and how a lack of support measures or rigid access criteria prevents carers of older people from reconciling care and paid work, or care and other family responsibilities.

Conclusion

The familialist regime of care for older people which, as shown, governs existing carer leave arrangements for older people in Slovenia faces several challenges in terms of its sustainability (Filipovič Hrast, Hlebec and Rakar, 2020). Building a work–life balance to meet the needs of working carers is becoming a critical issue not only in Slovenia but also in most European welfare states. However, most attention is paid to working parents, while public policies have rarely considered the reconciliation of work and responsibilities for the care of older relatives. Given the rapid ageing of the population, the simultaneous increase in the need for care, the rise in female labour force participation and the increase in the retirement age, the number of workers with care responsibilities will increase considerably in the future and become a critical problem for the sustainability of all types of care regimes, but especially familialist ones, as in the case of Slovenia. Following Saraceno's (2016) typology, Slovenia's care regime can be characterised as both familialism by default (where family care takes place in a context without formal care alternatives) and prescribed familialism (with legal obligations to provide care or contribute to the cost of care), which places an ever-increasing burden of caring for older people on families (see also Hlebec, Srakar and Majcen, 2016a; Filipovič Hrast, Hlebec and Rakar, 2020). Moreover, gender inequalities are an important issue in familialist regimes, as both legal obligations and public support for the family's caring role promote support in gendered ways, resulting in an extensive burden for women (Schmid, Brandt and Haberkern, 2012).

Therefore, the sustainability of care for older people in Slovenia's familialist care regime currently faces several challenges that need to be addressed adequately and quickly by policy makers. As Verbakel (2014) has discussed, in terms of the policy implications of addressing the expected growing pressures on family carers, the rising costs of formal long-term care are neither a sustainable nor an affordable option for future welfare states. Moreover, as attitudinal research in Slovenia shows (Rakar and Filipovič Hrast, 2018; Filipovič Hrast and Rakar, 2021), Slovenian citizens have high expectations of the welfare state in all areas of welfare, especially for older people. This may become more pronounced in the future, as the problems of institutional and especially home care will intensify with rapid demographic ageing, which could further challenge the sustainability of the Slovenian care regime (Filipovič Hrast, Hlebec and Rakar, 2020).

To help meet future challenges some of the good practices and measures introduced in Slovenia and in other European countries regarding childcare could also be applied to care for older people. For example, part-time work and other work flexibilities that are generally accepted in Europe in terms of work–life balance are still not present in relation to older people's care, especially in the countries of Central and Eastern Europe. Different leave policies or subsidised part-time schemes should apply to all dependent family members, and work–life balance issues need to be better defined in legislation to avoid leaving the matter to the decision of employers, for example, by making it simply a matter of goodwill on the part of employers (see Filipovič Hrast, Hlebec and Rakar, 2020). Adopting such approaches could narrow the gap between the increasing care needs of older people and the amount of publicly supported care in Slovenia, and lead to the Slovenian care regime moving towards defamilialisation. Such moves could sustainably develop support for 'ageing in place' and enable a greater welfare/care mix in which carers are supported and have more choice of (additional) care support (through formal home-based care workers as well as other forms). However, political consensus as well as high levels of civil dialogue are preconditions for long-awaited and sustainable long-term care.

Notes

[1]   The chapter is based on the legislation and its amendments up to July 2023.

[2]   *Zakon o dolgotrajni oskrbi* (*Official Gazette of the Republic of Slovenia*, no 196/21).

[3]   Health Care and Health Insurance Act (*Zakon o zdravstvenem varstvu in zdravstvenem zavarovanju*) (*Official Gazette of the Republic of Slovenia*, no 72/2006 – official consolidated text and subsequent amendments).

[4]   Guaranteed wage is defined in Minimum Wage Act (*Official Gazette of the Republic of Slovenia*, no 13/10, 92/15 in 83/18). It is a statutory national minimum and is calculated on a yearly basis according to the cost of living.

[5]   Social Assistance Act (*Zakon o socialnem varstvu*, *Official Gazette of the Republic of Slovenia*, no 3/07 – uradno prečiščeno besedilo, 23/07 – popr., 41/07 – popr., 61/10 – ZSVarPre, 62/10 – ZUPJS, 57/12, 39/16, 52/16 – ZPPreb-1, 15/17 – DZ, 29/17, 54/17, 21/18 – ZNOrg, 31/18 – ZOA-A, 28/19, 189/20 – ZFRO in 196/21 – ZDOsk).

[6]   *Zakon o dolgotrajni oskrbi* (*Official Gazette of the Republic of Slovenia*, no 196/21).

[7]   See Advocate of the Principle of Equality (2021). Also, an example of limitations as published by individual care homes, source: http://www.pristan.si/obiski/ and https://www.pristan.si/prepoved-obiskov/ [Accessed 20 December 2021].

[8]   Also see Advocate of the Principle of Equality (2021). The report lists how the government, the Ministry of Health, the Ministry of Labour, Family and Social Affairs and Equal Opportunities, the Human Rights Ombudsman and other stakeholders have prepared and issued several recommendations, information, specific orders and other ways for advising and managing the pandemic conditions in older people care homes.

[9]   Source: https://www.dnevnik.si/1042929774 [Accessed 2 December 2021].

[10]   Source: https://www.ssz-slo.si/pandemija-razgalila-posledice-dolgoletnega-zanemarja nja-skrbi-za-starejse-v-sloveniji/ [Accessed 12 August 2021].

[11]   Further, at the time of writing (May 2023) there are also problems in financing the increasing care for those placed in 'red zones' due to COVID-19, since the Health Insurance Institute of Slovenia (ZZZS) has not categorised their care as the highest possible rate. Source: https://www.ssz-slo.si/skupnost-socialnih-zavodov-slovenije/nov ice/ [Accessed 12 August 2021].

[12]   Protocols were given by Nacionalni inštitut za javno zdravje (NIJZ, translated as National Institute of Public Health), Source: https://www.nijz.si/sites/www.nijz.si/files/publ ikacije-datoteke/napotki_in_priporocila_covid-19_ranljive_skupine_final.pdf; also, some more extensive protocols were published by the government, Ministry of Labour, Family, Social Affairs and Equal Opportunities (MLFSA), on 1 March 2021. Available from: https://www.gov.si/teme/pomoc-na-domu/ [Accessed 12 August 2021].

[13]   Paid in three different amounts (€300, €230 and €130), depending on one's pension amount.

[14]   Source: Act Determining Intervention Measures to Assist in Mitigating the Consequences of the Second Wave of the COVID-19 Epidemic, articles 57 and 58a. Available from: http://www.pisrs.si/Pis.web/pregledPredpisa?id=ZAKO8190 [Accessed 3 September 2021].

[15]   Source: https://www.rtvslo.si/slovenija/druzinskim-pomocnikom-nakazani-visji-preje mki/612903 [Accessed 23 February 2022].

References

Advocate of the Principle of Equality (2021) 'Razmere v domovih za starejše v prvem valu epidemije'. Available from: http://www.zagovornik.si/wp-content/uploads/2021/05/Razmere-v-domovih-za-starejse-v-prvem-valu-epidemije-Covida-19.pdf [Accessed 14 January 2022].

Blum, S. and Dobrotić, I. (2021) 'Childcare-policy responses in the COVID-19 pandemic: Unpacking cross-country variation', *European Societies*, 23(S1): S545–S563.

Blum, S., Correia, S., Nygard, M., Rakar, T. and Wall, K. (2020) 'Social investment in an age of austerity: a comparison of family policy reforms in four European countries', *Revija za socijalnu politiku*, 27(3): 249–67.

Bohle, D. and Greskovits, B. (2007) 'Neoliberalism, embedded neoliberalism and neocorporatism: towards transnational capitalism in Central Eastern Europe', *West European Politics*, 30(3): 433–66.

Cantillon, B. (2011) 'The paradox of the social investment state: growth, employment and poverty in the Lisbon era', *Journal of European Social Policy*, 21(5): 432–49.

Chung, H., Filipovič Hrast, M. and Rakar, T. (2018) 'The provision of care – whose responsibility and why?' in P. Taylor-Gooby and B. Leruth (eds), *Attitudes, aspirations and welfare*, Basingstoke: Palgrave Macmillan, pp 183–214.

Confederation Syndicate European Trade Union (2019) 'Rebalance. Trade unions' strategies and good practices to promote work–life balance', Brussels. Available from: https://www.etuc.org/sites/default/files/publication/file/2019-10/743-Rebalance-long-EN-web.pdf [Accessed 20 January 2023].

Esping-Andersen, G. (1990) *The three worlds of welfare capitalism*, Princeton, NJ: Princeton University Press.

Eurofound (2020a) 'Living, working and COVID-19. First findings – April 2020'. Available from: https://www.eurofound.europa.eu/en/publications/2020/living-working-and-covid-19 [Accessed 4 April 2022].

Eurofound (2020b) 'Living, working and COVID-19 dataset'. Available from: https://www.eurofound.europa.eu/data/covid-19/working-teleworking [Accessed 8 May 2021].

Eurofound (2022) 'The pandemic's impacts on older people's lives and support', Luxembourg: Publications Office of the European Union. https://www.eurofound.europa.eu/publications/report/2022/covid-19-and-older-people-impact-on-their-lives-support-and-care [Accessed 3 May 2023].

Eurostat (2022) 'Eurostat data'. Available from: https://ec.europa.eu/eurostat/data/database [Accessed 5 May 2022].

Ferge, Z. (2001) 'Welfare and "ill-fare" systems in Central–Eastern Europe', in R. Sykes, B. Palier, and P.M. Prior (eds), *Globalization and European welfare states. Challenges and change*, Basingstoke and New York: Palgrave Macmillan, pp 127–52.

Filipovič Hrast, M. and Ignjatovič, M. (2012) *Country report on growing inequalities impacts in Slovenia*, GINI Report 2012, Ljubljana: Faculty of Social Sciences.

Filipovič Hrast, M. and Rakar, T. (2017) 'The future of the Slovenian welfare state and challenges to solidarity', in P. Taylor-Gooby, B. Leruth and H. Chung (eds), *After austerity: Welfare state transformation in Europe after the great recession*, Oxford: Oxford University Press, pp 115–35.

Filipovič Hrast, M. and Rakar, T. (2020) 'Restructuring the Slovenian welfare system: between economic pressures and future challenges', in S. Blum, J. Kuhlmann and K. Schubert (eds), *Routledge handbook of European welfare systems*, Abingdon and New York: Routledge, pp 483–501.

Filipovič Hrast, M. and Rakar, T. (2021) 'Care policy in Slovenia: divergent trends and convergent attitudes', *Revija za socijalnu politiku*, 28(3): 303–21.

Filipovič Hrast, M., Hlebec, V. and Rakar, T. (2020) ''Sustainable care in a familialist regime: coping with elderly care in Slovenia, *Sustainability*, 12(20): 1–15.

Flere, S. and Lavrič, M. (2003) 'Social inequalities in Slovenian higher education', *International Studies in Sociology of Education*, 13(3): 281–90.

Greve, B. (2011) 'Editorial overview: Introduction and conclusion', *Social Policy & Administration*, 45(4): 333–37.

Hemerijck, A. (2013) 'Fault lines and (still too few) silver linings in Europe's social market economy', in D.N. OSE (ed), *Social developments in the European Union 2013*, Brussels: ETUI, pp 29–55.

Hlebec, V. and Rakar, T. (2017) 'Aging policies in Slovenia: before and after "austerity"', in Ł. Tomczyk and A. Klimczuk (eds), *Selected contemporary challenges of ageing policy*, Kraków: Uniwersytet Pedagogiczny w Krakowie. pp 27–52.

Hlebec, V. and Šircelj, M. (2011) 'Population ageing in Slovenia and social support networks of older people', in A. Hoff (ed), *Population ageing in Central and Eastern Europe: Societal and policy implications (New perspectives on ageing and later life)*, Farnham and Burlington, VA: Ashgate, pp 115–31.

Hlebec, V., Srakar, A. and Majcen, B. (2016a) 'Care for the elderly in Slovenia: a combination of informal and formal care', *Revija za socijalnu politiku*, 23(2): 159–79.

Hlebec, V., Srakar, A. and Majcen, B. (2016b) 'Determinants of unmet needs among Slovenian old population', *Zdravstveno varstvo: Slovenian journal of public health*, 55(1): 78–85.

Hočevar, B. (2022) 'SDS po zakonih o vladi in RTV še nad dolgotrajno oskrbo', *Delo*, 28 July. Available from: https://www.delo.si/razno/sds-predl aga-referendum-o-zakonu-o-dolgotrajni-oskrba/ [Accessed 4 August 2022].

Ignjatović, M. (2011) 'Slowenien: Konsolidierung oder Erosion des Arbeitsmarktes', in W. Reiter and K.H. Müller (eds), *Arbeitsmärkte und Sozialsysteme nach der Krize: strukturelle Veränderungen und politische Herausforderungen*, Vienna/Wien: Echoraum, Bundesministerium für Arbeit, Soziales und Konsumentenschutz, pp 91–7.

Kajzer, A. (2011) 'Vpliv gospodarske krize na trg dela v Sloveniji in izzivi za politiko trga dela', *IB revija*, 4: 13–21.

Kolarič, Z., Kopač, A. and Rakar, T. (2009) 'The Slovene welfare system: gradual reform instead of shock treatment', in K. Schubert, S. Hegelich, and U. Bazant (Eds) *The handbook of European welfare systems*, New York: Routledge, pp 444–461.

Kolarič, Z., Kopač, A. and Rakar, T. (2011) 'Welfare states in transition: the development of the welfare system in Slovenia', in S. Dehnert and M. Stambolieva (eds), *Welfare states in transition: 20 years after the Yugoslav welfare model*, Sofia: Friedrich Ebert Foundation, pp 288–309.

Kresal Šoltes, K., Jensen, R.S., Poje, A., Skorupan, M., Alsos, K., Bajt Učakar, K. and Štamfelj, I. et al (2016) 'Reconciliation of professional and family life in collective agreements: role of social partners in the promotion of gender equality', Project GEQUAL, Ljubljana: Inštitut za delo, Pravna fakulteta.

Malnar, B. (2011) 'Trendi neenakosti v Sloveniji med statistiko in javnim mnenjem', *Teorija in praksa*, 48(4): 951–67.

MDDSZ (2022) 'Družinski pomočnik'. Republic of Slovenia GOV.SI'. Available from: https://www.gov.si/teme/druzinski-pomocnik/ [Accessed 7 May 2022].

MZ (2022) 'Dolgotrajna oskrba se z Ministrstva za zdravje seli na Ministrstvo za delo, družino in socialne zadeve'. Republic of Slovenia GOV.SI. Available from: https://www.gov.si/novice/2022-06-22-dolgotrajna-oskrba-se-z-ministrstva-za-zdravje-seli-na-ministrstvo-za-delo-druzino-in-socialne-zadeve/ [Accessed 23 July 2022].

OECD (2011) 'Economic surveys Slovenia'. Available from: www.oecd.org [Accessed 3 November 2023].

Official Gazette (2020) 'Ordinance on the temporary prohibition of the gathering of people at public meetings at public events and other events in public places in the Republic of Slovenia and prohibition of movement outside the municipality no. 52/20, 58/20 in 60/20'. Available from: http://www.pisrs.si/Pis.web/pregledPredpisa?id=ODLO2049 [Accessed 1 July 2022].

Oven, A. (2020) 'COVID-19 and long-term care in Slovenia: impact, measures and lessons learnt'. Country report, in LTCcovid.org, International Long-Term Care Policy Network, CPEC-LSE, 20 April, Ljubljana: Institute for long term care. Available from: https://ltccovid.org/wp-content/uploads/2020/04/COVID19-and-Long-Term-Care-in-Slovenia-impact-measures-and-lessons-learnt-21-April-2020.pdf [Accessed 6 April 2022].

Rakar, T. and Filipovič Hrast, M. (2018) 'The future of the Slovenian welfare state: a view from deliberative forums', *Revija za socialnu politiku*, 25(2): 157–73.

Rakar, T., Hlebec, V. and Filipovič Hrast, M. (2022) 'Challenges within care regime in Slovenia in the case of COVID-19 crisis', in V. Hlebec and T. Rakar (eds), *Quality of life in COVID-19 pandemic: A kaleidoscope of challenges and responses of various population groups during the crisis*, Ljubljana: Založba FDV, pp 5–47.

Rodrigues, R., Filipovič Hrast, M., Kadi, S., Hurtado Monarres, M. and Hlebec, V. (2022) 'Life course pathways into intergenerational caregiving', *The Journals of Gerontology. Series B, Psychological Sciences and Social Sciences*, 77(7): 1305–14.

Santini, S., Socci, M., D'Amen, B., Di Rossa, M., Casu, G., Hlebec, V. et al (2020) 'Positive and negative impacts of caring among adolescents caring for grandparents: results from an online survey in six European countries and implications for future research, policy and practice', *International Journal of Environmental Research and Public Health*, 17(18): 1–16.

Santini, S., D'Amen, B., Socci, M., Di Rossa, M., Hanson, E. and Hlebec, V. (2022) 'Difficulties and needs of adolescent young caregivers of grandparents in Italy and Slovenia: a concurrent mixed-methods study', *International Journal of Environmental Research and Public Health*, 19(5): 1–20.

Saraceno, C. (2016) 'Varieties of familialism: comparing four southern European and East Asian welfare regimes', *Journal of European Social Policy*, 26(4): 314–26.

Schmid, T., Brandt, M. and Haberkern, K. (2012) 'Gendered support to older parents: do welfare states matter?' *European Journal of Ageing*, 9(1): 39–50.

STA (2022) 'Obsoječi Zakon o dolgotrajni oskrbi iz vseh vidikov ni izvedljiv. Slovenska tiskovna agencija'. Available from: sta.si [Accessed 23 July 2022].

SURS (2022) 'SiStat database, Ljubljana: Republic of Slovenia Statistical Office'. Available from: https://pxweb.stat.si/SiStat/sl/Podrocja/Index/56/bdp-in-nacionalni-racuni [Accessed 3 May 2022].

Trbanc, M. (2020) 'Socialni položaj v Sloveniji 2018–2019'. Ljubljana: IRSSV.

UMAR (2017) 'Strategija dolgožive družbe'. Ljubljana: UMAR.

UMAR (2021) 'Poročilo o razvoju 2021', Ljubljana: UMAR.

van Aerschot, L., Kadi, S., Rodrigues, R., Filipovič Hrast, M., Hlebec, V. and Aaltonen, M. (2022) 'Community-dwelling older adults and their informal carers call for more attention to psychosocial needs: interview study on unmet care needs in three European countries', *Archives of Gerontology and Geriatrics*, 101: 1–8.

van Kersbergen, K., Vis, B. and Hemerijck, A. (2014) 'The Great Recession and welfare state reform: is retrenchment really the only game left in town?' *Social Policy & Administration*, 48(7): 883–904.

Vandenbroucke, F. and Vleminckx, K. (2011) 'Disappointing poverty trends: is the social investment state to blame?' *Journal of European Social Policy*, 21(5): 450–71.

Verbakel, E. (2014) 'Informal caregiving and well-being in Europe: what can ease the negative consequences for caregivers?' *Journal of European Social Policy*, 24(5): 424–41.

10

Poland

Jolanta Perek-Białas and Anna Ruzik-Sierdzińska

Introduction

The task of combining paid work and care duties for older or disabled relatives was not addressed by Poland's formal policy framework until the second decade of the 21st century (Hoff et al, 2014; Stypińska and Perek-Białas, 2014). Labour policy and care policy domains have been treated separately. Family members (mostly women) who had to work concurrently with caring for disabled people and older relatives were usually left without any legal or organisational measures which they could use effectively (Perek-Białas and Racław, 2014). According to a report by Eurofound (2015), Poland ranked last among the EU countries in terms of support for combining paid work and care. One of the aims of this chapter is to examine the extent to which improvements in support have occurred in the first two decades of the 21st century and the scope for further strengthening support for combined employment and care work.

Poland has several leave options available to working carers. Two new leaves, in accordance with Directive (EU) 2019/1158 of the European Parliament and of the Council of 20 June 2019 on work–life balance for parents and carers (European Parliament, 2019), were proposed by the Polish Government in February 2022 and implemented in April 2023. These new care leaves with adequate and tailored employment policies in Poland are a new chapter for labour market and care policies. Prior to their introduction, Poland also had in place a Care Benefit (introduced in 1999), which provides payment of 80 per cent of a carer's salary for 60 days.

To contextualise the recent changes that have occurred, we begin by discussing briefly the national social, economic and political context. This is followed by a description of policies and policy instruments that provide support for working carers in Poland. We then discuss the adequacy of care policies that allow workers to combine labour market participation and care duties in Poland. As legislation is not the only mechanism for providing care leave, and governments are not the only providers of support for carers, we also discuss support measures provided by employers, with some local examples. Finally, it is difficult to omit the impact of the COVID-19 pandemic on care policies in this country, so this is discussed in a separate section. The chapter ends with some conclusions and suggestions for measures that might lead to better organisation of care policies in Poland.

National context

Political context

With the dissolution of the Soviet Union in the 1990s came a profound shift in Poland's political context, from a socialist regime in which many social needs were satisfied by state (public) institutions and state-owned employers, to a more liberal welfare state with a more free market economy and greater personal responsibility. This shift accelerated when Poland joined the European Union (EU) in 2004. While many changes in social policy have occurred since Poland started this economic transition, today its system of social policy still uses measures from the previous socialist system. Responsibilities for providing social services and social security have been divided among various levels of national, regional (16 regions) and local (over 300 *poviats* [similar to a county or district] and 2,477 *gminas* [similar to a municipality]) governments, yet policy domains are linked across these levels of government. For instance, pensions are financed and coordinated at a national level, while access to health services and care services (including long-term care) is provided at the local level (*gmina*), with some differences in access between rural and urban locations. Support provided in the regions may differ due to scarcity of some services, resulting in variations in the mix of private and public providers.

Poland's political transition has resulted in the expectation that individuals and families will be responsible for meeting their own day-to-day needs, making family members the first line of defence in meeting care obligations. Only when family is not able to provide care will public institutions be available to meet these needs. Family carers are considered by many to be 'left behind', with inadequate public sector support (Perek-Białas and Racław, 2014; Bakalarczyk, 2021).

Economic context

Before economic liberalisation and the emergence of a free market system in the 1990s, almost every adult in Poland was employed. Following this transition, it became more difficult to find a job and the social safety net became less generous. Liberal reforms resulted in faster economic growth, with Poland's economy tripling in size during the early 2000s and the country's gross domestic product reaching an all-time high of US$679.07 billion in 2021 (O'Neill, 2023).

However, economic reforms also brought more instability and insecurity for workers, including periods of high unemployment. The unemployment rate peaked at nearly 20 per cent in 2002 but has declined steadily since then, with rates hovering around 3 per cent in the early 2020s (Statista, 2023b). The positive trend in unemployment rates slowed as a result of the COVID-19 pandemic, reaching a rate of 5 per cent in 2022, with regional disparities. In addition, job quality is generally poor in Poland: wage growth has not kept up with rapid productivity gains. Its share of temporary employment is among the highest in the Organisation for Economic Co-operation and Development, and temporary workers often suffer from lower wages, poor job security and limited job quality.

Polish labour policy in the 21st century has focused on the need to increase the employment rate, especially among those aged 50 and older (*Program Solidarity across Generations+* in 2013; OECD, 2014). A 1999 pension reform (implemented fully in 2009) resulted in the elimination of some early retirement possibilities. After joining the EU in 2004, additional efforts have been made to encourage an ageing workforce to work longer through active labour market policies targeting older workers. These efforts resulted in a slow increase in employment rates among older workers (age 55–64). In 2009, the employment rate among older workers stood at 32.3 per cent. By 2022, it had risen to a record high of 55 per cent, 67 per cent for men and 43 per cent for women aged 55–64 years (Eurostat, 2023). However, employment rates among older people vary by educational attainment. While employers have many options for supporting working carers, there is no mandate to support them if it is not viable, profitable or required by law.

Social context

There are 38 million inhabitants in Poland, making it the ninth-most populous country in the EU (Statista, 2023a). A key factor behind the future demand for care is the population's age distribution and its health status. Declining fertility and rising life expectancy have contributed to population ageing, as is the case in many European countries, though this process started later and has been faster in Poland than in other European countries (Hoff et al, 2011). The proportion of the population aged 65 years and over increased substantially from 2005 to 2021 (Statista, 2023c) and the population aged over 65 is projected to increase to 30.6 per cent by 2050, while the number of people aged 15–64 is projected to decrease by seven million (Eurostat, 2019).

While the health status of the population has been improving since the mid-1990s, the trend of living longer and healthier lives slowed in the second decade of the 21st century (GUS, 2021a, 2021b). Life expectancy was 72.6 years for men, and 80.7 years for women in 2020. Notably, healthy life expectancy was lower at 59.2 years for men and 63.1 years for women, a small decrease from 2019 (GUS, 2021a, 2021b). There remains substantial variation in health and longevity by age, gender and socioeconomic groups.

The main drivers of the demand for care are from those aged 75 and older and those in poorer health. Currently, almost 5 per cent (1.9 million) of the population in Poland are aged between 75 and 84 years and 2.1 per cent (0.8 million) are older than 84 years (Statistics Poland, 2021). Women live longer on average than men, so they are over-represented among older age cohorts. According to the 2021 national census of the population, 3.7 per cent of men and 6.1 per cent of women are aged 75–84 and 1.2 per cent of men and 2.9 per cent of women are aged 85 years or older (Statistics Poland, 2021). The proportion of people aged over 85 is projected to more than double from 2 per cent to 5.7 per cent in the period 2019–50 (Eurocarers, 2021).

Family carers provide the vast majority of long-term care to persons with physical or learning disabilities or functional limitations. This can be attributed to a convergence of traditionally strong family relations (including elderly parents residing with their children), traditional division of gender roles, insufficient supply of publicly funded care and a lack of affordable private care facilities. According to the 2016 European Quality of Life Survey, at least four million people provide family care on a regular basis in Poland, roughly 18 per cent of the working age population (Eurocarers, 2021). The need to care for older family members is a common reason for reduced labour market participation, especially among women aged 55 years and over (see, for example, Bakalarczyk, 2020).

Carer leave policies

In Poland, the reconciliation of work and family responsibilities has been addressed more often in the context of motherhood/parenthood and combining childcare with paid work (for example, Smoder, 2010) than in the context of care for older relatives. There are, however, short-term leaves as well as financial benefits available for a longer period for which carers may qualify if they cannot engage in paid work, or must leave their paid work, in order to provide care to an older person or person with disability. The Polish social security system distinguishes between short-term and long-term benefits for people who provide care. In the following sections we describe several of these cash benefits available for carers who withdraw from paid work, as well as benefits for care receivers.

Short-term leave and benefits

In February 2022, following protests by carers and supported by experts, and public and inter-ministerial consultations, the government proposed amendments to the Labour Code that would introduce additional possibilities for carers to combine care and work duties. On 26 April 2023, changes were implemented that bring Polish labour law into line with minimum EU standards for reconciliation of work and family responsibilities while ensuring protection against unequal treatment in employment (Gazeta Wyborcza, 2023). Changes include five days of unpaid leave annually to provide personal care or support to a person who is a relative (son, daughter, mother, father or spouse) or who lives in the same household and is in need of significant care or support for serious health reasons. In addition, an Emergency Leave was introduced to provide two days or 16 hours of leave from work to provide immediate care in the event of a family emergency. This leave is paid at 50 per cent of the employee's salary.

Longer-term benefits

While there are no longer-term carer leaves in Poland, long-term care benefits are available to those who cannot work because of their care responsibilities. These include a Care Benefit (*zasiłek opiekuńczy*), a Nursing Benefit (*świadczenie pielęgnacyjne*), a Special Attendance Allowance (*specjalny zasiłek opiekuńczy*) and a Caregiver Allowance (*zasiłek pielęgnacyjny*). These are regulated by the Act of 28 November 2003 on family benefits. If a carer is entitled and wants to receive any of the long-term care benefits they usually cannot work. The key characteristics of all benefits are described in the following sections.

Care Benefit (**zasiłek opiekuńczy**)

In addition to the two short-term leaves listed in Table 10.1, the Care Benefit is a long-term benefit to support those caring for sick family members who are *unable to participate in the paid labour force*. It is enabled by the Act of 25 June 1999 that provides for monetary benefits from social insurance in the event of sickness and maternity.[1] It applies to all employed or self-employed persons who make social security contributions and have sickness insurance. In 2019, around one million people received this benefit.

A worker can apply for the Care Benefit when not working because they must care for a healthy child (up to age eight), a sick or disabled child under age 18 or another sick family member other than their own child (spouse, parent, parent-in-law, grandparent, grandchild or sibling). Entitlement to the Care Benefit is granted when there are no other family members who can provide care. The care receiver must live in the same household as the carer during the period of care. A physician certifies the need for care based on a medical check of the health status of the person in need of care. The worker receiving the Care Benefit is compensated for their loss of earnings at 80 per cent of their base salary.

Table 10.1: Carer leave schemes, Poland (November 2023)

Leave details[2]		Eligibility				
Leave name and introduced	Time period	Compensation	Worker/employee status	Qualifying period	Person needing care	Evidence	Notice period and process
Care Benefit, 1999	Up to 60 days (longer periods reserved for carers of disabled children, 14 days for carers of other family members)	Paid at 80%	Employees	–	Healthy child up to age 8, sick child up to age 14, disabled child up to age 18, other sick family member	–	–
Carers' Leave, 2023	5 days per annum	Unpaid	Employees	–	Child, parent or spouse (or other person living in the same household)	–	A least one day in advance
Emergency Leave, 2023	2 days or 16 hours per annum	Paid at 50%	Employees	–	Emergency related to family or own sickness, accident and so on	–	Even on the first day of the leave

The benefit is paid for a maximum of 60 days per calendar year if caring for a sick or disabled child up to the age of 14, 30 days if caring for a disabled child aged 14–18 and 14 days if caring for a sick child over the age of 14 or for another sick family member. Regardless of the number of people entitled to the benefit, or the number of children or family members who require care, the total period of payment of the care benefit may not exceed 60 days in a calendar year. As this benefit is available to carers who pause working in order to care, we include it in Table 10.1 as a de facto carer leave.

Nursing Benefit (świadczenie pielęgnacyjne)

A Nursing Benefit is paid to individuals who look after a family member with a disability certificate and who are unable to hold down paid work because they need to provide care. The Nursing Benefit can be paid to a mother or father, guardian, foster family member or other person obliged to care for the dependent. Although a caregiver cannot work, registering with a labour office as a job seeker or having unemployment status does not affect eligibility for the Nursing Benefit. The Nursing Benefit is not income tested. In 2023, the Nursing Benefit amounted to PLN2,458 (about €520) per month. If caring for a child with a disability, a low-income carer may also be eligible for a supplement for the child's education and rehabilitation.

Special Attendance Allowance (specjalny zasiłek opiekuńczy)

Special Attendance Allowance is a benefit paid to those caring for children or adults with disabilities. This benefit is means tested; the household income of the family providing the care, and the person receiving the care, must be lower than PLN764 or about €167 per person per month. The allowance is awarded to carers if they cannot take up employment, or must resign from employment, to provide permanent care to a person who has been certified as having an eligible disability. This Special Attendance Allowance is a temporary benefit, granted for the period linked to the disability certificate of the dependent person. The benefit amount for 2023 was PLN620 (around €132) per month. The Special Attendance Allowance cannot be claimed in combination with other benefits, including retirement pension and the Nursing Benefit.

Caregiver Allowance (zasiłek pielęgnacyjny)

If the carer does not qualify for the Nursing Benefit or the Special Attendance Allowance, they may be eligible for the Caregiver Allowance. The Caregiver Allowance is intended to cover part of the expenses resulting from the need to provide care and assistance to another person due to their inability to live independently. As for the other benefits already described, the caregiver must be unable to work, or have resigned from employment in order to provide permanent care to a person with an eligible disability. It applies to a child with a disability, a person over the age of 16 if they have a moderate or severe disability or any person who is 75 years of age or older. It is not income tested. The amount for 2023 was PLN215.84 (around €45) per month. The allowance is a benefit that is strictly related to the person being cared for, therefore, when a carer works, the disabled person does not lose their right to the benefit in question.

Adequacy of carer leave policies and programmes

Aside from the recent introduction of five days' leave in line with the EU's Directive on Work–life Balance for Parents and Carers (2019/1158; European Parliament, 2019) and the option of two days of emergency, *'force majeure'* leave, Poland's solutions for enabling carers to combine care work and paid work apply primarily to those caring for (sick or disabled) children, largely ignoring employees caring for older or dependent members of the family. As such, existing solutions for carers have been viewed as inadequate (Stypińska and Perek-Białas, 2014; Bakalarczyk, 2021) and to negatively influence carers' quality of life (Abramowska-Kmon and Maciejasz, 2018).

There are, however, several benefit programmes, already described, that provide partial income replacement for carers who are unable to work because they are caring for a family member with high levels of care need. There is only one benefit in Poland that allows workers to combine work and care duties (the Care Benefit [*zasiłek opiekuńczy*]). In 2021, 1.172 million carers received this benefit. The 80 per cent income replacement rate of the Care Benefit is relatively generous compared to other countries represented in this book. Longer-term benefit options are also available only to carers who are unable to undertake paid work. In 2020, 164,000 Polish carers received Nursing Benefit (*świadczenie pielęgnacyjne*); 32,000 received Special Attendance Allowance (*specjalny zasiłek opiekuńczy*) and 906,500 received a Caregiver Allowance (*zasiłek pielęgnacyjny*) (GUS/ZUS, 2021).

Since the mid-2000s, researchers have indicated that family policy goals and objectives should focus increasingly on families with dependent older people (Błędowski 2004; Jurek 2015). Care for older people is left mostly in the hands of families and so-called informal caregivers, who often feel left behind (Racław, 2011; Rosochacka-Gmitrzak and Racław, 2015). However, demographic changes (lower fertility, longer life expectancy, migration) will make relying on families to provide elder care unsustainable in the future.

Because only carers who are unable to work are eligible for the Nursing Benefit (*świadczenie pielęgnacyjne*), Special Attendance Allowance (*specjalny zasiłek opiekuńczy*) and Caregiver Allowance (*zasiłek pielęgnacyjny*)

Table 10.2: Number of persons receiving various care benefits each year in the period 2018–21

Year	Short term	Long term		
	Care Benefit (*zasiłek opiekuńczy*)	Care Allowance (*zasiłek pielęgnacyjny*)	Nursing Benefit (*świadczenie pielęgnacyjne*)	Special Attendance Allowance (*specjalny zasiłek opiekuńczy*)
	Annual number	Average monthly number of recipients		
2018	1,003,047	911,300	131,200	42,400
2019	1,063,670	923,800	142,700	39,100
2020	1,440,526	906,500	164,100	31,800
2021	1,172,013	911,600	91,000	21,900

Source: GUS (2021b), authors' own presentation of data

programmes, there is no guarantee that an employee can return to work, and employers can be reluctant to continue employing, or to rehire, such workers. As a result, finding one's way back into the labour market after a break of several years is very difficult, thus increasing the risk of poverty (Bakalarczyk, 2021).

In 2014, after protests by carers of children with disabilities, the government increased the value of the Nursing Benefit, with inequitable results: a carer of a child with a disability received almost three times the assistance that carers of adults with a disability received. In the same year, the Polish Constitutional Court ruled that it is unconstitutional to differentiate among people with disabilities on the basis of age of onset of the disability. Since then, statistics (Table 10.2) show a gradual decrease in the number of carers applying for the lower special attendance allowance (from 42,400 in 2018 to 31,800 in 2020) and an increase in the number of carers receiving the much higher Nursing Benefit (from 131,200 in 2018 to 164,100 in 2020) (Table 10.2).

Experts and carers themselves have argued that changes to legislation are needed so that employers acknowledge the needs of workers who, at times, have dependents to care for at home (Bakalarczyk, 2021). Advocated changes include the need for recipients of the Special Attendance Allowance to be able to undertake gainful employment, possibly with limits on their earnings or hours of work. Expansion of the right to more flexible forms of work for people who are caring for older relatives has also been recommended, as have additional leave arrangements for people needing to combine care work with paid work. Another need emphasised by many experts, including those of the Commission of Older Persons under the Commissioner/Ombudsman for Civic Rights, is the promotion of and incentives for supportive employment practices, such as organising the working environment in a way that benefits employees who are also carers.

Other support measures

Flexible working arrangements enable workers to adapt their working patterns to their individual needs through teleworking, flexible working schedules (reduced working hours, individual working hours and interrupted working hours) and part-time work. Until very recently the right to request flexible work arrangements was guaranteed only to parents of children under eight years old. However, the January 2023 Labour Code amendments mentioned earlier extend the right to request flexible working arrangements to employees who have been working for a given employer for at least six months. Rejection of an application for flexible working arrangements requires written justification from the employer.

This means that employers in Poland theoretically could provide flexible working arrangements to their employees (Bakalarczyk, 2020). In practice, the most common assistance for reconciling work and caregiving roles has been available to people raising children, usually school aged, but not for employees caring for older relatives. Data on whether companies offer these solutions are not reported routinely to the national statistical office, so their prevalence is unknown. However, according to a 2018 survey of employees caring for either children or other family members (GUS, 2019),[3] almost half (48.9 per cent) of respondents reported that they had no ability to adjust their working hours. However, of this 48.9 per cent, 44.5 per cent were caring for children under age 15, 6 per cent were caring for other family members and 1 per cent were caring for both. Men were more likely than women (28.4 per cent and 24.6 per cent, respectively) to say that they were able to make use of such arrangements.

'Telecare' solutions – technologies that can be used to remotely monitor people receiving care – can also improve the well-being of carers combining work and care duties. These have been implemented or tested in several local authorities in Poland (at *gmina*/municipal level), but only in regions and in years when co-financing from public sources was available (Sierdziński and Ruzik-Sierdzińska, 2019). These community-based systems are provided by private firms, but it seems that their popularity is restricted by high costs without co-financing from the European Social Fund, a municipality's own budget for social policy or other public funds. Still, the Ministry of Family and Social Policy (MRiPS, 2021) urges that telecare services in *gminas* be treated as good practice.

Residential long-term care can also benefit family carers when care demands exceed their personal capacity. However, family care is considered the best care option for an older person in Poland, and acceptance of formal care in Polish society is relatively weak compared to other European countries (Eurofound, 2015). As a result, only two per cent of older people in Poland live in residential care. Some studies show that the demand for residential care is increasing, but low availability means that supply has not kept pace with increasing demand (Bielska et al, 2021).

COVID-19 pandemic response and implications for working carers

Consistent with pre-pandemic policies to support employed carers, response to the COVID-19 pandemic was more generous for childcare than for care of adults with disabilities or older people. Polish authorities extended the duration of the Care Benefit between March 2020 and February 2022, during periods when nurseries, children's clubs, kindergartens, schools or other similar facilities were closed, or when a nanny or day care provider could not provide care due to the pandemic. The period of payment of this additional allowance did not count towards the overall limit of 60 days per year for other carer benefits described earlier. An additional Care Allowance for carers of adults with disabilities was also offered when a facility could not provide care, for example when access was limited due to widespread coronavirus infections.

The situation of the COVID-19 pandemic was different in the case of carers of older people. Bakalarczyk and Kocejko (2021)[4] found that some carers had to increase their hours of care during the pandemic, in the absence of additional state support for family carers. Their survey also confirmed an overall decline in carers' quality of life but also revealed the varied impact of the pandemic on their professional situations. Sometimes employment situations did not change (for example, when the carer was already inactive). In other cases, the possibility of remote work, widespread during the pandemic, was seen as helpful for managing care and saving time (no commute, the ability to sleep longer). Older care recipients were also more likely to isolate themselves at home during the pandemic and required increased assistance. There were problems with access to preventive and direct health care in the first wave of the pandemic. Carers who did have to give up work applied for the same cash benefits as carers who could not work due to care duties.

Conclusion

The analysis presented in this chapter shows that existing policy solutions in Poland are not adequate to support working carers. While working parents caring for young children have more options for short-term and longer paid care breaks with a guarantee of returning to employment, family carers of older people usually have to give up work in order to receive cash benefits for an extended period. That often leads to early retirement, unemployment or prolonged labour market inactivity. Given the rapid ageing of the Polish population and the low availability of long-term care for older disabled people, it seems that facilitating the periodic suspension of employment to care for an older family member would be a helpful change in government policy.

In 2023, two new short (two and five days) care leave entitlements were introduced, in addition to the extension of the right to request flexible working arrangements (previously limited to those providing childcare) to all employees who have been employed by a given employer for at least six months. It is notable that these changes are being driven by EU policy, and it is too early to assess the efficacy of this leave in supporting people to combine work and care. Nonetheless, recently implemented and proposed amendments to facilitate better work–life balance for parents and other carers may help to shift thinking about supporting carers of older people as well.

Acknowledgements

Some inspiration for this chapter has comes from the earlier work of the authors, namely from project Erasmus+ KA2 – 2018-1-FR01-KA204-048210 CareEr: Empowering Informal Carers (2018-2020) – Jolanta Perek-Białas, Aleksandra Piłat, Natalia Krygowska-Nowak.

Notes

[1] Journal of Laws 1999 No 60 item 636, as amended.

[2] In accordance with the Labour Code, an employee with at least one child under 14 years old can take leave up to 16 hours or two days, fully paid; we do not include this leave here as it is a leave for parents, rather than carers, defined as 'unpaid individual[s], such as a family member, neighbour, friend or other significant individual, who takes on a caring role to support someone with a diminishing physical ability, a debilitating cognitive condition or a chronic life-limiting illness' (IACO, nd).

[3] Survey respondents were aged 18–64, caring either for children below 15 or for other family members.

[4] This was an online study of 73 survey respondents and 20 individual in-depth interviews. Respondents cared for a person over age 65 at least eight hours per day and more than once a week. They also had internet access and were digitally literate. The authors recommend that results be considered exploratory rather than presenting the opinions of all carers. The person most often cared for was a parent (68 per cent) or a spouse/partner (15 per cent). Nearly half (45 per cent) of respondents were residents of cities with a population of over 500,000, while rural residents accounted for 15 per cent of respondents.

References

Abramowska-Kmon, A. and Maciejasz, M. (2018) 'Subjective quality of life of informal caregivers aged 50–69 in Poland', *Studia Demograficzne*, 2(174): 37–65.

Bakalarczyk, R. (2020) *Godzenie pracy zawodowej z opieką nad osobami zależnymi wyzwaniem dla dialogu społecznego i polityki publicznej różnych szczebli*, Warsaw: KDS KIG.

Bakalarczyk, R. (2021) *Starość po polsku. Propozycja reformy systemu opieki nad osobami starszymi, Centrum Analiz Klubu Jagiellońskiego, Senior Hub.* Krakow–Warsaw: Instytut Polityki Senioralnej.

Bakalarczyk, R. and Kocejko, M. (2021) *Sytuacja opiekunów rodzinnych osób starszych w czasie pandemii Covid-19 – raport z badania*, SENIOR.HUB.

Bielska, I., Błędowski P., Golinowska, S., Łuczak, P., Mrożek-Gąsiorowska, M., Sowa-Kofta, A. et al (2021) *Bezpieczeństwo zdrowotne w opiece długoterminowej w kontekście pandemii COVID-19*, Alert Zdrowotny 3.

Błędowski, P. (2004) 'Polityka rodzinna wobec zadania organizacji systemu opieki nad ludźmi starymi', in J.T. Kowaleski and P. Szukalski (eds), *Nasze starzejące się społeczeństwo. Nadzieje i zagrożenia*, Łódź: Wydawnictwo Uniwersytetu Łódzkiego, pp 267–278.

Eurocarers (2021) *Towards carer-friendly societies, Eurocarers country profiles: Poland*. Available from: https://eurocarers.org/country-profiles/poland/ [Accessed 26 January 2024].

Eurofound (2015) 'Working and caring: reconciliation measures in times of demographic change', Publications Office of the European Union, Luxembourg.

European Parliament (2019) 'Directive (EU) 2019/1158 of the European Parliament and of the Council of 20 June 2019 on work–life balance for parents and carers and repealing Council Directive 2010/18/EU', Brussels: European Parliament. Available from: https://eur-lex.europa.eu/legal-cont ent/EN/TXT/?uri=celex%3A32019L1158 [Accessed 30 June 2023].

Eurostat (2019) *Eurostat population projections*, 2019. Available from: https:// ec.europa.eu/eurostat/web/population-demography/population-projecti ons/database [Accessed 20 November 2023].

Eurostat (2023) 'Employment rates by sex, age, educational attainment level and citizenship, [LFSA_ERGAEDN]'. Available from: https://ec.europa. eu/eurostat/databrowser/view/LFSA_ERGAEDN__custom_5789742/ default/table?lang=en [Accessed 26 January 2024].

Gazeta Wyborcza (2023) 'Urlopy rodzicielskie. Tak rząd PiS deformuje równościową politykę UE'. Available from: https://wyborcza.pl/ 7,75968,29392152,urlopy-rodzicielskie-tak-rzad-pis-deformuje-rownosci owa-polityke.html [Accessed 26 January 2024].

GUS (2019) 'Praca a obowiązki rodzinne w 2018 r.', GUS Warszawa. Available from: https://stat.gov.pl/obszary-tematyczne/rynek-pracy/pracuj acy-bezrobotni-bierni-zawodowo-wg-bael/praca-a-obowiazki-rodzinne- w-2018-roku,25,3.html [Accessed 26 January 2024].

GUS (2021a) 'Świadczenia na rzecz rodziny w 2020 r.', GUS Warszawa. Available from: https://stat.gov.pl/obszary-tematyczne/dzieci-i-rodzina/ rodzina/swiadczenia-na-rzecz-rodziny-w-2020-roku,4,4.html [Accessed 26 January 2024].

GUS (2021b) 'Trwanie życia w zdrowiu w 2020 r.', GUS Warszawa. Available from: https://stat.gov.pl/wyszukiwarka/?query=tag:trwanie+%C5%BCy cia [Accessed 26 January 2024].

GUS/ZUS (2021) 'Family benefits in 2020'. Available from: https://stat. gov.pl/files/gfx/portalinformacyjny/en/defaultaktualnosci/3640/2/4/1/ family_benefits_in_2020.pdf [Accessed 26 January 2024].

Hoff, A. (ed) (2011) *Population ageing in Central and Eastern Europe: Societal and policy implications*, Farnham: Ashgate Publishing.

Hoff, A., Reichert, M., Hamblin, K.A., Perek-Bialas, J. and Principi, A. (2014) 'Informal and formal reconciliation strategies of older peoples' working carers: the European carers@ work project', *Vulnerable Groups & Inclusion*, 5(1): 24264.

IACO (International Association of Carers Organizations) (nd) 'Recognising carers'. Available from: https://internationalcarers.org/carer-facts/ [Accessed 16 November 2023].

Jurek, Ł. (2015) 'Polityka łączenia pracy zawodowej z opieką nad osobą starszą, Acta Universitatis Lodziensis', *Folia Oeconomics*, 2(312): 95–110.

Martinez-Fernandez, C., Weyman, T., Perek-Białas, J., Sagan, I., Szukalski, P. and Stronkowski, P. (2013) 'Demographic transition and an ageing society: Implications for local labour markets in Poland', OECD. Available from: https://www.oecd-ilibrary.org/industry-and-services/demographic-transition-and-an-ageing-society_5k47xj1js027-en [Accessed 26 January 2024].

MRiPS (2021) 'Informacja o sytuacji osób starszych w Polsce za 2020 r.', Warszawa.

OECD (2014) 'Poland: Solidarity between Generations', in OECD, The Missing Entrepreneurs 2014: Policies for Inclusive Entrepreneurship in Europe, OECD Publishing, Paris. Available from: https://doi.org/10.1787/ 9789264213593-34-en [Accessed 26 January 2024].

OECD (2022) 'Employment rate by age group 55–64 year olds, % in same age group', Q4 2022 or latest available. Available from: https://data.oecd. org/emp/employment-rate-by-age-group.htm [Accessed 26 January 2024].

O'Neill, A. (2023) 'Gross domestic product (GDP) in Poland 2027'. Available from: Available from: https://www.statista.com/statistics/263588/gross-domestic-product-gdp-in-poland/ [Accessed 26 January 2024].

Perek-Białas, J. and Racław, M. (2014) 'Transformation of elderly care in Poland', in M. León (ed), *The transformation of care in European societies*, Basingstoke: Palgrave Macmillan, pp 256–75.

Racław, M. (2011) 'Publiczna troska, prywatna opieka'. Warszawa: Instytut Spraw Publicznych.

Rosochacka-Gmitrzak, M. and Racław, M. (2015) 'Opieka nad zależnymi osobami starszymi wrodzinie, ryzyko i ambiwalencja', *Studia Socjologiczne*, 2(217): 23–47.

Sierdziński, J. and Ruzik-Sierdzińska, A. (2019) 'Rozwiązania telemedyczne w usługach społecznych', *Polityka Społeczna*, 8(545): 17–24.

Smoder, A. (2010) 'Równowaga praca-rodzina – wybór czy konieczność?' *Polityka Społeczna*, 4: 12–16.

Statista (2023a) 'Poland: total population from 2017 to 2027'. Available from: https://www.statista.com/statistics/263750/total-population-of-poland/ [Accessed 26 January 2024].

Statista (2023b) 'Poland: unemployment rate from 1999 to 2021'. Available from: https://www.statista.com/statistics/263705/unemployment-rate-in-poland/#:~:text=The%20statistic%20shows%20the%20unemployment,amounted%20to%20about%203.37%20percent [Accessed 26 January 2024].

Statista (2023c) 'Share of population aged 60 and more in total population in Poland from 2005 to 2021'. Available from: https://www.statista.com/statistics/1089510/poland-share-of-population-aged-60-and-more/#:~:text=Every%20fourth%20person%20in%20Poland,increased%20in%20the%20observed%20period [Accessed 26 January 2024].

Statistics Poland (2021) *National Census*, 2021. Available from: https://stat.gov.pl/en/national-census [Accessed 21 November 2023].

Stypińska, J. and Perek-Białas, J. (2014) 'Working carers in Poland: successful strategies of reconciliation of work and care of an older adult', *Anthropological Notebooks*, 20(1): 87–103.

Trading Economics (2023) 'Poland – employment rate of older workers, age group 55–64', https://tradingeconomics.com/poland/employment-rate-of-older-workers-age-group-55-64-eurostat-data.html [Accessed 26 January 2024].

11

Critical comparative analysis: similarities, differences and lessons learned

Kate Hamblin, Jason Heyes and Janet Fast

Introduction

The contributors to this book have provided overviews of leave policies available to working carers in nine countries with varied social, political and economic contexts. They have also examined the available evidence regarding the outcomes of carer leave measures, including their inclusivity and, in turn, their implications for equality and equity and their adequacy with regard to job protection and income security. In this concluding chapter we offer a summary and critical comparative analysis of the commonalities and differences in carer leave policies and related policy instruments, and their outcomes. We close with a discussion of the capacity for findings to inform international policy transfer.

Our introductory chapter discussed why we sought to compare different nations' carer leave policies – essentially as '[w]e gain knowledge through reference' (Dogan and Pelassy, 1990: 3); this chapter now begins by outlining how we will do this. For Rose (1991), there are three questions to ask of the data when conducting comparative policy analysis:

1. To what extent are countries similar?
2. When do differences occur?
3. What are the consequences of these observed differences?

We begin by exploring similarities and differences in terms of the contexts within which carer leaves and associated policies have been introduced in the nine countries. We then return to the care and employment regimes literature explored in the introductory chapter (and referenced in various contributions on specific countries). As discussed there, we do this not to suggest that these literatures offer causal models, but to facilitate comparison between nations that might be expected to adopt similar or different approaches to supporting working carers. We next examine similarities and differences in the carer leave policies themselves, and in other support for working carers. We consider consequences, exploring the implications of carer leave policies for income and job security, and equality and equity, as well as other supports for working carers, and we close with potential insights for policy and research.

Contextual and motivating factors: commonalities and differences

Policies are not developed, implemented or administered in a vacuum: economic, political and social contexts matter. While this book does not offer a causal analysis of the factors that have influenced the convergence or divergence of national carer leave policies across the globe, it is important to draw together some key contextual factors that are common to the countries that have been covered or, indeed, that present stark differences.

As noted in Chapter 1, the countries included in this book face common challenges to their health and long-term care systems. Although populations are ageing faster in some countries (for example, Japan, Finland, Germany) than in others (for example, Canada), in all the countries represented in this book, concerns about demographically driven increases in demand for care are shifting attention towards support for carers. Interest has also grown because of the increased participation of women in the labour market; concerns relating to the ability to maintain a dual-breadwinner model of labour force participation; a reduction over time in average family size; and an increased tendency for family members to live at a substantial distance from older relatives. All of these present challenges to the sustainability of family care on which the 'formal' or statutory care sector depends so heavily (Dykstra and Djuneva, 2020).

As discussed in Chapter 1, the countries included have been categorised in the literature on employment and care regimes according to how welfare and care are organised and conceptualised (Esping-Andersen 1990, 1999; Langan and Ostner, 1991; Lewis, 1992; Anttonen and Sipilä, 1996; Lewis, 1997; Millar, 1999; Pfau-Effinger, 1999; Yeandle, 1999; Leitner, 2003; Pfau-Effinger, 2005a, 2005b; Gallie, 2007; Kröger, 2011). The literature on care regimes has paid attention to the roles played by families, communities, national, local and regional governance structures and the market in providing care.

In the introduction to this book, we explained that we had drawn on the care and employment regimes literature in selecting the countries for study and in ordering their presentation in this book. We grouped Finland and Sweden together as nations characterised by a strong historical focus on gender equality and universal state provision of care that has supported female engagement in the labour market (Lewis, 1992; Anttonen and Sipilä, 1996; Millar, 1999; Pfau-Effinger, 1999; Leitner, 2003). In contrast, statutory care provision in Australia, the UK and Canada is often depicted as liberal and residual, with an emphasis on the market and strong reliance on carers (Anttonen and Sipilä, 1996; Pfau-Effinger, 1999; Yeandle, 1999; Leitner, 2003; Fine and Davidson, 2018; Stall, 2019). Germany and Japan have traditionally focused on the family as the provider of care, respectively through the principles of subsidiarity and filial piety; in these countries the introduction of long-term care insurance systems has more recently, some argue, resulted in a more active role for the state (Anttonen and Sipilä, 1996; Lewis, 1997; Leitner, 2003; Soma and Yamashita, 2011; Peng and Yeandle, 2017). In Slovenia and Poland, both former socialist states, 'implicit familialism' or 'family-by-default' arrangements remain dominant (Radziwinowiczówna and Rosińska, 2022) and state intervention in care remains limited.

The country chapters show that efforts to contain the projected costs of health and long-term/social care appear to be producing convergence in policy approaches to care between previously very different countries. In countries previously distinct in their approaches (Finland, Japan, Slovenia), policy makers' attention appears to be shifting back to families as the main providers of care through retrenchment of public provision, creating the conditions for the 're-familialisation' of care (Leitner, 2003; and in this volume see: Leinonen, Chapter 2; Ikeda, Chapter 8; and Rakar, Filipovič, Hrast and Hlebec, Chapter 9). Chapters 2 (Finland) and 7 (Germany) in this volume show that policies designed to support older adults to 'age in place', outside of residential care facilities, are redistributing care and placing a greater emphasis on provision by family members. In Sweden too (Chapter 3), a move towards more needs-based approaches is indicated, in which only those with the highest needs are eligible to receive publicly provided, funded or subsidised services. A similar development is evident in Slovenia (Chapter 9) and Poland (Chapter 10), albeit for different reasons influenced by a past in which social services were provided exclusively by the state in a context that emphasised 'traditional' family values. By contrast, in Canada, Germany, Australia and the UK (Chapters 6, 7, 4, 5), a long-standing emphasis on individual and family responsibility for care has continued to dominate, alongside an increased focus on the provision of care via the market.

As a counterpoint, all contributors to the book report growing debate and action regarding carer leaves and other policies to support working carers, despite (in most countries) according carers' needs low priority in debates about how best to address the 'crisis of care' and demographic ageing. A variety of contextual factors have put carers' needs on the policy agenda in the nine countries. In Australia and the UK, carers' organisations have often been actors in the policy process, playing a significant role in promoting carer leave and keeping carers' rights on the policy agenda, with some notable impacts on policy reforms (O'Loughlin and Williams, Chapter 4; Hamblin et al, Chapter 5). In some countries, organisations representing employers and trade unions have been influential. Thus, in Sweden carer leave provisions are negotiated in central agreements between national unions and employers. In Germany, however, lobbying by employers' associations had an adverse effect on the scope of carer leave policy, with small and medium-sized enterprises (SMEs) exempt from requirements in the Care Leave and Family Care Leave policies (Knauthe and Hoff, Chapter 7).

Wider contextual factors have also played a role in creating the conditions for policy convergence. For European Union (EU) member states, policy making at EU level is a driving force for change and an important contextual factor. The European Parliament and Council's Directive 2019/1158 on Work–life Balance for Parents and Carers and subsequent European Care Strategy (EC, 2022) created a further imperative for action on carer leave in many European countries (although Sweden already had carer leave policies that covered the five days mandated by the Directive; Aldman et al, Chapter 3). International labour standards are also important reference points for national policy making, in particular the International Labour Organization's (ILO) Convention on Workers with Family Responsibilities, 1981 (C156) and accompanying Recommendation (R165), which outline the responsibility of member countries to ensure that workers with family responsibilities do not experience discrimination in employment or, 'to the extent possible', conflict between their employment and family responsibilities. Investment in, and support for, care are also central to the ILO's 2019 Declaration for the Future of Work and its recent 'global call to action for a human-centred recovery from the COVID-19 crisis that is inclusive, sustainable and resilient'.

During 2020, the COVID-19 pandemic raised the profile of the challenges carers face, focusing attention on the sustainability and adequacy of care systems. Most national governments' responses to the pandemic included restrictions that led to higher unemployment (notably in the leisure and hospitality sectors) while simultaneously contributing to rising demand for labour in the health and care sector. Some workers remained in their jobs, working from home, finding their work more difficult to manage due to the home schooling of children and care of adult family members. Closures and restrictions affecting formal care services, and stressful conditions in residential facilities, placed additional burdens on many carers. The nine countries discussed in this book responded to these pressures in various ways, including providing special financial benefits (or extending existing ones). Most, at the time of writing (November 2023), have since been suspended (along with the COVID-19 restrictions), with the consequence that, for the longer term, despite the higher profile of care and carers during the pandemic, few changes introduced to increase their support have been retained.

Comparing carer leave policies

The key characteristics of leave policies in the nine countries represented in this book are summarised in Tables 11.1 and 11.2.

The carer leaves available in the nine nations include both short- (lasting ten days or less) and longer-term leaves (more than ten days)[1] for working carers (except in the UK, whose government mandates only short leaves). Poland has a five-day carer leave, reflecting the European Parliament and Council's 2019 Directive, and a two-day/16-hours '*force majeure*' emergency leave. The EU could also be argued to have provided the impetus for reform in the UK, which (although no longer part of the EU) began the process of developing carer leave prior to Brexit, with the national carers' movement and policy makers with an interest in caring maintaining political momentum. Of the countries in the book that offer at least one short-term leave option, only Sweden, Germany and Poland mandate that (some of) these are paid.

Most of the eight countries offering longer-term leave options (Finland, Sweden, Australia, Canada, Germany, Japan, Slovenia and Poland) provide income replacement through their employment insurance or benefits systems (Germany's offer includes an interest-free loan). Some nations offer flexibility, with the possibility of dividing periods of carer leave into shorter blocks of time (Canada, Japan, Poland); sharing the leave with other family members or among members of a caring network (Germany, Sweden, Canada); and the option to 'bank' entitlements (Australia).

In all countries, eligibility criteria narrow the options to include only specific groups of working carers. Similarities here include restricting care leave to employees (that is, people with an employment contract), leaving other workers (on temporary contracts or with casual arrangements) unprotected. Of note is the disparity in how length of service with the employer affects eligibility, ranging from 'day one' of employment in Australia to Finland's requirement of a 20-year work record for its Job Alternation Leave option.

In determining eligibility for carer leave, some countries define 'family' rather inclusively (Finland, Sweden, Canada), while in others (Slovenia, Poland) only those caring for a co-resident spouse or child are eligible for short-term carer leave. In most countries care need must arise from an illness or disability (severity of the condition varies). In Sweden, Germany and Canada, longer-term leaves are available only to those caring for someone at the end of life or who has a serious condition requiring a high level of care. In Poland, the longer-term leave distinguishes between care provided for children versus other adults, with the maximum of 60 days per calendar year reserved for those caring for a sick child up to the age of 14, in contrast to 14 days for another sick family member. Similarly, in Sweden there is a more generous support

Table 11.1: Short-term leave options compared

Short-term leave (<11 days)	Finland	Sweden	Australia	UK	Canada	Germany	Japan	Slovenia	Poland
Leave name	a. Absence for compelling family reasons, 2001 b. Absence for taking care of a family member or someone close to the employee, 2011 c. Carers Leave, 2022	a. Leave for urgent family reasons, 1998 b. Contact days, 1993	a. Unpaid Personal/Carer's Leave, 2009 b. Compassionate leave, 2009	a. Emergency Leave b. Carers' Leave, 1999	Family Responsibility Leave, 1995	Short-Term Prevented Work Absence, 2012	Short-Term Care Leave, 2009	–	a. Carers' Leave, 2023 b. Emergency Leave 'force majeure', 2023
Time period	a. and b. Unspecified but intended to be short-term c. 5 days per annum	a. Unspecified but short-term b. 10 days per annum	a. 2 days/4 half days per annum b. 2 days per annum	a. Unspecified but short-term b. 5 days per annum	Varies across provinces – typically 3–5 days per annum	10 days per annum	5 days per annum (or 10 for 2+ family members)	–	a. 5 days per annum b. 2 days or 16 hours
Compensation	a–c. Unpaid	a. Varies between 0 and 100% b. 80% of pay	a. Unpaid b. Paid but not for casual workers	a. and b. Unpaid	Unpaid	90% of pay through Carer Support Allowance	Unpaid	–	a. Unpaid b. Paid at 50%
Worker/ employee status	a–c. All with employment contracts	a. and b. Employees	a. Employees including casual b. All but not paid for causal workers	a. and b. Employees	Workers in specific industries	All employees	All employees (but not day labourers)	–	a. and b. Employees
Qualifying period	–	a. – b. Earnings threshold, six months of work history	–	None	Varies across provinces	– (but size of company a factor)	Working individuals in a labour-management agreement not eligible; 6 months	–	–

Table 11.1: Short-term leave options compared (continued)

Short-term leave (<11 days)	Finland	Sweden	Australia	UK	Canada	Germany	Japan	Slovenia	Poland
									of employment with employer; works more than 2 days a week
Person needing care	a. Family member b. and c. Family member or someone close	a. Unspecified b. Children with disability/serious illness	a. Family b. Family/household	a. A 'dependant' (spouse, partner, child, grandchild, parent or someone who depends on person for care) b. Anyone who relies on person for care	Child or other immediate family members	Close relative	Spouse, parents, children, parents-in-law, grandparents, siblings or grandchildren	–	a. Child, parent or spouse (or other person living in the same household) b. Emergency related to family or own sickness, accident and so on
Evidence	a–c. Employer can ask for medical certification	a. Employers can request a medical certificate b. –	a. and b. Employer can ask for medical certification	Not required	–	Need for care/no care degree	–	–	–
Notice period and process	a–c. Notify employer ASAP	a. Notify employer ASAP b. –	a. Have to have exhausted paid carers' leave entitlement b. Notify employer ASAP	a. Not required. b. Twice the length of time being requested as leave + one day	Varies across provinces	Notify employer ASAP	Notice given in advance in writing or over the telephone on the day in emergencies	–	1. A least one day in advance 2. –

Table 11.2: Long-term leave options compared

Long-term leave (>10 days)	Finland	Sweden	Australia	UK	Canada	Germany	Japan	Slovenia	Poland
Leave name	Job Alternation Leave, 2003	a. Compassionate Care Leave, 1988 b. Temporary parental benefits, 1993/2010	Personal/Carer's Leave, 2005	N/A	a. Compassionate Care Leave, 2004 b. Critical Illness Leave for Adults, 2017 c. Critical Illness Leave for Children, 2017	a. Care Leave, 2008 b. Family Care Leave, 2015	Long Term Care Leave, 1995	Leave to care for sick family members, 1992	Care benefit, 1999
Time period	100–180 days	a. 100 days (or 240 days for a family member/significant other with HIV) b. 10–120 days	10 days per annum but accrues[a]	N/A	a. Varies across provinces but 8–28 weeks per annum b. 17 weeks per annum c. 37 weeks per annum	a. Full or partial leave up to six months b. Reduce working time for up to 24 months	93 days per annum which can be split into up to three separate blocks	Varies but typically 10 days' leave (or 20 for children under 7/those with additional care needs). There is no annual limit on how many periods of leave can be taken[b]	Up to 60 days per annum[c]
Compensation	70% of one's unemployment benefit for a maximum of 180 days	a. approx. 80% of pay b. Paid	Yes, at base salary	N/A	a–c. Eligible for partial income replacement through EI; 55% of usual earnings to max	a. and b. Interest-free loan (BAFzA)	Unpaid but can receive up to 67% of salary through employment insurance system	80% of wages	80% of wage

Table 11.2: Long-term leave options compared (continued)

Long-term leave (>10 days)	Finland	Sweden	Australia	UK	Canada	Germany	Japan	Slovenia	Poland
Worker/employee status	Contracted employees working at least 75%	a. and b. Employees	Full-time/part-time employees, not casual workers	N/A	a–c. All	a. All employees of companies with 15+ employees b. All employees of companies with 25+ employees	All employees (but not day labourers); limited-term contract workers need a certain period left on their contract before the leave starts	All insured persons	Insured employees
Qualifying period	20 year work history; 13 months with employer	–	Accrues from day one	N/A	a–c. 600 insured hours of work in the 52 weeks before the start of their claim	–	1 year with current employer; minimum period left on contract; works more than 2 days a week		–
Person needing care	Family member or someone close	a. Family member, relative, friend or neighbour with a life-threatening illness b. Children with disability/serious illness	Family/household member	N/A	a. Family member for whom the employee is caring be diagnosed with a serious medical condition with a significant risk of death within 26 weeks b. Family member or 'like family' c. Child under 18 who is a family member or 'like family'	a. Close relatives b. Close relatives who are minors	Family member[d]	Immediate co-resident family member (spouse and children, biological or adopted)	Healthy child up to age 8, sick child up to age 14, disabled child up to age 18, other sick family member

(continued)

Table 11.2: Long-term leave options compared (continued)

Long-term leave (>10 days)	Finland	Sweden	Australia	UK	Canada	Germany	Japan	Slovenia	Poland
Evidence	Employer can ask for a medical certificate	a. Medical certificate required b. Medical certificate, plus additional paperwork	Employer can ask for medical certification	N/A	a–c. Medical certificate	a. and b. Proof of care need	–	Medical certificate required	–
Notice period and process	Notify employer ASAP	a. – b. Notify employer ASAP	Notify employer ASAP	N/A	a–c. Varies across provinces	a. 10 days, written agreement with employer b. Eight weeks, written agreement with employer	Application in writing to their employer at least two weeks before the planned start date of leave	–	N/A

Notes:

[a] The inclusion of this leave as a 'long-term' scheme reflects the ability to accrue leave and that often particular sectors offer more than ten days.

[b] Ten days of leave may be taken for each episode of illness per family member in need of care; 20 days for children under seven and those with special needs; and in exceptional cases the period may be extended up to 40 days (in case of children under seven years and those with special needs) or up to 20 days for other close family members; in extreme cases, up to six months' leave is possible. There are no regulations that limit the duration of the annual entitlement, only for each episode of leave taken. For this reason, we include this leave as a long-term measure.

[c] A maximum of 60 days per calendar year if caring for a sick child up to the age of 14, 30 days per calendar year if caring for a disabled child aged 14–18 and 14 days in a calendar year if caring for a child over the age of 14 or for another sick family member.

[d] Includes a partner (including a common-law partner), parents, children (in a legal parent–child relationship, including adopted children), parents of the partner, grandparents, siblings and grandchildren.

system for parents caring for children covered by the Law on Special Support and Service to Certain Persons with Disabilities, as compared to carers of, for example, older adults. In all countries it is illegal for the employer to terminate the employment of someone taking carer leave (or to otherwise discriminate against an employee who accesses either short- or longer-term leave). In some countries (for example, Finland) employers are permitted to decline a request for leave without providing a justification for doing so.

Implications of carer leave policies

A striking feature of our nine-country comparison of the country-specific chapters is the absence of data on use of carer leave policies. This is a notable gap. In some countries data are collected (nationally) on uptake of other benefits available to carers (Poland, UK, Canada), but not on use of carer leave. Japan and Canada collect data on use of carer leave policies centrally (respectively, through their Ministry of Health, Labor and Welfare, and Employment Insurance Commission), but in the other nations no data, recent or otherwise, are collected. For example, there are no recent data collected in Finland on the use of short-term leave options although the numbers of people receiving the Job Alternation Allowance are recorded; in Germany, data were collected on the use of the Short-term Prevented Work Absence and the interest-free loan, but not since 2017 (and the results were disappointing for the government). Similarly, countries have not formally evaluated the impact of carer leave policies on working carers, making answering our third question regarding the consequences of similar or markedly different policy approaches difficult. Not only is it apparent (from the country-specific chapters) that evaluation and data on the uptake and impact of carer leave policies and policy instruments are rare; authors of the chapters in this book also note that the academic and grey literature is almost equally thin. Contributors to the book have nevertheless assessed the implications for income and job security, and for equality and equity of the legislated developments in their countries. We focus on these core areas, as set out in the Introduction, as acute issues that working carers face (Boise and Neal, 1996; Dentinger and Clarkberg, 2002; Daly and Rake, 2003; Anderson et al, 2013; Matthews and Fisher, 2013; Do et al, 2014; Carr et al, 2018; Cohen et al, 2017, 2019; Stanfors et al, 2019; Urwin et al, 2023).

Income and job security

Job protection and income security are crucial for most employed carers contemplating taking a carer leave. Income security is enhanced when earnings lost in taking a care-related leave of absence are fully or partially replaced. This happens in most of the countries discussed in this book, at least where longer-term leave arrangements are in place. The adequacy of earnings-replacement payments during longer-term leave nevertheless remains an issue, as these rarely cover all of a working carer's earnings, ranging between 55 per cent (Canada), 67 per cent (Japan), 70 per cent (Finland), 80 per cent (Sweden, Slovenia and Poland) and 'base rate' salary (Australia). During periods of short-term carer leave, some groups of working carers are partially paid or compensated in Australia, Germany, Poland and Sweden; in the other countries (Finland, UK, Canada and Japan), they receive no pay or compensation when taking this leave.

The extent to which usual earnings are replaced for carers taking leave affects their immediate and longer-term financial situation, and for some leads to significant financial hardship. This makes it likely that working carers with lower household incomes will be reluctant to take the carer leave to which they are entitled. Some will instead take time off as (their own) sick leave, during which most will receive usual earnings. Carers in low-paid jobs may feel they cannot afford to take unpaid care leave. As noted in Chapter 2, on Finland, not only are female workers more likely to be carers than male workers, but they are also more likely to face lower incomes when taking available carer leave options. There are thus real risks implicit in many carer leave provisions of exacerbating inequalities (discussed in more detail later). Long-term income security is also threatened when care interrupts accrual of pension benefits, as these are often calculated on hours worked and duration of employment. Although pension protection is available to some carers, including in the UK, Finland and Germany, during a period of carer leave carers in other countries will not accrue any pension entitlements, with negative consequences for their income security in later life.

In all countries included in this book, discrimination on the basis of family status is prohibited; this means that employers cannot legally dismiss, or otherwise penalise, employees for using carer leaves for which they are eligible, providing working carers with a degree of job protection. In most cases, these protections are explicitly legislated or covered in national legislation on human rights. By contrast, Poland's approach includes several financial benefits to carers *unable to work* because of their care responsibilities, making no promise that the carer can return to their original job, or indeed to any employment, once their caring role has ended or their caring situation allows them to engage in paid work again.

Equality and equity

The differing eligibility criteria applicable to carer leave in the nine countries (discussed earlier) show that not all groups of working carers are covered by carer leave policies and supports, leaving some excluded and unprotected. In this section we consider in more detail how, inadvertently or otherwise, carer leave policies may create or reinforce inequalities. Wider contextual factors (decentralised governance and infrastructure; persistent gender disparities in pay; divisions of paid and unpaid labour) and the conditions attached to carer leave in some countries also have implications for equality and equity. As O'Loughlin and Williams observe (Chapter 4), whatever the nominal leave provisions might be, they '[do] not always translate into equitable practices in all workplaces'.

In most of the nine countries, governments claim to strive to achieve equality and equity, yet decentralised government structures (as in Canada, Australia and Sweden) have produced different carer leave policy instruments within country, and different entitlements apply in some parts of the same country. Canada and Australia have decentralised government structures in which federal and state/provincial jurisdictions overlap in some policy domains, meaning that leaves from paid work are under the jurisdiction of multiple levels of government. In Sweden, Poland and Finland, responsibility is devolved in various ways to these countries' municipal and regional governments. This results in numerous within-country differences in the types and characteristics of carer leave available to working carers. Finland has recently sought to reduce such geographical disparities by targeting equality of access to health, care and social welfare provision (Leinonen, Chapter 2). Geographical inequalities in provision are particularly evident in Canada (Fast and Eales, Chapter 6), where the length of leave and eligibility criteria vary between 13 provinces and territories, and across Sweden's various regions and municipalities (Aldman et al, Chapter 3). In Australia, long-term leave arrangements are complicated by both geography and industrial sector, as different schemes apply to public and private sector employees in different states or territories (O'Loughlin and Williams, Chapter 4).

Further inequities in available carer leave options can arise from collective bargaining agreements between national trade unions and employers. Sweden has a national minimum standard for carer leaves; collective bargaining, in some industries, has resulted in these being paid. Eligibility for some carer leave can also vary by employer size, as in Germany where workers in SMEs are excluded from some schemes. In Germany, over half of all private sector employees work in SMEs, leaving many workers excluded from carer leave (the Care Leave ['*Pflegezeit*'] applies only to employees in companies with 16 or more employees; Family Caregiver Leave ['*Familienpflegezeit*'] applies only to companies with 26 or more employees) (Statista, 2022; Knauthe and Hoff, Chapter 7).

Many countries also distinguish between 'employees' (usually subject to a contract of employment) and 'workers' (engaged in labour on a more temporary, casual or flexible basis), as already noted. As with other employment rights, carer leave schemes are typically available only to the former. 'Workers', thus defined, are a large group in the labour market in Australia (~19 per cent,

ABS, 2021; O'Loughlin and Williams, Chapter 4); women are also more likely both to be carers and to be in casual forms of work. The UK has an estimated 3.9 million people in insecure employment (TUC, 2023) and in Japan almost a third of workers aged 16–64 are in non-permanent employment,[2] while over half of women work in non-regular employment (Statistics Bureau of Japan, and Ministry of Internal Affairs and Communications, 2023).

Comparison of the nine countries' policies does indicate that equity is generally supported by inclusive definitions of 'family' and the inclusion of a wide range of relationships in the eligibility criteria for carer leaves. In Sweden and Canada, however, carer leave explicitly target parents caring for children with health conditions or disabilities, but excludes carers of adults with care needs; Poland too offers longer periods of Care Benefit to parents of sick and disabled children than for carers of other family members. In Sweden the support available to carers varies according to the health conditions of the person cared for, with fewer options available to those caring for people with mental health problems. There are also differences in provision for carers of people with disabilities aged 65 and over, and for Canada's Compassionate Care Leave scheme the person receiving care must suffer from a 'life-threatening' condition, creating further variation in the way different categories of 'carer' are supported. This is also a point of tension between national policy in Sweden and the EU Directive 2019/1159 on Work–life Balance for Parents and Carers (European Parliament, 2019); the Swedish Government felt its existing leaves already exceeded the Directive's requirements but, as shown in Chapter 3, restrictions related to the health of the person cared for mean that some are not in practice entitled to these leaves (Aldman et al, Chapter 3).

This book has shown that, in the countries studied, contemporary carer support policies, including carer leave schemes, are being made available to both men and women. This was not always the case; previous international analyses have shown that some of the earliest policies for carers applied specifically to women or to wives (Yeandle et al, 2013). Policies and policy instruments that appear 'neutral' may, in their operation, nevertheless reinforce gender inequities, as they are inevitably affected by related issues: persistent gender pay gaps; continuing gendered divisions in unpaid labour and formal labour markets; and uneven access to available leave options and other workplace support for carers. Leinonen (Chapter 2) has shown that Finland's unpaid carer leave policies may be amplifying inequalities related to caring, as these operate in the context of a gender-segregated labour market with a substantial gender pay gap. In Canada (Chapter 6), where some workers taking carer leave receive only partial income replacement (typically 55 per cent), households often decide that the female partner should access the leave, as her pay is typically lower; in 2019–20, women were by far the main users of the Compassionate Care Leave, Critical Illness Leave for Children and Critical

Illness Leave for Adults (Canada Employment Insurance Commission, 2021). Data from Canada also show that working carers over age 45 disportionately access available carer leaves, and thus are more affected by the negative outcomes of these for pension accrual and later life income.

Eligibility criteria, often based on length of employment (as in Finland, Sweden, Canada, Germany and Japan), can lead to inequality and inequity. This is highlighted in data from Finland, where an increase in 2016 in the number of years in employment required to access the Job Alternation Leave saw numbers of applications (previously mostly from women) drop dramatically (Finnish Social Insurance Institution, 2016; The Federation of Unemployment Funds in Finland, 2022; Leinonen, Chapter 2). In cases where policies use 'deservingness criteria' (van Ooschot, 2000) based on employment contributions to make carer leave decisions, it is often workers who are carers who find it most challenging to accrue enough years of employment to access the very leave options that might help them retain their connection with the labour market.

Wider gender equality issues are also relevant to how working carers are supported. As Leinonen highlights in her discussion of Finland (Chapter 2), despite legal prohibition of discrimination on the basis of caring and mandatory 'gender equality' policies, gender-related labour market segmentation, gender pay gaps, the expectation that families will support 'ageing in place' and unequal divisions of parental care all persist (Mesiäislehto et al, 2022). In Sweden – another country that has prioritised gender equality – the division of care remains highly gendered; women both provide more care hours and do the most demanding care tasks. Nonetheless, as Aldman et al (Chapter 3, citing Vicente et al, 2022) highlight, men are more likely to be offered support with caring. For them, caring remains gendered partly due to wage differentials between men and women, which make it 'logical' that women are mainly the ones who reduce their working hours to provide care. In the UK and Canada, too, women's disproportionate participation in part-time work is linked to their greater contributions to caring and domestic labour (Zamberlan et al, 2021; Hamblin et al, Chapter 5; Fast and Eales, Chapter 6). In many countries, uneven divisions of care became more pronounced during the COVID-19 pandemic. Without wider policy interventions to address gender equalities, care is likely to remain a site of inequity between men and women that carer leave arrangements alone will be insufficient to ameliorate.

Other policies to support working carers

In some countries, other policies offer further support to working carers. For working people with caring responsibilities, flexibility is among the most sought-after features of employment arrangements (Brimblecombe et al, 2018; Bainbridge and Townsend, 2020; Spann et al, 2020). In the UK and Finland, flexible working is 'mainstreamed' and used widely across the workforce, rather than a policy specific to carers. The UK's 'right to request' legislation on flexible working began with a focus on working parents and was extended later to all employees with six months' service and is due to be expanded further in 2024 to become a 'day one right' to those in employment. Such approaches often have a wider impact, affecting not only working carers; one survey of employees in Finland found 64 per cent had a 'working time bank' system at their workplace, while 71 per cent had flexible hours available (Keyriläinen, 2021). Finnish data nevertheless indicate that while flexibility at work is almost universally available there, gender differences remain, with men more likely than women to take advantage of these opportunities (Leinonen, Chapter 2), and the negative repercussions of choosing flexible work felt more keenly by women (Kauppinen and Silfver-Kuhalampi, 2015). The legal right to request flexible working arrangements in Australia is limited to specific groups, including carers, but used most by parents of school-age or younger children (Fair Work Commission, 2021b: 8); survey data show that requests are generally granted (Fair Work Commission, 2021b) and O'Loughlin and Williams (Chapter 4) report that these measures are still widely seen as 'something for women'.

Lessons learned and ways forward

The 'invisibility' of carers is a recurring theme in this book. In Sweden, Aldman et al (Chapter 3) argue that the assumption that the state is the provider of welfare from the 'cradle to the grave' obscures the central and increasing role carers play in the provision of care. Elsewhere, in countries where the subsidiarity principle (as in Germany) or familialism dominates, caring has traditionally been viewed as mainly a private matter. In all nine countries, policy discourses are beginning to acknowledge the dual importance of supporting carers in their caring role and to engage in paid employment.

The increasing attention paid to working carers' needs should be understood in relation to the wider context of care provision. In several of the country chapters 'ageing in place' and retrenchment or inadequacies in formal care provision have contributed to the 'refamilialisation of care' (Leinonen, Chapter 2; Ikeda, Chapter 8; Kodate and Timonen, 2017). How the 'ageing in place' measures in the contested Long-Term Care Act 2021 in Slovenia (Rakar et al, Chapter 9) will play out, if implemented, remains to be seen. It is clear, however, that a sustainable approach to care must consider the interests and well-being of both those who provide and those who receive care (Keating et al, 2021).

Several of our chapters show that, often, employers are still unaware of the implications of having carers in their workforce and the benefits of supporting them (Aldman et al, Chapter 3; Fast and Eales, Chapter 6; Lero et al, 2012). Measures to support carers in some countries have been opposed by organisations representing the interests of employers. Thus, in Germany, some employers' organisations blocked the introduction of carers leave in SMEs and refused to endorse the recommendations on paid carer leave made by the official Independent Advisory Board for the Reconciliation of Caregiving and Employment (Knauthe and Hoff, Chapter 7). In the UK, some employers and most carers' organisations argue there is a strong 'business case' for supporting working carers, highlighting the costs of replacing those who exit the labour market to care and the added value they bring to organisations (Carers UK and HM Government, 2013; Carers UK, 2019; Austin and Heyes 2020). Further research and engagement with employers and their representative organisations could be an important way forward to ensure support for carers is present in a wide range of workplaces (Kelliher et al, 2002; Swanberg, 2006; Lilley et al, 2007; Lero et al, 2009; Ireson et al, 2018).

Too often, carers themselves remain unaware of available supports and many do not identify with the term 'carer' or are reluctant to do so, some fearing they will subsequently be treated unfavourably by their employers (Eales et al, 2015). A survey of working carers (n=450) in Finland found low levels of awareness of the amendment to the Employment Contracts Act (allowing for a temporary absence to provide care – less than 15 per cent knew about this) (Kauppinen, 2013). A survey in Sweden found that, of the wide range of supports and leaves available, only 'information' was offered to, or received by, over 20 per cent of working carers (Vicente et al, 2022; Aldman et al, Chapter 3). It is thus essential that greater efforts are made to raise carers' (and employers') awareness of existing forms of support, and also, as Lloyd (2023) argues, to encourage employers and other stakeholders such as health professionals to identify carers within their workforces, reducing the onus on carers alone to self-identify.

A further issue, related to awareness, is that in many countries carers are neglected in official statistics. This can be both a cause and an effect of carers' invisibility. Many countries rely on estimates of the total number of carers in their population, as they do not measure this in official surveys; some attempt to place a value on the contributions carers make. Finland estimates that 1.4 million people are carers (Vilkko et al, 2014), with over 700,000 employees combining paid work with family care (Carers Finland, 2022), concluding that providing this care would otherwise cost the Finnish state €2.8 billion per year (Kehusmaa, 2014). In the UK, the latest estimate of the value of the care provided by carers in England and Wales is £162 billion per year (Petrillo and Bennett, 2023; Hamblin et al, Chapter 5). Researchers in

Australia have estimated replacement care costs at AU$77.9 billion per year, if the formal care sector undertook the tasks done by carers (Deloitte Access Economics, 2020; O'Loughlin and Williams, Chapter 4). Such estimates are increasingly used to bring issues of care onto policy agendas.

A striking conclusion of our comparative analysis is that data on the use of carer leave policies, in terms of absolute numbers using these and their impact, is absent almost everywhere. Governments in the countries we have considered seem not to have commissioned evaluation studies of the carer leave policies they have introduced (Yeandle, 2017) and there are few alternative sources of data. The UK, for example, does not require employers to record and report use of the unpaid carer leave introduced in the Employment Rights Act 1996 or flexible working requests. Even in countries where data are available on uptake, numbers seem low, perhaps reflecting barriers to the use of leave and other policies to support carers. In Finland, for example, the numbers of people accessing the Job Alternation Allowance had fallen to only 5,000 by 2021 (The Federation of Unemployment Funds in Finland, 2022). In Germany, in 2018, only 867 people were granted the interest-free loan to compensate for wages lost while on carer leave (INTERVAL, 2018; FMFSWY, 2019).

This book has broken new ground in providing detailed accounts, by national experts, of a wide range of carer leave options, explaining their specific provisions and discussing implementation issues. We believe policy makers, trade unions, employers and carers' advocacy organisations in many countries, within and beyond the nine considered here, will find the book valuable as they develop and refine their own approaches. Contributors to the book have provided a range of ideas on how present policies could be improved: by reducing or eliminating within-country jurisdictional/ geographic variability, to improve equity and inclusiveness; by allowing employees who support a family member needing care to share longer-term leaves; by enabling carers to split the permitted maximum duration of carer leave into smaller increments; and through options to accumulate and to 'bank' leave entitlements over time. Such measures could result in fairer treatment of working carers as well as increased flexibility in care provision. They could also help working carers to cope better with changes and fluctuations in their caring roles over the lifecourse, due to the ebb and flow of caring demands throughout their lives (Fast et al, 2020). Without statutory job protection, carer leave cannot be effective in facilitating integration of work and care responsibilities across the lifecourse. It seems certain too that whether carer leave is paid/compensated or unpaid really matters. An abiding concern is that workers and employees in low-paid or insecure jobs are disadvantaged by most current leave arrangements. The message of this book is clear: carer leave needs to be paid leave if it is to make a significant contribution to care provision in years to come.

Notes

1 Australia's Personal/Carer's Leave is included in the long-term leaves, as working carers are able to accrue their days; Slovenia too allows for ten days of leave per caring episode, with the possibility of extension in some circumstances, with no annual limit.

2 Including part-time workers, temporary full-time and part-time workers and dispatched full-time and part-time workers from temporary labour agencies.

References

Anderson, L.A., Edwards, V.J., Pearson, W.S., Talley, R.C., McGuire, L.C. and Andresen, E.M. (2013) 'Adult caregivers in the United States: characteristics and differences in well-being, by caregiver age and caregiving status', *Preventing Chronic Disease: Public Health Research*, 15:10:E135. https://doi.org/10.5888/pcd10.130090

Anttonen, A. and Sipilä, J. (1996) 'European social care services: is it possible to identify models?' *Journal of European Social Policy*, 6(2): 87–100.

Austin, A. and Heyes, J. (2020) *Supporting working carers: How employers and employees can benefit*, CIPD/University of Sheffield.

Australian Bureau of Statistics (ABS) (2021) 'Characteristics of employment, Australia'. Available from: https://www.abs.gov.au/statistics/labour/earni ngs-and-working-conditions/characteristics-employment-australia/latest-release [Accessed 19 January 2024].

Bainbridge, H.T. and Townsend, K. (2020) 'The effects of offering flexible work practices to employees with unpaid caregiving responsibilities for elderly or disabled family members', *Human Resource Management*, 59(5): 483–95.

Bettio, F. and Plantenga, J. (2004) 'Comparing care regimes in Europe', *Feminist Economics*, 10(1): 85–113.

Boise, L. and Neal, M. (1996) 'Family responsibilities and absenteeism: Employees caring for parents versus employees caring for children', *Journal of Managerial Issues*, 8(2): 218–38.

Brimblecombe, N., Fernandez, J.L., Knapp, M., Rehill, A. and Wittenberg, R. (2018) 'Review of the international evidence on support for unpaid carers', *Journal of Long-Term Care*, (September): 25–40.

Canada Employment Insurance Commission (2021) 'Employment insurance monitoring and assessment report for the fiscal year beginning April 1, 2019 and ending March 31, 2020.' Available from: https://www.canada. ca/en/employment-social-development/programs/ei/ei-list/reports/mon itoring2020.html [Accessed 3 May 2021].

Carers Finland (2022) 'Omaishoidon tietopaketti. Ansiotyö ja omaishoito' ['Information package of family care. Employment and family care']. https://omaishoitajat.fi/omaishoidon-tietopaketti/ansiotyo-ja-omaisho ito/ [Accessed 31 January 2022].

Carers UK (2019) *Juggling work and unpaid care: a growing issue, policy report*. Available from: https://www.carersuk.org/media/no2lwyxl/juggling-work-and-unpaid-care-report-final-web.pdf [Accessed 19 January 2024].

Carers UK and HM Government (2013) 'Supporting working carers: the benefits to families, business and the economy'. Available from: https://www.gov.uk/government/publications/supporting-working-carers-the-benefits-to-families-business-and-the-economy [Accessed 30 May 2023].

Carr, E., Murray, E.T., Zaninotto, P., Cadar, D., Head, J., Stansfeld, S. and Stafford, M. (2018) 'The association between informal caregiving and exit from employment among older workers: Prospective findings from the UK household longitudinal study', *The Journals of Gerontology: Series B*, 73(7): 1253–1262. https://doi.org/10.1093/geronb/gbw156

Cohen, S.A., Cook, S.K., Sando, T.A., Brown, M.J. and Longo, D.R. (2017) 'Socioeconomic and demographic disparities in caregiving intensity and quality of life in informal caregivers: a first look at the National Study of caregiving', *Journal of Gerontological Nursing*, 43(6): 17–24.

Cohen, S.A., Sabik, N.J., Cook, S.K., Azzoli, A.B. and Mendez-Luck, C.A. (2019) 'Differences within differences: gender inequalities in caregiving intensity vary by race and ethnicity in informal caregivers', *Journal of Cross-Cultural Gerontology*, 34: 245–63.

Crompton, R. and Lyonette, C. (2006) 'Work–life "balance" in Europe', *Acta Sociologica*, 49(4): 379–93.

Daly, M. and Rake, K. (2003) *Gender and the welfare state: Care, work and welfare in Europe and the USA*, Hoboken, NJ: John Wiley & Sons.

Deloitte Access Economics (2020) *The value of informal care in 2020, report commissioned by Carers Australia*. Available from: https://www2.deloitte.com/au/en/pages/economics/articles/value-of-informal-care-2020.html [Accessed 19 January 2024].

Dentinger, E. and Clarkberg, M. (2002) 'Informal caregiving and retirement timing among men and women: gender and caregiving relationships in late midlife', *Journal of Family Issues*, 23, 857–79. https://doi.org/10.1177/019251302236598

Do, E.K., Cohen, S.A. and Brown, M.J. (2014) 'Socioeconomic and demographic factors modify the association between informal caregiving and health in the Sandwich Generation', *BMC Public Health*, 14: 1–8.

Dogan, M. and Pelassy, D. (1990) *How to Compare Nations. Strategies in Comparative Politics*, Chatham: Chatham House.

Dykstra, P.A. and Djundeva, M. (2020) 'Policies for later-life families in a comparative European perspective', in R. Nieuwenhuis and W. Van Lancker (eds), *The Palgrave handbook of family policy*, Cham: Palgrave Macmillan, pp 331–66.

Eales, J. Keating, N., Donalds, S. and Fast, J. (2015) 'Assessing the needs of employed caregivers and employers', Edmonton: Research on Aging, Policies and Practice and Alberta Caregivers Association. Available from: https://rapp.ualberta.ca/wp-content/uploads/sites/49/2018/04/Assessing-needs-of-employed-caregivers-and-employers-Final-Report_2015May25.pdf [Accessed 24 January 2024].

Esping-Andersen, G. (1990) *The three worlds of welfare capitalism*, Cambridge: Polity Press.

Esping-Andersen, G. (1999) *Social foundations of postindustrial economies*, Oxford: Oxford University Press.

European Commission [EC] (2022) *Communication from the Commission to the European Parliament, the Council, the European Economic and Social Committee and the Committee of the Regions*, Brussels: European Commission. Available from: https://ec.europa.eu/social/BlobServlet?docId=26014&langId=en [Accessed 30 June 2023].

European Parliament (2019) *Directive (EU) 2019/1158 of the European Parliament and of the Council of 20 June 2019 on work–life balance for parents and carers and repealing Council Directive 2010/18/EU*, Brussels: European Parliament. Available from: https://eur-lex.europa.eu/legal-content/EN/TXT/?uri=celex%3A32019L1158 [Accessed 30 June 2023].

Fair Work Commission (2021a) 'General Manager's report into individual flexibility arrangements under s.653 of the Fair Work Act 2009 (Cth): 2015–18', Canberra: Commonwealth of Australia.

Fair Work Commission (2021b) 'General Manager's report into the operation of the provisions of the National Employment Standards relating to requests for flexible working arrangements and extensions of unpaid parental leave under s.653 of the Fair Work Act 2009 (Cth): 2015–18', Canberra: Commonwealth of Australia.

Fast, J., Eales, J., Keating, N., Lee, Y. and Kim, C. (2020) 'Trajectories of family care over the life course: evidence from Canada', *Ageing and Society*, 41(5): 1145–62.

Fine, M. and Davidson, B. (2018) 'The marketization of care: global challenges and national responses in Australia', *Current Sociology*, 66(4): 503–16.

Finnish Social Insurance Institution (2016) 'Vuorotteluvapaan ehdot muuttuvat' ['Eligibility criteria for job alternation leave will be changed']. Available from: https://www.kela.fi/-/vuorotteluvapaan-ehdot-muuttuv-1?inheritRedirect=true [Accessed 29 March 2022].

FMFSWY (2019) *First report of the German Independent Advisory Board on Work–Care Reconciliation*, Berlin.

Gallie, D. (2007) 'Production regimes, employment regimes, and the quality of work', in D. Gallie (ed), *Employment regimes and the quality of work*, Oxford: Oxford University Press, 1–33.

International Labour Organization (ILO) (1985) *ILO's Convention on Workers with Family Responsibilities Convention, 1981 (C156)*. Available from: https://www.ilo.org/century/history/iloandyou/WCMS_213324/lang--en/index.htm [Accessed 29 November 2023].

ILO (2019) *ILO Centenary Declaration for the Future of Work, 2019*. Available from: https://www.ilo.org/global/about-the-ilo/mission-and-objectives/centenary-declaration/lang--en/index.htm [Accessed 29 November 2023].

INTERVAL (2018) *Abschlussbericht zur Untersuchung der Regelungen des Pflegezeitgesetzes und des Familienpflegezeitgesetzes in der seit 1 Januar 2015 geltenden Fassung unter Einbeziehung der kurzzeiteigen Arbeitsverhinderung und des Pflegeunterstützungsgeldes (unveröffentlicht).*

Ireson, R., Sethi, B. and Williams, A. (2018) 'Availability of caregiver-friendly workplace policies (CFWPs): an international scoping review', *Health & Social Care in the Community*, 26(1), e1–e14.

Kauppinen, K. (2013) 'Omais- ja läheishoitovapaan käytön tilanneselvitys' ['The situation of the use of family care leaves and absence for compelling family reasons'] Helsinki: Finnish Institute of Occupational Health.

Kauppinen, K. and Silfver-Kuhalampi, M. (2015) 'Työssäkäynti ja läheis- ja omaishoiva – työssä jaksamisen ja jatkamisen tukeminen' ['Employment and family care. How to support well-being and continuation in working life']. Helsinki: University of Helsinki.

Keating, N., McGregor, J.A. and Yeandle, S. (2021) 'Sustainable care: theorising the wellbeing of caregivers to older persons', *International Journal of Care and Caring*, 5(4): 611–30.

Kehusmaa, S. (2014) *Hoidon menoja hillitsemässä. Heikkokuntoisten kotona asuvien ikäihmisten palvelujen käyttö, omaishoito ja kuntoutus [Controlling the costs of care. The use of services, family care and rehabilitation of frail older persons living at home]*, Tampere: Juvenes Print.

Kelliher, C., Gore, J. and Riley, M. (2002) 'Functional flexibility: implementation and outcomes', in I.U. Zeytinoglu (ed), *Flexible work arrangements: Conceptualizations and international experience*, New York: Kluwer Law International, pp 65–76.

Keyriläinen, M. (2021) *Working life barometer 2020*, Helsinki: Ministry of Economic Affairs and Employment of Finland. Available from: https://julkaisut.valtioneuvosto.fi/bitstream/handle/10024/163200/TEM_2021_36.pdf?sequence=1&isAllowed=y [Accessed 18 February 2022].

Kodate, N. and Timonen, V. (2017) 'Bringing the family in through the back door: the stealthy expansion of family care in Asian and European long-term care policy', *Journal of Cross-Cultural Gerontology*, 32: 291–301.

Kröger, T. (2011) 'Defamilisation, dedomestication and care policy: Comparing childcare service provisions of welfare states', *International Journal of Sociology and Social Policy*, 31(7/8): 424–40.

Langan, M. and Ostner, I. (1991) 'Gender and welfare: towards a comparative framework', in G. Room (ed), *Towards a European welfare state?* Bristol: SAUS, pp 127–50.

Leitner, S. (2003) 'Varieties of familialism: The caring function of the family in comparative perspective', *European Societies*, 5(4): 353–75.

Lero, D.S., Richardson, J. and Korabik, K. (2009) *Cost-benefit review of work–life balance practices –2009*, Canadian Association of Administrators of Labour Legislation.

Lero, D., Spinks, N., Fast, J. and Tremblay, D.-G. (2012) 'The availability, accessibility and effectiveness of workplace supports for Canadian caregivers', Final report to Human Resources and Skills Development Canada, Gatineau, PQ.

Lewis, J. (1992) 'Gender and the development of welfare regimes', *Journal of European Social Policy*, 2(3): 159–73.

Lewis, J. (1997) 'Gender and welfare regimes: further thoughts', *Social Politics: International Studies in Gender, State & Society*, 4(2): 160–77.

Lilly, M.B., Laporte, A. and Coyte, P. (2007) 'Labour market work and home care's unpaid caregivers: a systematic review of labour force participation rates, predictors of labour market withdrawal, and hours of work. *Milbank Quarterly* 85(4): 641–90.

Lloyd, L. (2023) *Unpaid care policies in the UK: Rights, resources and relationships*, Bristol: Policy Press.

Matthews, R.A. and Fisher, G.G. (2013) 'The role of work and family in the retirement process: a review and new directions', in M. Wang (ed), *The Oxford handbook of retirement*, New York: Oxford University Press, pp 354–70.

Mesiäislehto, M., Elomäki, A., Närvi, J., Simanainen, M., Sutela, H. and Räsänen, T. (2022) *The gendered impacts of the Covid-19 crisis in Finland and the effectiveness of the policy responses. Findings of the project 'The impact of the Covid-19 crisis in Finland'*, Helsinki: Finnish Institute of Health and Welfare.

Millar, J. (1999) 'Obligations and autonomy in social welfare', in R. Crompton (ed), *Restructuring gender relations and employment: The decline of the male breadwinner*, Oxford: Oxford University Press, pp 26–40.

Peng, I. and Yeandle, S.M. (2017) *Eldercare policies in East Asia and Europe: Mapping policy changes and variations and their implications*, UN Women's Discussion Paper Series, United Nations Entity for Gender Equality and the Empowerment of Women (UN Women), New York: United Nations.

Petrillo, M and Bennett, M. (2023) 'Valuing Carers 2021: England and Wales'. London: Carers UK.

Pfau-Effinger, B. (1999) 'The modernization of family and motherhood', in R. Crompton (ed), *Restructuring gender relations and employment: The decline of the male breadwinner*, Oxford: Oxford University Press, pp 60–80.

Pfau-Effinger, B. (2005a) 'Culture and welfare state policies: reflections on a complex interrelation', *Journal of Social Policy*, 34(1): 3–20.

Pfau-Effinger, B. (2005b) 'Welfare state policies and the development of care arrangements', *European Societies*, 7(2): 321–47.

Radziwinowiczówna, A. and Rosińska, A. (2022) 'Neoliberalization of familialism by default: the case of local organization of elder care in Poland', in L. Näre and L. Widding Isaksen (eds), *Care loops and mobilities in Nordic, Central, and Eastern European welfare states*, Cham: Springer International Publishing, pp 41–62.

Soma, N. and Yamashita, J. (2011) 'Child care and elder care regimes in Japan', *Journal of Comparative Social Welfare*, 27(2): 133–42.

Spann, A., Vicente, J., Allard, C., Hawley, M., Spreeuwenberg, M. and de Witte, L. (2020) 'Challenges of combining work and unpaid care, and solutions: a scoping review', *Health & Social Care in the Community*, 28(3): 699–715.

Stall, N. (2019) 'We should care more about caregivers', *Canadian Medical Association Journal*, 191(9): E245–E246.

Stanfors, M., Jacobs, J.C. and Neilson, J. (2019) 'Caregiving time costs and trade-offs: Gender differences in Sweden, the UK, and Canada', *SSM-Population Health*, 9: 100501.

Statista (2022) *Kleine und mittlere Unternehmen (KMU) in Deutschland.* Available from: https://de.statista.com/statistik/studie/id/46952/dokum ent/kleine-und-mittlere-unternehmen-kmu-in-deutschland/ [Accessed 24 January 2024].

Statistics Bureau of Japan, and Ministry of Internal Affairs and Communications (2023, 31 January) *Share of employees working in non-regular employment in Japan from 2003 to 2022, by gender [Graph]. In Statista.* Available from: https://www.statista.com/statistics/1126055/japan-share-employees-non-regular-employment-by-gender/ [Accessed 4 November 2023].

Swanberg, J.E. (2006) 'Making it work: informal caregiving, cancer, and employment', *Journal of Psychosocial Oncology*, 24(3): 1–18.

The Federation of Unemployment Funds in Finland (2022) 'Muut kassojen maksamat etuudet, vuorottelukorvaus' ['Other benefits paid by the unemployment funds, job alternation allowance']. Available from: https://www.tyj.fi/tilastot/muut-kassojen-etuudet/#vuorottelukorvaus [Accessed 16 March 2022].

Trade Union Congress (TUC) (2023) *Insecure work in 2023.* Available from: https://www.tuc.org.uk/sites/default/files/insecureworkin2023.pdf [Accessed 16 November 2023].

Urwin, S., Lau, Y.S., Grande, G. and Sutton, M. (2023) 'Informal caregiving and the allocation of time: implications for opportunity costs and measurement', *Social Science and Medicine,* 334: 116164.

van Oorschot, W. (2000) 'Who should get what, and why? On deservingness criteria and the conditionality of solidarity among the public', *Policy & Politics*, 28(1): 33–48.

Vicente, J., McKee, K., Magnusson, L., Johansson, P., Ekman, B. and Hanson, E. (2022) 'Informal care provision among male and female working carers: findings from a Swedish national survey', *PLoS ONE*, 17(3): e0263396. https://doi.org/10.1371/journal.pone.0263396

Vilkko, A., Muuri, A., Saarikalle, K., Noro, A., Finne-Soveri, H. and Jokinen, S. (2014) 'Läheisavun moninaisuus' ['The diversity of informal care and informal help'], in M. Vaarama, S. Karvonen, L. Kestilä and P. Moisio (eds), *Suomalaisten hyvinvointi 2014 [The wellbeing of Finnish people in 2014]*, Tampere: Suomen yliopistopaino, pp 222–37.

Yeandle, S. (1999) 'Women, men, and non-standard employment: breadwinning and caregiving in Germany, Italy and the UK', in R. Crompton (ed), *Restructuring gender relations and employment: The decline of the male breadwinner*, Oxford: Oxford University Press, pp 80–105.

Yeandle, S. (2017) 'Work-care reconciliation policy: legislation in policy context in eight countries.' Report prepared for the German Bundesministeriumfür Familie, Senioren, Frauen und Jugend. Available from: http://circle.group.shef.ac.uk/wp-content/uploads/2018/11/yeandle-WCR-v2.pdf [Accessed 24 January 2024].

Yeandle, S. and Kröger, T. with Cass, B., Chou, Y.-C., Shimmei, M. and Szebehely, M. (2013) 'The emergence of policy supporting working carers: developments in six countries' in T. Kröger and S. Yeandle (eds), *Combining paid work and family care: Policies and experiences in international perspective*, Bristol: Policy Press, pp 23–50.

Zamberlan, A., Gioachin, F. and Gritti, D. (2021) 'Work less, help out more? The persistence of gender inequality in housework and childcare during UK COVID-19', *Research in Social Stratification and Mobility*, 73: 100583.

Index

References to figures appear in *italic* type; those in **bold** refer to tables. References to notes are the page number followed by the note number (17n1).